REFINED CARBOHYDRATE FOODS and DISEASE

Some Implications of Dietary Fibre

Edited by

D. P. BURKITT
CMG, MD, FRCSEd,
DSc (Hon), FRCSI (Hon), FRS
Medical Research Council
External Scientific Staff

H. C. TROWELL
OBE, MD, FRCP
Former Consultant
Physician, Uganda

Both formerly of Makerere University and Mulago Hospital,
Kampala, Uganda

Foreword by

Sir RICHARD DOLL

OBE, DSc, MD, FRCP, FRS
Regius Professor of Medicine
University of Oxford

1975

ACADEMIC PRESS

London   New York   San Francisco

A Subsidiary of Harcourt Brace Jovanovich, Publishers

ACADEMIC PRESS INC. (LONDON) LTD.
24/28 Oval Road,
London NW1

United States Edition published by
ACADEMIC PRESS INC.
111 Fifth Avenue
New York, New York 10003

Library of Congress Catalog Card Number: 74-18522
ISBN: 0-12-144750-2

Printed in Great Britain by Whitstable Litho Ltd.,
Whitstable, Kent.

REFINED CARBOHYDRATE
FOODS and DISEASE

Some Implications of Dietary Fibre

List of Contributors

A. K. ADATIA, Consultant Dental Surgeon, United Bristol Hospitals. Consultant Senior Lecturer in Dental Medicine, University of Bristol Dental School, Lower Maudlin Street, Bristol, BS1 2LY, England.
Formerly: Hon. Lecturer in Dental Surgery and Anatomy, Makerere University Medical School, Kampala, Uganda.

D. P. BURKITT, External Scientific Staff, Medical Research Council, 172 Tottenham Court Road, London, W1P 9LG, England.
Formerly: Surgeon, Uganda Government and Department of Surgery, Makerere University, Uganda.

D. W. HAYDEN, Research Assistant III, Department of Pathobiology, University of Connecticut, Storrs, Connecticut 06268, U.S.A.

K. W. HEATON, Consultant Senior Lecturer in Medicine, University of Bristol, Department of Medicine, Bristol Royal Infirmary, Bristol, BS2 8HW, England.

R. W. LEADER, Professor and Head, Department of Pathobiology, University of Connecticut, Storrs, Connecticut 06268, U.S.A.

N. S. PAINTER, Senior Consultant Surgeon, Manor House Hospital, North End Road, London, NW11 7HX, England.

F. I. TOVEY, Consultant Surgeon, Basingstoke District Hospital, Basingstoke, Hants, RG24 9NA, England.
Formerly: Holdsworth Memorial Hospital, Mysore, South India.

H. C. TROWELL, Windhover, Woodgreen, Fordingbridge, Hants, SP6 2AZ, England. *Formerly:* Physician, Uganda Government and Department of Medicine, Makerere University, Uganda.

Preface

During our twenty and thirty years' service in surgical and medical work, respectively, in Africa, we could not fail to be impressed by the contrasts between the patterns of disease in that continent and those of Europe and North America. Differing incidences of infective diseases were to be expected, and these had largely been explained on the basis of the presence of pathogenic organisms and the availability of suitable vectors, contaminated food or drink, or other means of transmission. It was the contrasts in prevalence of non-infective diseases that attracted our attention. One of us (D. B.) was able to demonstrate in at least one form of cancer, now generally known as Burkitt's lymphoma, that even incomplete epidemiological data could provide valuable clues as to the pathogenesis of disease. The experience of the other (H. T.) led him to write *Non-infective Disease in Africa*, published in 1960. Our combined experience suggests that relatively imprecise information can be of epidemiological value and much of the evidence set out in this book may be considered in that category.

With the recent exception of cancer and a growing interest in ischaemic heart disease, little information has been published on the epidemiology of non-infective disease. We decided therefore to pool our experience and review the literature on this subject in order to gather together epidemiological information on diseases normally divorced from one another by geographical boundaries or medical specialization.

Our interest was subsequently raised from the plane of merely recognizing geographical contrasts to that of investigating possible explanations for the phenomena observed by what we consider to be perceptive genius in the work of Surgeon Captain T. L. Cleave to whom we wish to pay particular credit and acknowledge a profound debt. His concept became widely known through the book *Diabetes, Coronary Thrombosis and the Saccharine Disease*, which is repeatedly referred to in the chapters of this book. A more recent and in some cases amended presentation of Cleave's hypothesis under the title *The Saccharine Disease* was published too late for more than occasional reference in this book.

We decided to examine the geographical distribution and historical emergence of the characteristically western diseases which we considered might be, at least in part, accounted for on a common dietary basis. By this we do not imply the direct action of only a single aetiological factor,

vii

but rather one that might play a part in all the diseases considered, though of differing degrees of importance in each, together with other environmental and genetic factors. As we have sifted the evidence and acquired new information we have repeatedly had to change our viewpoint and modify our emphasis, and we realize that any conclusions we have reached will certainly have to be modified, indeed radically changed, or even be disproved, as new evidence emerges.

Some of the epidemiological data from developing countries will be questioned by medical statisticians, especially as regards diseases which are common in older people. We hope that our work may stimulate others to collect by approved methodology more precise data in terms of age, sex, socio-economic background and variations in time and place, which will contribute to the correction of error and substantiation of truth necessary to convert hypotheses into theories and theories into facts.

We hope too that this work will help to forge stronger links between epidemiologists and experimental workers and demonstrate to those lacking opportunities for laboratory studies that clinical observation is usually the basis of an hypothesis on which experimental programmes are later constructed.

We wish to thank many doctors in countries overseas who have supplied facts and figures on which the epidemiological evidence is based; some of them work in teaching hospitals and medical schools, but the majority work in smaller rural and often isolated units. All have made a great contribution.

We are most grateful to Sir Richard Doll for his foreword.

Our contributors, experts each in his own field, have often read other sections of the book and their criticisms have been most helpful.

Mrs Priscilla Milton has typed and re-typed much of the manuscript most meticulously and Miss Sandra Osborn, in addition to secretarial assistance, has done much careful checking and enlivened the chapters with her diagrams. Miss Maria Tunstall has analysed and summarized the information received regularly from well over 130 hospitals in some 30 countries. We owe a particular debt to Miss Ella Wright for her thoughtful suggestions, and for the patience and care with which she has coordinated all the contributions, so that the book reads as a uniform whole.

One editor (H. T.) wishes to thank the British Heart Foundation for a grant to meet the expenses of his investigation of the literature.

Denis Burkitt
Medical Research Council
172 Tottenham Court Road
London, W1P 9LG

Hugh Trowell
Woodgreen
Fordingbridge
Hants SP6 2AZ

Foreword

Once every 10 years or so a new idea emerges about the cause of disease that captures the imagination and, for a time, seems to provide a key to the understanding of many of those diseases whose aetiology was previously unknown. Such ideas have included the concepts of hormone deficiency and excess, inborn errors of metabolism, vitamin deficiency, septic foci, psychosomatic disease, stress, and auto-immunity. To these we may now add a deficiency of dietary fibre. But whether it will be as seminal an idea as that of vitamin deficiency or as sterile as that of stress, we shall probably not know for another 10 years.

Many of the ideas that are put forward and discussed so clearly by Burkitt and Trowell and their collaborators in this book can be traced back to investigators who were impressed by the changes they saw taking place in the incidence of individual diseases 30 or 40 years ago. The suggestions that were then made about, for example, the aetiology of appendicitis attracted little attention and they tended to be dismissed either because they were too simple or because of inadequate proof that the change in incidence was indeed a real phenomenon and not just an artefact due to improved diagnosis. That they have been revived now is due primarily to the imagination and enthusiasm of Surgeon Captain Cleave, who was impressed by the changes that had taken place in the diet of industralized countries during the last 150 years and by the fact that many diseases that are common in Europe and North America are relatively rare in underdeveloped countries. Cleave argued that common diseases could not be due primarily to genetic factors, but were most likely to be due to new factors in the environment to which man had not yet had time to adapt. One such factor, which impressed him with its ubiquity in modern society, was the processing of food which resulted in the consumption of large quantities of pure sugar and starch. This, he contended, led to disease because man was evolutionarily adjusted to eating smaller amounts of carbohydrate intimately mixed with fibre and protein.

Cleave's hypothesis did not attract many scientists, who tended to be distrustful of broad all-embracing theories and were sceptical of the reliability of many of his figures for disease incidence. Burkitt and Trowell, however, knew from their own experience that the broad differences in pathology to which Cleave had drawn attention were true and indeed they had reported many themselves independently. They were impressed by the way certain diseases tended to group themselves not only in the same areas but in the same individuals, and they were sufficiently open-minded to be able to face up to the possibility that the diet which we, in England, had become accustomed to think was "normal" might not be metabolically ideal. They, therefore, decided to review the evidence for themselves and to bring together in a book the results of what they had found, pinpointing, in particular, the gaps in knowledge which needed to be filled in before the general hypothesis could be accepted, modified, or rejected. Their findings make an exciting medical adventure story. Starting from Cleave's hypothesis the authors are led to the conclusion that the refining of food is indeed a significant cause of disease; but not so much because it results in excess consumption, as because it removes fibre which, it is suggested, has many hitherto unsuspected physiological functions.

This idea, and the facts from which it is derived, cannot fail to lead to much research. If these researches show that the fibre hypothesis is relevant to only very few of the diseases discussed—or even disprove it altogether—that will detract very little from the value and interest of the book, as we can hardly fail to gain from trying to answer the questions that it poses. Personally, however, I have little doubt that the fibre hypothesis will be found to have established for itself a permanent place in the structure of medical knowledge.

Sir Richard Doll, F.R.S.
Regius Professor of Medicine
University of Oxford

Contents

List of Contributors v

Preface vii

Foreword ix

Part I   Disease and environment

Chapter 1.   Relating disease to environment in a search for causative factors.
DENIS BURKITT 3

Chapter 2.   Significance of relationships.
DENIS BURKITT 9

Part II   Refined carbohydrate foods

Chapter 3.   Refined carbohydrate foods and fibre.
HUGH TROWELL 23

Chapter 4.   Some historical aspects of milling cereals and refining sugar.
HUGH TROWELL 43

Chapter 5.   Dietary changes in modern times.
HUGH TROWELL 47

Part III   Refined carbohydrate foods in the gastrointestinal tract

Chapter 6.   The effects of carbohydrate refining on food ingestion, digestion and absorption.
KENNETH HEATON 59

Chapter 7.   Gastrointestinal transit times; stool weights and consistency; intraluminal pressures.
DENIS BURKITT and NEIL PAINTER 69

Part IV   Diseases of the large intestine

Chapter 8.   Appendicitis.
DENIS BURKITT 87

Chapter 9. Diverticular disease of the colon.
NEIL PAINTER and DENIS BURKITT   99

Chapter 10. Benign and malignant tumours of large bowel.
DENIS BURKITT   117

Chapter 11. Ulcerative colitis and Crohn's disease.
HUGH TROWELL   135

Part V Other diseases associated with constipation and
straining at stool

Chapter 12. Varicose veins, deep vein thrombosis and haemorrhoids.
DENIS BURKITT   143

Chapter 13. Hiatus hernia.
DENIS BURKITT   161

Part VI Other disorders related to refined carbohydrate
foods

Chapter 14. Gallstones and cholecystitis.
KENNETH HEATON   173

Chapter 15. Ischaemic heart disease, atheroma and fibrinolysis.
HUGH TROWELL   195

Chapter 16. Diabetes mellitus and obesity.
HUGH TROWELL   227

Chapter 17. Dental caries and periodontal disease.
ABDUL ADATIA   251

Part VII
Chapter 18. Duodenal ulcer and diet.
FRANK TOVEY   279

Part VIII
Chapter 19. Some diseases characteristic of western civilization
prevalent in wild and domestic animals.
ROBERT LEADER and DAVID HAYDEN 311

Part IX
Chapter 20.   Disorders of unknown aetiology showing certain epidemiological associations.
IIUGH TROWELL 319

Part X
Chapter 21.   Concluding considerations.
HUGH TROWELL and DENIS BURKITT . . . 333
Index 347
Postscript 353

Dedicated to

Surgeon Captain T. L. Cleave, R.N. (retd)

Part I

Disease and environment

Chapter 1

Relating disease to environment in a search for causative factors

DENIS BURKITT

I. Harmful environmental factors 3
II. Genetically determined susceptibility 4
III. Multiple factors 4
IV. Environmental factors characteristic of specific areas, countries, communities and individuals 5
    A. Geographical areas 5
    B. Countries, communities and groups 5
    C. Individuals 5
V. Alteration in environmental factors 6
    A. Increased risk 6
    B. Decreased risk 7
    C. Absence of harmful environmental factors 7
    D. Adaptation to harmful environmental factors 7
VI. Value of environment–disease relationships 8
References 8

Throughout the world environment plays an important part in the varying incidence of some diseases; indeed it is the primary cause of most. Genetic endowment also plays a role and may determine the susceptibility of individuals, or of different organs or structures in individuals, to particular environments. This could explain why, within a given environment, not only will some people be affected and others escape, but amongst those affected there may be different disease manifestations.

I. Harmful environmental factors

Infection by bacteria, viruses or parasites is responsible for a large proportion of all diseases. Injuries of all kinds, whether by physical agents,

3

extremes of temperature or corrosive chemicals, are the result of environmental hazards. Radiation, whether from sun, X-rays or atomic explosions, can produce serious tissue changes. Poisonous chemicals from snakes, insects, plants and fish can be dangerous, even fatal. Climate—intense heat or intense cold—may cause profound pathological changes as well as local injury, especially in people who are not adapted to such extremes. Arctic explorers are liable to develop frostbite, and visitors to tropical countries may suffer from heat exhaustion.

Deficiencies in dietary necessities such as protein, various minerals and vitamins, produce their own characteristic disease syndromes. In fact a wide range of pathological effects may result from inadequate or unbalanced diets, or even from excessive food. Even the foetus is vulnerable to environmental changes, as is witnessed in the tragic deformities resulting from rubella infection or from the administration of thalidomide during pregnancy.

II. Genetically determined susceptibility

Obvious examples of genetically determined diseases are provided by conditions such as xeroderma pigmentosum, which readily gives rise to a skin epithelioma on exposure to sunlight; and albinism, which in tropical countries commonly results in the development of cancer in skin unprotected by pigment. Sickle-cell trait, which has a beneficial effect in diminishing susceptibility to malaria, is an example of genetically determined protection from disease.

III. Multiple factors

A single environmental factor which is unlikely to produce disease on its own may, when associated with another environmental factor, be highly pathogenic. For example, measles (or some other infection) when associated with gross malnutrition may result in cancrum oris. In experimental animals the incidence of virus-induced leukaemia or other forms of cancer has been greatly increased after X-ray radiation.

The cause of many, if not most, diseases is multifactorial. Not only is there a relationship between environmental factors and host defence mechanisms, but disease manifestations are usually the cumulative effect of many interacting factors. Psychological changes may increase symptoms of disease caused by physical agents or they may actually induce physical disease. Hence the designation "psychosomatic".

IV. Environmental factors characteristic of specific areas, countries, communities and individuals

A. Geographical areas

Particular environmental factors may be peculiar to, or unusually prevalent within, specific geographical areas. Much fruitful epidemiological study has consisted of determining the geographical distribution of a disease and subsequently relating it to environmental factors. These studies have usually involved several areas, relating the recorded experience of one country with another, or even making generalizations for continents or sub-continents. Such inter-territorial comparisons need to be complemented by detailed studies within each territory which are often more important but have tended to be less emphasized (Burkitt and Hutt, 1966). Political boundaries seldom coincide with pathological frontiers. Specific areas, in which the frequency of a particular disease is unduly high or low, may straddle political demarcations, and may evade detection when comparisons are limited to records of the two adjacent countries (Hutt and Burkitt, 1965; Burkitt and Hutt, 1966).

B. Countries, communities and groups

Pathological changes related to cultural and socio-economic conditions may be peculiar to certain countries or to specific communities within a country. Those associated with affluence and modern economic development are most prevalent in western countries, and rare in developing countries, particularly among their less technically advanced rural communities.

Particular groups of people in the same geographical area may be susceptible in varying degrees to certain environmental factors which relate to their occupation or other circumstances. Some of the most notable examples have been the recognition by Sir Percival Pott in 1775 that cancer of the scrotum was particularly common in chimney sweeps, and the observation relating skin cancer to certain cotton-mill workers whose clothes became impregnated with oil. These were probably the first observations which related cancer to specific environmental factors and to hydrocarbons in particular. Subsequently, aniline dye workers were shown to be especially prone to bladder cancer.

C. Individuals

Within a community people may be exposed to specific environmental hazards usually on account of either personal habits or addictions, the most obvious examples being the relationship between cigarette smoking and lung cancer, bronchitis and ischaemic heart disease. An almost identical situation exists in the close association between buccal cancer and the chewing of a "quid" containing tobacco, lime and other ingredients, in India and other parts of the East. The prevalence of dental caries is closely associated with eating sweets and confectionery between meals, and the lack of dental hygiene.

V. Alteration in environmental factors

A. Increased risk

When a community changes its customs, or is influenced by a different environment, some previously unknown diseases may appear and others may increase in frequency. The period elapsing between the altered environment and the manifestation of pathological effects depends on the duration and intensity of exposure required to produce a particular disease. In the case of infectious diseases such as poliomyelitis or cholera this interval of time will be short. In cancer it may cover several decades: for example the skin cancer in early workers with X-rays only became manifest many years after the introduction of this new environmental hazard, and the rise in incidence of lung cancer followed the increase in cigarette smoking after a considerable time interval.

When searching for some environmental agent which may, over a particular period, be responsible for an increased incidence of a certain disease, one must first consider environmental changes which could be related to this increase. In the case of infectious disease the suspect should be some organism recently introduced into the environment. In cancer and diseases characteristic of later life, a factor introduced 20 or more years previously could be the likely culprit. Environmental factors that have remained fairly static during or prior to the rise in incidence of a disease are unlikely to be of major aetiological importance.

When individuals or groups move to another area, they may for the first time become significantly exposed to new environmental factors responsible for particular diseases which they will then be more likely to develop. For example, malaria and trypanosomiasis, both diseases characteristic of parts of Africa, took a heavy toll of early pioneers from Europe and America. The incidence of certain diseases has increased considerably among Japanese immigrants to Hawaii who have adopted western customs of food and living.

B. *Decreased risk*

A decrease in the incidence of a particular disease following the diminution or elimination of the causative environmental factor is of no less epidemiological significance than is a rise in incidence associated with the introduction of a new factor.

Although a decrease in the incidence of a disease suggests a change in environment, such a decrease could also be brought about by the introduction of protective measures against the environmental hazard, which may remain unchanged. Both prophylactic immunization and protection of drinking water from contamination will diminish the risk of contracting cholera. Both the routine administration of anti-malarial drugs and attempted elimination of or protection from infected mosquitos will reduce the risk of developing malaria.

The reduction in incidence of these diseases which followed the first attempts to eradicate the factors presumed to be responsible, confirmed the incrimination of certain causative agents.

C. *Absence of harmful environmental factors*

In epidemiological studies the value of negatives has been insufficiently stressed. It may be more important to detect where a disease is rare than where it is common. When a disease is prevalent throughout a continent, country or community it is the particular areas or groups of people found to be unusually exempt that demand special attention.

Sir Harold Himsworth has frequently quoted Sherlock Holmes' remark to his assistant, Dr Watson, that in a certain case it was the dog's behaviour that had attracted his attention. When Watson replied that the dog had done nothing, Sherlock Holmes explained that that, in fact, was the important clue. This lesson is immensely relevant to epidemiological studies.

D. *Adaptation to harmful environmental factors*

Cleave (Cleave *et al.*, 1969) has made a great contribution to the understanding of disease–environment relationships by his emphasis on the importance of evolutionary adaptation and he has shown how man, given sufficient time, can adapt to certain environmental factors, including changes in diet. It is probable that the Eskimos and certain pastoral tribes in Africa such as the Masai, adapted to their very high-fat low-carbohydrate diet many thousands of years ago. The Masai appear to have adapted well to a high dietary intake of cholesterol, and their plasma cholesterol levels do not rise as much as those of other ethnic groups on milk-rich diets (Mann *et al.*, 1972). Little is known about man's adaptation to harmful environmental factors. People exposed to the sun develop protective pigment in the skin, but there are no signs that man can adapt to X-ray radiation. If a harmful environmental factor produces disease only in middle-aged and elderly persons it is difficult to see how evolutionary adaptation secures the survival of the fittest. Man's ability or failure to adapt to new environmental factors has considerable relevance to the main theme of this book, which concerns the emergence of certain chronic diseases owing to lack of adaptation to the consumption of a large amount of fibre-depleted carbohydrate foods.

VI. Value of environment–disease relationships

Only what is looked for is seen, and only what is listened for heard. In order to establish the frequency or more especially the absence of a particular disease in a given area or community, it must be specifically looked for. Epidemiological studies based on the analysis of regular reports from doctors in numerous hospitals in many countries who have over a long period been on the lookout for a limited selection of diseases, have provided much of the evidence in support of hypotheses discussed in this book.

Historically, the observed relationships between certain diseases and the environments in which they are most prevalent frequently provided the bases of hypotheses as to possible causative factors. The subsequent experimental testing of such hypotheses has in many instances confirmed the suggested cause of the disease.

The ultimate goal in establishing a relationship between an environment and a disease is to be able to reduce or eliminate the disease-causing factor, or at least to provide protection against it.

Experimental work is likely to be most fruitful when it is an endeavour to test a hypothesis which is consistent with epidemiological evidence.

References

BURKITT, D. and HUTT, M. S. R. (1966). *International Pathology* **7**, 1.
CLEAVE, T. L., CAMPBELL, G. D. and PAINTER, N. S. (1969). "Diabetes, Coronary Thrombosis and the Saccharine Disease", 2nd edition. John Wright, Bristol.
HUTT, M. S. R. and BURKITT, D. (1965). *British Medical Journal* **2**, 719.
MANN, G. V., SPOERRY, A., GRAY, M. and JARSAHOW, D. (1972). *American Journal of Epidemiology* **95**, 26.

Chapter 2

Significance of relationships

DENIS BURKITT

I. Types of relationships 9
II. Associated effects of a common cause 9
III. Types of disease association 10
   A. Geographical areas 10
   B. Particular groups 10
   C. Individuals 11
   D. Time and order of emergence 12
IV. Related causes 13
V. Association as a possible guide to causative factors . . . 15
VI. A group of diseases associated with western civilization . . . 17
References 19

I. Types of relationships

The importance of determining the geographical distribution of a particular disease in certain communities, or in particular groups within a community, has been emphasized in Chapter 1. After a distribution pattern has been determined a search must be made for environmental factors peculiar to, or prominent in, all areas or groups having a high frequency of that disease, and absent, or of low intensity, in those in which the disease is rare or unknown. A second form of relationship which might assist in the search for disease causation is that which may exist between the distribution of one disease and that of another.

II. Associated effects of a common cause

All the effects of a single common cause will tend to be associated together wherever this cause operates (Fig. 2.1), and absent if the cause is not present. Before the insistence on smokeless fuel in London and other cities, blackened masonry, dusty windows and smog were all more prevalent than they are today, since they resulted from a common factor: a smoke-laden atmosphere. The same principle applies in the field of medicine: diseases observed to be frequently associated with one another may be suspected of having some causative factor in common (Burkitt, 1969, 1970a, b).

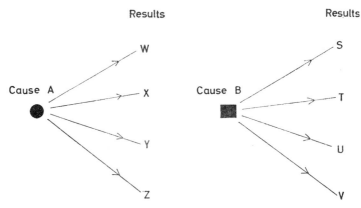

FIG. 2.1. The different results of a common cause will tend to be associated with one another.

III. Types of disease association

A. Geographical areas

An example of geographical association between diseases reflecting dependence on a common environmental factor is the observation that excessive exposure to the sun leads to a high prevalence of skin epithelioma, basal-cell carcinoma and loss of skin elasticity, all of which conditions are particularly common in eastern Australia, where white-skinned people are much exposed to the sun (Fig. 2.2).

B. Particular groups

Two or more diseases may be found associated with one another in groups of individuals who are unduly exposed to some harmful environmental factor. Yachtsmen, for example, may be unduly prone to the skin diseases associated with excessive exposure to the sun as mentioned above (Fig. 2.2). A community dependent on a polluted water supply could be subjected to diseases caused by faecal contamination of its drinking water, for instance enteritis of various forms, typhoid fever, and possibly in some circumstances cholera. In both these examples a number of different diseases might tend to be associated with one another within particular sub-groups of the population.

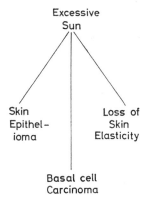

FIG. 2.2. The association between different skin diseases each of which is related to excessive exposure to the sun.

C. Individuals

If two or more diseases are causally related to a single environmental factor, individuals exposed to this common factor would be prone to develop several of the diseases. These diseases will therefore be more frequently associated with one another in single patients than would otherwise be expected.

The various effects of severe exposure to cigarette smoke provide an example. Bronchitis, lung cancer and stained fingers tend to be associated in the same individuals though all need not necessarily be present in any one person (Fig. 2.3).

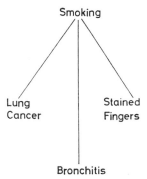

FIG. 2.3. The association between conditions each of which is related to smoking cigarettes.

Before the causative spirochaete of syphilis had been identified, the association in individual patients of several manifestations of this disease must have suggested a common cause. Palate perforation, sub-periosteal bone deposits and a previous history of a characteristic skin rash and penile sore would have been observed to be associated in a single patient.

In the case of Burkitt's lymphoma it was the recognition of an association in individuals between tumours in different but characteristic anatomical sites which led to the conviction that these were in fact all different results of a common cause (Burkitt, 1958). It was the subsequent recognition that these clinical manifestations were associated geographically in the same areas that initiated the studies which led to the hypothesis that a virus might be implicated in the cause of the disease and the subsequent identification of the E.B. virus.

D. Time and order of emergence

A harmful environmental factor often produces several diseases; some appear quickly, others develop slowly. Much depends on the severity and duration of the exposure that is required to produce the disease and, in addition, persons react in a variable manner. Cigarette smoking may produce laryngitis in an adolescent ("early arrival"), bronchitis in middle-age ("mid-arrival") and lung cancer in later life ("late arrival"). If a new and harmful environmental factor starts to affect a community, the order of appearance of certain diseases as important clinical problems has a characteristic pattern of emergence. In order to explain this concept diagrammatically a model will be used to illustrate certain principles.

1. Threshold level of exposure

A disease does not appear below a certain threshold of exposure to causative factors. This threshold is represented by the height of a flask standing in the rain which represents the harmful environmental factor. When the flask is filled, water is spilled; this represents the disease (Fig. 2.4).

2. Period of exposure

Different periods of exposure are required to produce various diseases. This is depicted by flasks of different heights: short flasks fill more easily and "early arrival" diseases appear in youth; "mid-arrival" diseases of middle-age appear several years later; the "late arrivals" of later life are the last to appear (Fig. 2.5). The characteristic pattern of disease emergence involves the order in which the diseases appear as common clinical problems, and the age-groups affected by different varieties of disease. The diseases of childhood, "early arrivals", appear first, then come the disorders of middle-age, "mid-arrivals" and finally those of later life, "late arrivals" (Fig. 2.5).

It follows that communities, such as those in developing countries, may be found to have only "early arrival" diseases but no "late arrival" disorders. Other communities, such as the technologically advanced countries, with long exposure to this harmful environmental factor, may show "early", "mid" and "late arrivals". No community should show

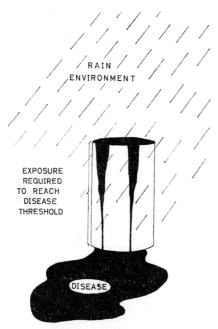

FIG. 2.4. The height of a jar representing the required exposure to an environment before a particular disease, represented by the overflow, is caused.

only "late arrival" diseases. If this characteristic pattern of emergence of certain diseases occurs in communities previously almost exempt from these disorders, this suggests a common causative factor or associated causative factors. Such a hypothesis is strengthened if this characteristic order of emergence of diseases as important clinical problems appears uniform in all communities examined whether they have been exposed to the posulated causative factor or associated factors for a short or long period of time.

IV. Related causes

If two causes are directly related to one another the effects of each tend also to be associated with one another (Fig. 2.6). In underdeveloped

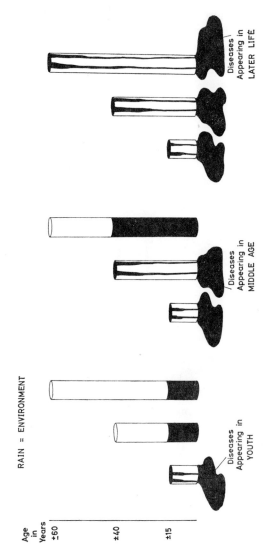

FIG. 2.5. Jars of different heights representing the varying extents of exposure to an environment required before different diseases appear.

countries education and economic sufficiency tend to be associated, for the educated man usually earns enough to meet his basic needs and anyone with financial means ensures that his family is educated. Basically, education results in the ability to read and write, as well as some technical and general knowledge, while economic sufficiency usually means that modern western diets are purchased. It follows that some or all the

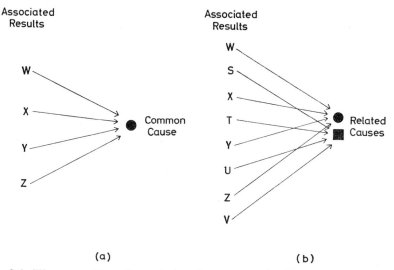

(a)   (b)

FIG. 2.6. The recognition of associations between results (diseases) points to the possibility that they may each be due to (a) common or (b) related causes.

results of these related causes tend to be associated within higher socio-economic groups, whilst all are rare or absent among the poor and illiterate members of underdeveloped countries.

Bantu labourers who have moved to work in South African mines have more money to purchase sugar and cigarettes than they had in the villages of the nearby homelands from which they were recruited. Since sugar and tobacco are associated with one another in the mine environment their effects will also tend to be associated in the resultant diseases. It is therefore likely that former miners who develop lung cancer in Natal villages will have lost more teeth from dental caries than their neighbours who have never left their home environment. The association of these diseases in individuals would thus reflect long previous exposure to two associated but different causes.

V. Associations as a possible guide to causative factors

If two or more diseases are the result of a single common cause, they will be unduly prevalent not only in specific countries and communities in which the causative factor operates but also in individuals who are severely exposed. They will therefore tend to be found in association in individual patients more often than would be expected from their independent incidence in the community as a whole. Similarly, if two or more different diseases are found in association geographically, or in communities or in individuals, this suggests that they may result from a single common cause or related causes (Fig. 2.6) (Burkitt, 1969, 1970a, b, 1971a).

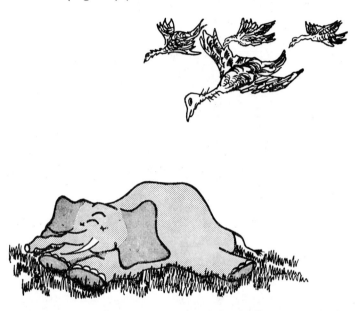

FIG. 2.7. Vultures are more readily detected than dead animals; the former are consequently a helpful guide to the latter.

When two diseases are observed to be consistently associated and the cause of one is identified, this known causative factor or factors may throw light on the obscure aetiology of the other disease. Moreover, if two or more diseases of obscure aetiology are closely associated it is more prudent to search first for the causative factors of the common or more readily recognized disorder. Having identified these factors, the possibility that they may also play a causative role in the case of the other disease can be investigated. In the African bush this principle can be applied when looking for the carcass of a dead animal, the position of which can easily be located by searching the sky for tell-tale vultures overhead, rather than by parting the grass with one's eyes to the ground, which would probably prove fruitless (Fig. 2.7). The separation of medicine into narrowly confined specialities precludes investigations which depend on clues provided by different fields (Burkitt, 1971a).

VI. A group of diseases associated with western civilization

Modern western civilization brings certain injuries due to obvious causes that arise in modern technological society, examples being motor car accidents and industrial pollution. In addition, there are in modern

	Diverticulosis	Colon cancer	Adenomatous polyps	Varicose veins	D.V.T.	Haemorrhoids	Ischaemic heart disease	Gallstones	Obesity	Diabetes	Hiatus hernia
Diverticulosis		+	+	+	+	+	+	+	+	+	+
Colon cancer	+		+	+	+	+	+	+	+	+	+
Adenomatous polyps	+	+		+	+	+	+	+	+	+	+
Varicose veins	+	+	+		+	+	+	+	+	+	+
D.V.T.	+	+	+	+		+	+	+	+	+	+
Haemorrhoids	+	+	+	+	+		+	+	+	+	+
Ischaemic heart disease	+	+	+	+	+	+		+	+	+	+
Gallstones	+	+	+	+	+	+	+		+	+	+
Obesity	+	+	+	+	+	+	+	+		+	+
Diabetes	+	+	+	+	+	+	+	+	+		+
Hiatus hernia	+	+	+	+	+	+	+	+	+	+	

FIG. 2.8. The geographical associations between each of the diseases listed. + represents a positive association.

technological society diseases of unknown causation which are rare or unknown in countries or communities which have departed least from their traditional way of life. These diseases tend to have intermediate levels of prevalence in countries and groups of people who have diverged only to a moderate degree from their customary diet and manner of life (Burkitt, 1972). Another characteristic of this group of diseases is that they are

	Diverticulosis	Colon cancer	Adenomatous polyps	Varicose veins	D.V.T.	Haemorrhoids	Ischaemic heart disease	Gallstones	Obesity	Diabetes	Hiatus hernia
Hiatus hernia	19							19	19		///
Diabetes	10						2, 15	2, 10, 14, 12	3, 18	///	
Obesity	19			16	5, 6		1	3, 11, 13	///	3, 18	19
Gallstones	19						2, 3, 14, 17	///	3, 11, 13	2, 10, 14, 12	19
Ischaemic heart disease	4, 9	20				5	///	2, 3, 14, 17	1	2, 15	
Haemorrhoids					5	///	5				
D.V.T.				5, 6	///	5			5, 6		
Varicose veins	7			///	5, 6				16		
Adenomatous polyps		8, 21	///								
Colon cancer		///	8, 21				20				
Diverticulosis	///			7			4, 9	19	19	10	19

1. Kannel et al., 1967
2. Bergman et al., 1968
3. Gross, 1929
4. Hughes, 1969
5. Lancet leader, 1971a
6. Kakkar et al., 1970
7. Latto et al., 1973
8. Morson and Bussey, 1970
9. Goldgraber and Kirsner, 1964
10. Schowengerdt et al., 1969
11. Robertson, 1945
12. Lieber, 1952
13. Burnett, 1971
14. Watkinson, 1967
15. Epstein, 1967
16. Mekky et al., 1969
17. Breyfogle, 1940
18. Lancet leader, 1971b
19. Muller, 1948
20. Wynder and Shigematsu, 1967
21. Bockus et al., 1961

FIG. 2.9. Recognized associations between diseases in individual patients (several require confirmation).

rare in wild animals which live on their traditional diets and follow their natural pattern of life, but certain of these diseases appear to be commoner in domestic animals fed food which differs considerably from that taken in their natural environment. For example, obesity and diabetes are commoner in domesticated dogs than in many other animals.

It is probable that diseases common in sophisticated communities and domesticated animals, and rare or unknown in people and animals that have retained their traditional manner of life and diet, are related to man-made environmental factors. Cleave and Campbell (1966) and Cleave *et al.* (1969) produced much epidemiological evidence that such diseases constitute a definite group including diabetes, obesity, dental caries, varicose veins, haemorrhoids, coronary heart disease and diverticular disease; they attributed them to the excessive consumption of unrefined carbohydrate foods—especially sugar—and the removal of fibre. This work was the immediate stimulus to my own study, with emphasis placed on the reduction of fibre as the common causative factor in the increased incidence of diseases of the colon (Burkitt, 1973), diverticular disease (Painter and Burkitt, 1971), cancer of the colon (Burkitt, 1971b) and appendicitis (Burkitt, 1971c). Fibre decreased transit times and increased stool weights (Burkitt *et al.*, 1972).

In this book these diseases are considered first, then the metabolic disorders—gallstones, ischaemic heart disease, diabetes and obesity, followed by the relationship of dental caries to diet. The possible influence of diet on the prevalence of duodenal ulcer and on certain auto-immune diseases is next discussed, after which a chapter is devoted to the vulnerability of animals to these diseases, which appear to emanate from a "man-made" environment.

The inter-relationships between some of these diseases both in their geographical distribution and in individual patients, as depicted in Fig. 2.8 and Fig. 2.9, suggest that some causative factor is common to each disease.

References

BERGMAN, F., VAN DER LINDEN, W. and SÖDERSTRÖM, J. (1968). *Acta pathologica et microbiologica scandinavica* **73**, 559.

BOCKUS, H. L., TACHDJIAN, V., FERGUSON, L. K., MOUHRAN, Y. and CHAMBERLAIN, C. (1961). *Gastroenterology* **41**, 225.

BREYFOGLE, H. S. (1940). *Journal of the American Medical Association* **114**, 1434.

BURKITT, D. P. (1958). *British Journal of Surgery* **46**, 218.

BURKITT, D. P. (1969). *Lancet* **2**, 1229.

BURKITT, D. P. (1970a). *Lancet* **2**, 1237.

BURKITT, D. P. (1970b). *International Pathology* **11**, 3.

BURKITT, D. P. (1971a). *Journal of the National Cancer Institute* **47**, 913.

BURKITT, D. P. (1971b). *Cancer* **28**, 3.

BURKITT, D. P. (1971c). *British Journal of Surgery* **58**, 695.

BURKITT, D. P. (1972). *In* "Medical Annual" (R. B. Scott and R. M. Walker, eds), p. 5. John Wright, Bristol.

BURKITT, D. P., WALKER, A. R. P. and PAINTER, N. S. (1972). *Lancet* **2**, 1408.

BURKITT, D. P. (1973). *Clinical Radiology* **24**, 271.

BURNETT, W. (1971). *Tijdschrift voor Gastroenterologie* **14**, 79.

CLEAVE, T. L. and CAMPBELL, G. D. (1966). "Diabetes, Coronary Thrombosis, and the Saccharine Disease", John Wright, Bristol.

CLEAVE, T. L., CAMPBELL, G. D. and PAINTER, N. S. (1969). "Diabetes, Coronary Thrombosis and the Saccharine Disease", 2nd edition. John Wright, Bristol.

EPSTEIN, F. H. (1967). *Journal of the American Medical Association* **201**, 795.

GOLDGRABER, M. B. and KIRSNER, J. B. (1964). *Diseases of the Colon and Rectum* **7**, 336.

GROSS, D. M. B. (1929). *Journal of Pathology and Bacteriology* **32**, 503.

HUGHES, L. E. (1969). *Gut* **10**, 336.

KAKKAR, V. V., HOWE, C. T., NICOLAIDES, A. N., RENNEY, J. T. G. and CLARKE, M. B. (1970). *American Journal of Surgery* **120**, 527.

KANNEL, W. B., LEBAUER, E. J., DAWBER, T. R. and McNAMARA, P. M. (1967). *Circulation* **35**, 734.

Lancet leader (1971a). *Lancet* **2**, 693.

Lancet leader (1971b). *Lancet* **1**, 381.

LATTO, C., WILKINSON, R. W. and GILMORE, O. J. A. (1973). *Lancet* **1**, 1089.

LIEBER, M. M. (1952). *Annals of Surgery* **135**, 394.

MEKKY, S., SCHILLING, R. S. F. and WALFORD, J. (1969). *British Medical Journal* **2**, 591.

MORSON, B. C. and BUSSEY, H. J. R. (1970). Predisposing causes of intestinal cancer. *In* "Current Problems in Surgery". Year Book Medical Publishers, Chicago.

MULLER, C. J. B. (1948). *South African Medical Journal* **22**, 376.

PAINTER, N. S. and BURKITT, D. P. (1971). *British Medical Journal* **2**, 450.

ROBERTSON, H. E. (1945). *International Abstracts of Surgery* **80**, 1.

SCHOWENGEROT, C. G., HEDGES, G. R., YAW, P. B. and ALTEMEIER, W. A. (1969). *Archives of Surgery* **98**, 500.

WATKINSON, G. (1967). Relationship between gallstones and other medical diseases. *In Proceedings of 3rd World Congress of Gastroenterology, Tokyo.* 1966, Vol. 4, pp. 125–130. Karger, Basel.

WYNDER, E. L. and SHIGEMATSU, T. (1967). *Cancer* **20**, 1520.

Part II

Refined carbohydrate foods

Chapter 3

Refined carbohydrate foods and fibre

HUGH TROWELL

I. Refined and unrefined carbohydrate foods 23
   A. Definition 23
   B. Refined cereals 24
   C. Refined sugar 25
   D. Unrefined starchy roots, tubers and fruit 26
   E. Unrefined legumes 27
II. Dietary fibre 27
   A. Definition 27
   B. Analysis of fibre 30
   C. Composition 32
III. History of medical thought on refined carbohydrates . . . 35
   A. Sugar 35
   B. Refined cereals 36
   C. Cleave's hypothesis 37
References 39

I. Refined and unrefined carbohydrate foods

A. Definition

Refined carbohydrate foods are defined as refined sugar and refined starchy foods, a practical, if not a scientific definition. A fundamental division is made between sucrose, which is broken down by enzymes to glucose and fructose at the brush border membrane of the villi in the small intestine, and starch, which is broken down by pancreatic α-amylase largely within the lumen of the small intestine into maltose and a little glucose. Amylase may also act at the border of the villi of the small intestine breaking down soluble starch into glucose (Dawson, 1968).

Man invariably eats processed food, which is always prepared and

23

purified. Refinement of food is not inherently wrong, but we must consider how far this can be done without impairing health.

B. Refined cereals

The processing of cereal foods (Kent, 1970a) starts by removing the chaff. At the mill wheat is cleaned and then milled to various degrees of extraction. Wholemeal (100% extraction) (known in the U.S.A. as wholewheat flour) is milled by grinding the whole of the wheat kernel. Wholemeal is brownish in colour, and rich in protein, vitamins, essential fatty acids, mineral salts and crude fibre (2·0%) as well as starch. Brown bread, of which there are many varieties, must by British law contain a minimum of crude fibre (0·6%), but is often brown largely because it has been coloured by caramel. White flour and bread (70% extraction) contain little crude fibre (0·1%), and less protein, mineral salts or vitamins. In Britain by law white flour is enriched with thiamin, niacin, iron and chalk. In the U.S.A. the addition of chalk is optional, but that of riboflavin is compulsory. A low extraction rate of 70% means that from 100 parts of whole wheat grain 70 parts of white flour have been extracted, and the remaining 30 parts, containing most of the fibre and much of the protein, vitamins and mineral salts have been discarded.

Oatmeal (crude fibre 1·1%) or rolled oats (crude fibre 0·9%) are lightly milled products prepared from oats. Oatmeal is prepared as a meal, not as a flour, thereby signifying that much fibre-rich bran has been retained with the starchy endosperm. This fibre does not have a detrimental effect on the quality or flavour. Although the milling of rye is similar to that of wheat, it is more difficult to remove the fibre-rich bran from the starchy endosperm. Whole rye products, as in Scandinavian crisp-bread, are rich in crude fibre (2·0%), especially the hemicelluloses, and even the low extraction rye flour (70%) contains moderate amounts of crude fibre (0·5%). Bread in both Germany and Scandinavia may contain a mixture of wheat and rye flour. Barley, which was the cereal of the Stone Age, was still the staple cereal of British peasants up to the fifteenth century, whereas the nobility ate wheaten bread.

Maize (corn) is grown extensively in North and South America, India, parts of southern Europe and Africa. Low-fibre breakfast cereals, such as corn flakes, are made from it. If maize is milled by modern methods, the hull (outer coat) and germ are removed. The latter is a rich source of essential fatty acids, especially linolenic and oleic acids. In many rural areas of Africa maize is pounded as whole grain, or taken as lightly milled maize meal as by the Bantu of the southern countries of Africa. This meal is still rich in crude fibre, 80% extraction containing 1·2% and 60% extraction 0·7%. Millet was the traditional cereal of Africa and many countries of the Middle East. Millet meal is also rich in crude fibre, the wholemeal containing 3·0% and the lightly processed millet flour 1·8%.

Rice is the main cereal of the East. Over half that grown is lightly processed and eaten on the small-holdings on which it is planted. Rice, like barley and oats, retains its husk after threshing, when it is called paddy rice. This can be put through a sheller which removes the woody husk, leaving "brown" or "whole" rice, which is comparable to whole wheat grain, for it contains pericarp, and the underlying aleurone layer surrounds the starchy endosperm. Parboiled rice is prepared by an ancient method of steeping the paddy rice in hot water, so that even after the subsequent removal of the husk, most of the vitamins and a moderate amount of crude fibre (0·7%) are retained. Modern methods of milling initially remove most of the bran, leaving unpolished rice (crude fibre 0·5%), and it is often further processed in a brush machine, removing the last layers of the vitamin-rich aleurone layer, to produce "polished" rice with only 0·2% fibre content. Various schemes of vitamin fortification have replaced the vitamins lost in milling, but no attempt has been made to restore the fibre.

C. Refined sugar

Sixty per cent of refined sugar is manufactured from sugar cane, and 40% from sugar beet. Sugar cane is chewed by some country peasants in tropical regions and the pith then rejected. The chemical composition of refined sugar is almost the same as that of the unrefined, dirty greenish juice expressed from the crushed sugar cane; the latter contains only a trace of fibre. Many impurities are removed during refinement. The consumption of refined white sugar, which is the cheapest source of energy (calories), increases rapidly as soon as sophistication comes to an underdeveloped community, and the level of consumption usually rises quickly to approach the western level of some 50 kg/year. In the U.S.A. sugar consumption had reached its plateau by 1920, and in Britain by 1957 (Fig. 3.1). In both countries there was a steep rise from about 10 kg/year in 1850 to the present levels of over 50 kg. As far as it is known the main danger from sucrose is the possibility of over-consumption. It is a concentrated form of energy (400 kcal/100 g) and it contains no protein, vitamins or fibre. In any consideration of obesity it is probable that sugar, white flour, fats, oils and milk must all be considered. None of these contains any fibre, except a trace in refined flour. In terms of history the common man in western society had little milk or butter until the agricultural revolution of the eighteenth century made it possible to feed cattle during the winter, and in the nineteenth and twentieth centuries improved

wages for industrial workers meant that they could purchase these com-
modities. The presence of raised serum lipid levels in adult life brings up
the question of western man's adaptation to high-fat diets in recent
centuries.

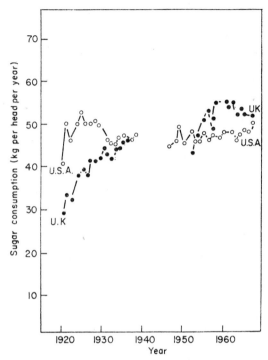

Fig. 3.1. Average sugar consumption in U.S.A. and U.K. (Gap 1939 onwards
during period of rationing.) (Yudkin, 1972.)

D. Unrefined starchy roots, tubers and fruit

These starchy foods have a high water content (75%) and store less well
than do drier cereal grains. The "Irish" potato is the only starchy tuber
commonly eaten in the western world. In proportion to its calories it
contains almost as much crude fibre (5·2 g/1000 kcal) as does wholemeal
bread (5·4 g/1000 kcal).

In the rural communities of Africa, Asia and tropical America, starchy
roots such as cassava and yam, which can be stored as dried flours, are
important sources of energy. All are rich in fibre. The tough outer skin
of starchy tubers was at one time considered to contain all the "goodness",
as in the case of the vitamin-rich outer layers of all cereals. There appears,
however, to be little foundation for the concept that "protein-stripping"

(Cleave *et al.*, 1969) occurs when these foods are prepared by peeling. Raw old potato for example contains protein 2·1 g/100 g, which is only slightly less than the 2·5 g/100 g contained in the peel.

Starchy roots, tubers and fruit probably represent the oldest foods known to man, who picked them and dug them up from tropical regions during the million or more years that he was a food-gatherer. Some tubers, and many fruits, especially in the tropics, contain a fair amount of sucrose: for example bananas 16%, sweet potatoes 9%, beetroot 10%, grapes 16%, dates 64%, dried figs 53% and dried apricots 44%. Prehistoric man sucked these and other fruits and spat out the pithy portion. Man has probably become adapted to receive moderate amounts of dissolved sucrose into his alimentary tract, but the problem with modern refined sugar is its ease of consumption.

E. Unrefined legumes

In many countries in the drier parts of Asia, the Middle East and Africa, leguminous seeds are eaten not as soft, immature vegetables, such as the green peas of any western nation, but as mature, dried, stored seeds. They make important contributions to both protein (20–30 g/100 g) and energy (300–400 kcal/100 g) and are the richest in fibre of all vegetable foods (4–7 g/100 g), containing from two to three times as much as does wheat wholemeal bread. After the inedible outer coverings are removed from these dried leguminous seeds, they are seldom milled but merely pounded into a coarse meal and consumed unrefined.

II. Dietary fibre

A. Definition

Dietary fibre has been defined as the remnants of the plant cell-wall that are not hydrolysed by the alimentary enzymes of man (Trowell, 1972a, b). It is composed largely of celluloses, hemicelluloses and lignin (Southgate, 1973). Dietary fibre is not the same as crude fibre which is often called merely fibre, and reported as such in food tables. Crude fibre is composed of a portion of the celluloses, adherent traces of hemicelluloses and lignin; it contains little of the hemicelluloses. The first reference to any specific use of the term dietary fibre was made by Hipsley (1953), who stated that it consisted of cellulose, lignin and hemicellulose.

McCance and Lawrence (1929) in their classic study *The Carbohydrate Content of Foods* adopted this chemical definition of fibre: "Fibre [is] defined as insoluble residue left after treating plant material with water, dilute acids and alkalis, alcohol and ether and it represents the most resistant parts of the skeletal framework of the plant". It was considered to contain cellulose, lignin and some resistant hemicelluloses (pentosans). These workers referred in considerable detail to the basic studies of Rubner (1885, 1901) on "cell-membranes", defined chemically as the residue of plant cell-walls after extraction by water, diastase, chloral hydrate and ether. Rubner's "cell-membranes" appear to be largely the same as dietary fibre. McCance and Lawrence recognized, as had Rubner, that the "cell-membranes" or total "fibre" from cereals were far more laxative than those of vegetables and fruit. Chemists no longer use terms such as hemicellulose and pectic substances, which can be compared to old-fashioned phrases like "fat-soluble vitamins" as opposed to "water-soluble vitamins" that preceded the isolation and chemical definition of the individual vitamins. Chemists speak of various groups of substances in the "hemicelluloses" such as xylans and arabinans, which are homopolysaccharides. These, however, occur less commonly in "fibre" than do the heteropolysaccharides such as the arabinoxylans which are commonly found in cereal grains and are water soluble. It is no longer possible to define the hemicelluloses merely in terms of a group of substances extracted by alkali.

Many years previously Atwater (1902) had elaborated the concept of the "availability" of various nutrients. Thus the "available" nitrogen was the nitrogen derived from the protein in the food, minus the nitrogen in the faeces. It was assumed that the "available" nitrogen had been completely absorbed, and the "unavailable" nitrogen, or fat, had been passed in the stool. The term and concept of "unavailable carbohydrate", meaning carbohydrate in food minus carbohydrate in faeces, was never used, largely because starch and sugar appeared to be completely, or almost completely, digested. This term was given an entirely new slant and definition when McCance and Lawrence (1929) divided the carbohydrates in food into those which were known to be hydrolysed by human alimentary enzymes, such as starch, amylopectin, dextrin and sugar, which they referred to collectively as "available carbohydrate"; and the remainder of the carbohydrates, that is the crude fibre (celluloses and lignin), hemi-celluloses and pectic substances, which were not hydrolysed, were put into the other group, the "unavailable carbohydrates". These investigators were concerned to define the group of substances that could be digested and were available to contribute energy. As a result a group of workers, based largely on Cambridge, have continued to publish studies on the "unavailable carbohydrates", but these have been almost disregarded by nutritionists, many of whom failed to recognize that "unavailable carbo-hydrate" had anything to do with "fibre". Until recently even gastro-enterologists have failed to recognize the extent to which unavailable carbohydrates can alter either the function of the small intestine where they remain unhydrolysed, or that of the large bowel, where many of them are profoundly altered, being degraded by bacteria (Cummings, 1973).

A further confusion arose from the fact that few books of nutrition or standard food tables stated clearly that the available carbohydrate portion of foods was seldom measured by direct determination. The protein, as nitrogen, and the fat were estimated by direct determination, but the carbohydrate content of foods was assessed "by difference". That is to say

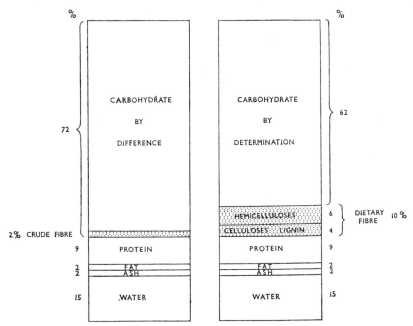

FIG. 3.2. Approximate analysis of wheat wholemeal 100% extraction. (Fraser, 1958; Kent, 1970b.)

the food was analysed for moisture, ash, fat and protein (calculated from the total nitrogen) and it was assumed that if the sum of all these fractions was deducted from the total weight, the difference represented the carbohydrate content, which was reported as monosaccharide (Fig. 3.2). In most food tables this included the crude fibre, but in others this was excluded (Platt, 1971). In most American and European food tables "carbohydrate by difference" is equated with the total carbohydrate content of foods. This is a reasonably rapid procedure for estimating the amount of digestible carbohydrate for many animals, especially ruminants. Since celluloses, lignins and hemicelluloses are not hydrolysed by human alimentary enzymes, this method is inappropriate for estimating available carbohydrate in man. British workers (McCance and Lawrence, 1929; Southgate, 1969a) have preferred direct methods of determination and the British

Food Composition Tables (McCance and Widdowson, 1960) record values for available carbohydrate thus measured.

The term "unavailable carbohydrate" is not acceptable, for three reasons.

(1) If unavailable nitrogen is the difference between nitrogen (as protein) eaten and nitrogen in the faeces, then the term unavailable carbohydrate might be surmised to be the difference between carbohydrate eaten and that present in the faeces.

(2) Unavailable carbohydrate is partially degraded by bacteria in the colon (Southgate and Durnin, 1970) and makes a definite even if small contribution to absorbed energy.

(3) The "unavailable carbohydrate" was found to be associated with lignin, which is not a carbohydrate. The concept of dietary fibre is, on the other hand, physiologically valid (Cummings, 1973).

B. Analysis of fibre

1. Unavailable carbohydrate and lignin—the dietary fibre

At the present time it is difficult to estimate by direct determination the various polysaccharides and lignins that comprise dietary fibre. All analytical procedures represent a compromise between ideal procedures based on the known properties of the polysaccharides and practical laboratory procedures. All methods are time-consuming and must be checked at several stages by other qualitative information obtained possibly by thin-layer chromatography.

The various schemes of analysis proposed (Williams and Olmsted, 1935; Fraser et al., 1956) have been limited to certain classes of foodstuff and were not generally applicable to all foods or to homogenates of a mixed diet. More recently Southgate (1969b) has proposed methods for the analysis of the main groups of substances present in the unavailable carbohydrate and lignin, that is to say celluloses, lignin, hemicelluloses, and also water-soluble polysaccharides which are seldom found in commonly eaten foods but are present as inulin in Jerusalem artichokes, galactan from agar, and gum from gum arabic. Van Soest and McQueen (1973) in the United States have proposed other methods of analysis; they have isolated the plant cell-wall structures with solutions containing detergents.

2. Crude fibre

The method of estimating crude fibre has been defined meticulously by international agreement of the Association of Official Agricultural Chemists and this supplies the figures for "fibre", more correctly called crude fibre in food tables (see Table 3.1). In outline it consists of obtaining from the carbohydrate food the residue that resists extraction by boiling first with 0·255 N sulphuric acid and subsequently with 0·313 N sodium hydroxide (Kent-Jones and Amos, 1967). The crude fibre content of cereal foods is a totally inadequate guide to the dietary fibre content, that

TABLE 3.1. Crude fibre and calorie content of food (per 100 g edible portion)

		Crude fibre (g/100 g)	Calories (kcal/100 g)
CEREALS	(Platt, 1971; Kent-Jones and Amos, 1967; McCance et al., 1945)		
barley,	whole dehusked	2·0	363
	pearled	0·8	351
maize,	whole	2·0	363
	meal, 96% extraction	1·5	362
	meal, 60% extraction	0·7	354
	cornflour	0·2	352
millet,	bulrush, whole	2·0	363
	meal	1·0	365
millet,	finger, whole	3·0	336
	meal	2·4	332
oats,	oatmeal	0·9	350
rice,	brown	2·0	360
	white, skinned	0·7	354
	polished	0·25	352
rye,	meal 85–90% extraction	1·5	350
sorghum,	whole	2·0	355
wheat,	wholemeal 100% extraction	1·6–2·1	344
	85% extraction	0·4–0·9	346
	70% extraction	trace–0·2	350
	bran	10·5–13·5	300
STARCHY ROOTS, TUBERS AND STARCHY FRUITS			
cassava,	fresh	1·0	153
	flour	1·5	342
plantain, and banana		0·3	128
potato,	Irish	0·4	75
	sweet	1·0	114
sago,	flour	trace	352
yam,	fresh	0·5	104
sugar cane, stem		2·1	50

Table 3.1—*continued*

	Crude fibre (g/100 g)	Calories (kcal/100 g)
GRAIN LEGUMES (Platt, 1971)		
chick pea	2·8	368
fenugreek	7·2	335
groundnut, dry	3·0	579
horse gram	5·3	338
kidney bean	4·0	339
lathyrus pea	15·0	293
lentil	4·0	339
lima bean	5·0	326
mung bean	4·5	329
pea, mature	4·5	337
immature	1·0	70
pigeon pea	7·0	328
soya bean, mature	4·5	382
OIL SEEDS AND NUTS		
most varieties	2–5	500–700
VEGETABLES AND FRUITS (Platt, 1971)		
most vegetables	0·5–1·5	30–50
most fruits	0·5–1·5	50–150
dates, dried	2·4	303
figs, dried	11·0	269

FIBRE-FREE FOODS
all meat, fish, eggs, fats, milk, cheese, sugar,
beverages and alcoholic drinks

is the unhydrolysed cell-wall remnants. Thus the crude fibre content of whole wheat is recorded as approximately 2·0 g/100 g (Platt, 1971). Two recent analyses of polysaccharides in the cell-wall of whole wheat are presented in Table 3.2. In whole cereals dietary fibre may exceed crude fibre by five times.

C. Composition

Gathering together different attempts to analyse the unavailable carbohydrates and lignin, it is possible to present data (Table 3.3) on the estimated composition of the plant cell-wall polysaccharides (Southgate,

1969b). These data agree well with those published by other workers (Jermyn and Isherwood, 1956; Thornber and Northcote, 1961a, b).

TABLE 3.2. Whole wheat dietary fibre (g/100 g)

	Celluloses	Lignins	Hemicelluloses	Total
Southgate (1969b)	1·1	2·6	7·5	11·2
Fraser (1958)	4·4		6·4	10·8

Fraser (1958) reported hemicelluloses 5·8 g/100 g, but this has been expressed as monosaccharide 6·4 g/100 g to bring it into line with the data of Southgate (1969b).

TABLE 3.3. Estimated composition of dietary fibre (after Southgate, 1969b) g/100 g of total unavailable carbohydrate and lignin

Constituent	Wheat	Rye	Potato	Apple	Pea	Cabbage	Plantain
"Cellulose"	10	12	36	42	64	69	14
"Hemicellulose"	65	78	32	32	29	24	84
Lignin	23	10	32	25	7	6	2

1. *Cellulose* (Aspinall, 1970a)

Cellulose is the most plentiful organic compound on earth, being widely distributed as a skeletal substance in all plant cell-walls which, however, vary considerably in their cellulose content. To the chemist and the crystallographer, cellulose is a polymer of linear chains of 1⟶ 4′ linked β-D-glucopyranose residues. The material exists as extremely thin long threads, some 100–200 Å in diameter. These threads contain a central crystalline core that is "pure" cellulose, but surrounded by a coat of mixed polysaccharide chains including xylans and mannans (two hemicelluloses) so tightly bound that they cannot be removed by chemical means without completely breaking the cellulose (R. D. Preston, p.c. 1972).

The special properties of cellulose result from the association of bundles of microfibrils of individual molecules held together in a highly ordered structure, which differs according to its source. The microfibrils are of almost infinite length. Cellulose is not hydrolysed by human alimentary enzymes and this fine network, in the meshes of which lie hemicelluloses and small amounts of partially digested cellular contents, travels intact down the small intestine. It has been assessed that some 15%

undergoes bacterial degradation in the large bowel (Southgate and Durnin, 1970).

2. *Hemicelluloses* (Pentosans) (Aspinall, 1970b)

This is an inaccurate, if not an obsolete term, which was used at one time to describe all the polysaccharides other than crude fibre. Indeed it was erroneously believed that hemicellulose was a precursor of cellulose; actually many of the polysaccharides in the plant cell-wall are present as a gel-matrix in which the cellulose fibrils are laid down (Southgate, 1973). Originally the term hemicellulose referred only to those polysaccharides which could be extracted from plant cell-walls with alkaline reagents, but not with water. In recent years classification has been based on chemical structure of the different polysaccharides. Thus the xylan group includes not only those soluble in alkalis but also the water-soluble arabinoxylans, commonly found in cereal grains. The "hemicellulose" fraction of the plant cell-wall possesses marked water-binding properties and produces soft stools. It has been assessed that some 85% undergoes bacterial degradation in the large bowel (Southgate and Durnin, 1970).

(a) *Xylans*, from the pentose sugar D-xylose, are a major component of all lignified land plant cell-wall structures and comprise 20–30% of grain hulls. Those derived from cereals have side-chains of more than one sugar unit. Partial degradation by mild acid hydrolysis or by enzymes has allowed some study of their complexity.

(b) *Arabinans*, from the pentose sugar L-arabinose, are found in association with the pectic substances in many plants, such as peanuts and sugar beet, and in the pectins of citrus fruits.

(c) *Galactans*, from the sugar galactose, of which the commoner forms D-galactose, D-galacturonic acid and L-arabinose, are the main constituents of a group of polysaccharides commonly referred to as the pectic substances or pectins, which contain considerable gelatinizing properties.

(d) *Mannans*, from the sugar D-mannose, either alone or in combination with other sugars, are common plant cell-wall polysaccharides. With D-galactose, as galactomannans, they are common in leguminous seeds. There is considerable complexity since the main chain of mannopyranose residues carries single unit side-chains based on varying proportions of galactopyranose residues.

(e) *Glucans*, from the sugar D-glucose, may occur as linear or branched glucans, and both varieties may be met in the same polysaccharide. Linear β-D-glucans are water-soluble polysaccharides which occur in oats and barley.

(*f*) *Glycuronans*, formerly called polyuronides, are composed exclusively or mainly of hexuronic acid residues. There are two varieties, alginic acid, found commonly in algae (seaweeds), and the pectic substances.

(*g*) *Other complex polysaccharides.*

3. Lignin

This is not a carbohydrate but an extremely complex aromatic polymer based on phenylpropane units such as coniferyl alcohol and sinapyl alcohol (Aspinall, 1970c). Lignin, which is not hydrolysed by strong acids or alkalis, nor perhaps degraded by bacteria in the colon (McCance and Lawrence, 1929), is the most resistant of all the plant cell-wall structures. Many foods eaten by man have not been analysed for their lignin content; this may increase considerably as the plant grows or the seed matures.

III. History of medical thought on refined carbohydrates

A. Sugar

The fear that sugar may be injurious is as old as the written history of this sweet food. In India about A.D. 100, soon after the cultivation of sugar cane had come from New Guinea (Deerr, 1949), Charaka Samhita ascribed not only obesity but even diabetes to this new article of diet (Tulloch, 1962). Emerson and Larimore (1924), having traced the reported rise in diabetic mortality in New York since 1866, ascribed it to increasing consumption of sugar, as did Stocks (1944), having considered the reported increased diabetic mortality in England and Wales from 1861 to 1942. Stocks was almost the first in Britain to draw attention to the marked decline in diabetic mortality in two World Wars, which he linked with war-time rationing and decreased consumption of sugar. This data, together with that of Himsworth (1949), was re-examined and amplified by Cleave and Campbell (1966), who stressed an apparent association in England and Wales between a decline in sugar consumption during both World Wars and a decline in diabetes mortality. Yudkin (1957, 1972) in a series of communications has maintained that diabetes, obesity and ischaemic heart disease are associated with a high consumption of sucrose.

Weighty criticisms have, however, been levelled against this postulated role of high sucrose consumption in the pathogenesis of ischaemic heart disease (Keys, 1971; Walker, 1971). This hypothesis has seldom been supported by epidemiological studies in various countries, or by individual case records of the consumption of sucrose in those who have sustained myocardial infarction, or by prospective studies of persons who reduced their intake of sugar. Grande (1967) summarized the experimental evidence when he stated that the effect of sucrose "on serum cholesterol in normal man was very limited". If sucrose in large amounts (60% calories) is fed experimentally to man or to animals, fasting serum lipids, especially triglycerides, rise, but there is little evidence that this occurs to a significant degree at normal dietary levels of consumption (under 20% calories) (Macdonald, 1972). Although there have been few long-term studies of the influence of sucrose (15–20% calories) on the production of obesity in man, many clinical workers still believe that sucrose consumption does influence obesity.

B. Refined cereals

It is considerably more difficult to summarize the history of medical thought concerning the possible ill-effects of refining cereals. Standard medical teaching, which is challenged in this study, has stated that bran "is a disadvantage" (Wright, 1962). Such teaching has suggested, until recently, that fibre intake should be reduced in the treatment of all diseases of the colon, a therapeutic approach that has recently been entirely reversed (Chapter 9). It has been demonstrated that fibre reduces the absorption of energy (calories), protein and fat from the gastrointestinal tract. This was formerly deemed to be a disadvantage, but it must now be asked whether it would not reduce development of obesity (Chapter 16).

The fact that the refining of wheat flour became more widespread in the eighteenth century (Chapter 5) could explain why Graham (1837) in the United States and Allinson (undated) early in the present century in Britain should extol the health-giving properties of wholemeal bread. Both these investigators had a mystical reverence for all "natural food", and their advocacy of teetotalism, and regrettably even opposition to vaccination, understandably estranged them from many members of the medical profession. Hay (1935), who strongly advocated "natural foods in their natural form", was the first to propound the notion that danger lay in concentration, and consequently lampooned "concentrated starches". As the notion of concentration is still discussed, it should be noted that in terms of bulk white flour 70% extraction (349 kcal/100 g) is only a little more concentrated than wholemeal flour 100% extraction (333 kcal/100 g) (McCance and Widdowson, 1960). Sugar is only slightly more concentrated (400 kcal/100 g), but refined fats and oils are much more so (900 kcal/100 g).

In Asia the refining of rice into polished rice led to an increased incidence of beri-beri. It is impossible to summarize here the epidemiological and experimental studies that related this disease to the removal of thiamin from the rice in the process of polishing. These investigations included the fundamental studies of McCarrison (1921, 1943), who during 7 years' work as a medical officer in the Punjab had noticed the excellent physique of those who ate whole cereals, milk and vegetables. He conducted numerous animal experiments designed to demonstrate that deficiency diseases could be produced if highly milled cereals were consumed. These studies preceded the unravelling of the vitamin B complex.

In Britain there has been a prolonged debate concerning the respective merits of wholemeal and white bread, which in 1956 was comprehensively reviewed up till that time by McCance and Widdowson. Their studies suggested that the reinforcement of white flour with essential vitamins and mineral salts prevented any deficiency of these absorbed nutrients. They did not discuss whether or not an unabsorbed constituent, fibre, was essential to the health of the host.

C. Cleave's hypothesis

From time to time a number of workers, mainly in the United States and Britain, have analysed bran, demonstrated its laxative effect and advocated its use (Williams and Olmsted, 1935, 1936). Dimock (1936) successfully treated 100 patients suffering from constipation with bran and recorded its apparent benefit in irritable colon, chronic colitis of unspecified type, and haemorrhoids, and cited some 75 references.

Cleave (1941) stated that he had treated naval personnel for constipation with "unprocessed bran". Reflecting on his experience he was led eventually to elaborate his concept of a single saccharine disease (Cleave, 1956) under which heading he included most of the diseases discussed in this book, along with some others, all of which he attributed to the excessive consumption of refined carbohydrate foods and of sugar in particular. These seminal ideas might be called Cleave's hypothesis. It is impossible to do justice to it here; suffice it to say that whatever defects may exist in the initial charting of this unmapped territory, the concept that man has adapted poorly to refined carbohydrates has proved for every writer in this book a mental catalyst.

Cleave (1957), who at first extolled the virtues of natural foods, considered that machinery "concentrated" carbohydrate foods, especially sugar, "stripping" them of protein, and decreasing the content of fibre. Ischaemic heart disease, diabetes and obesity were ascribed to increased consumption of sugar which he believed also led to an enhanced growth of *Bacillus coli* in the intestines, with a consequent increase of "infective conditions" such as appendicitis, cholecystitis and diverticulitis.

Cleave et al. (1969) further amplified one aspect of the already formulated Cleave's hypothesis, that is the effect of removal of fibre from food. This was believed to result in delayed intestinal transit times, resulting in constipation, diverticular disease, haemorrhoids, even varicose veins (Cleave, 1960), likewise dental caries (Cleave et al., 1969).

These broad generalizations, couched in terms of Darwinian evolution, appeared incredible to many. More attention might have been paid to them if Cleave (1957) had not dismissed completely the role of saturated animal fats in ischaemic heart disease, on the grounds that these were natural fats. There were, however, those whose independent studies had prepared them to consider that some aspect of Cleave's hypothesis might enlighten certain unsolved problems. Thus Painter (1964), who by his own observations had demonstrated high intraluminal pressures in the contracting colon of diverticular disease, did much to revolutionize its treatment by adding wheat bran to the diet; he challenged accepted concepts regarding its cause.

Heaton, in a series of publications culminating in the monograph on bile salts (Heaton, 1972), had appreciated the role of refined carbohydrate foods in the formation of gallstones. Tovey (1962) had studied the epidemiology of peptic ulcer in India and was stimulated to verify the evidence that impelled Cleave (1962) to relate this disease to refined carbohydrate foods. Burkitt (1970), from his experience as a surgeon in East Africa, recognized that the surgical diseases mentioned in Cleave's hypothesis were rare among Africans until they ate western diets. Stimulated by the previous work in South Africa of Walker (1947, 1949), Burkitt has studied bowel transit times and stool weights in relation to fibre in the diet (Burkitt et al., 1972) and he stressed the role of fibre in the aetiology of appendicitis (Burkitt, 1971a), cancer of the large bowel (Burkitt, 1971b), varicose veins, haemorrhoids, deep vein thrombosis (Burkitt, 1972) and hiatus hernia (Burkitt and James, 1973).

Trowell in his study of non-infective disease in Africans in 1960 was ignorant of the initial statement of the hypothesis of Cleave (1956). In his *Non-infective Disease in Africa* (1960) he gathered together his own experience as a physician for 30 years in East Africa and the existing medical literature from that continent. In 1971 he became aware that almost all the diseases listed by him as rare in Africans were among those mentioned by Cleave in the later amplifications of his concept of "the saccharine disease" (Cleave et al., 1969). Trowell's list fell largely into two groups: (1) diseases of the colon (diverticular disease, ulcerative colitis, carcinoma, haemorrhoids and irritable colon); these had been ascribed to the protective action of high-fibre diets, and (2) diabetes, ischaemic heart disease, gallstones and obesity. Trowell (1960) could suggest no explanation for the rarity of the latter diseases in Africans. He had first heard of the postulated role of fibre from Walker, who had, in numerous communications from South Africa (Walker, 1947, 1949, 1961, 1966; Bersohn et al., 1956) stressed its possible importance as a factor in many diseases. Trowell revisited Uganda in 1970 and realized that the pattern of non-infective diseases was changing; he therefore decided to examine critically the existing literature in the light of Cleave's hypothesis concerning sugar and fibre. The first essential was to define the term "fibre" which has been attempted in this chapter.

References

ALLINSON, T. R. (undated), "The Advantage of Whole Meal Bread." London.

ASPINALL, G. O. (1970). "Polysaccharides." Pergamon Press, Oxford. (a) pp. 43–53; (b) 69–221; (c) 43–44.

ATWATER, W. O. (1902). Connecticut (Storrs) Agriculture Experimental Station 14th Annual Report, 1901.

BERSOHN, I., WALKER, A. R. P. and HIGGINSON, J. (1956), *South African Medical Journal* **30**, 411.

BURKITT, D. P. (1970). *Lancet* **2**, 1237.

BURKITT, D. P. (1971a). *British Journal of Surgery* **58**, 695.

BURKITT, D. P. (1971b). *Cancer* **28**, 3.

BURKITT, D. P. (1972). *British Medical Journal* **1**, 556.

BURKITT, D. P. and JAMES, P. A. (1973). *Lancet* **2**, 128.

BURKITT, D. P., WALKER, A. R. P. and PAINTER, N. S. (1972). *Lancet* **2**, 1408.

CLEAVE, T. L. (1941). *British Medical Journal* **1**, 461.

CLEAVE, T. L. (1956). *Journal of the Royal Naval Medical Service* **40**, 116.

CLEAVE, T. L. (1957). "Fat Consumption and Coronary Disease." John Wright, Bristol.

CLEAVE, T. L. (1960). "On the Causation of Varicose Veins." John Wright, Bristol.

CLEAVE, T. L. (1962). "Peptic Ulcer." John Wright, Bristol.

CLEAVE, T. L. and CAMPBELL, G. D. (1966). "Diabetes, Coronary Thrombosis and the Saccharine Disease", pp. 15–60. John Wright, Bristol.

CLEAVE, T. L., CAMPBELL, G. D. and PAINTER, N. S. (1969). "Diabetes, Coronary Thrombosis and the Saccharine Disease", 2nd edition, pp. 89–94. John Wright, Bristol.

CUMMINGS, J. H. (1973). *Gut* **14**, 69.

DAWSON, A. M. (1968). *In* "The Scientific Basis of Medicine Annual Reviews", pp. 186–205. Athlone Press, London.

DEERR, N. (1949). "The History of Sugar", p. 14. Chapman and Hall, London.

DIMOCK, E. M. (1936). "The Treatment of Habitual Constipation by the Bran Method." M.D. Thesis, Cambridge.

EMERSON, H. and LARIMORE, L. D. (1924). *Archives of Internal Medicine* **34**, 587.

FRASER, J. R. (1958). *Journal of the Science of Food and Agriculture* **9**, 125.

FRASER, J. R., BRENDON-BRAVO, M. and HOLMES, D. C. (1956). *Journal of the Science of Food and Agriculture* **7**, 577.

GRAHAM, S. (1837). "A Treatise on Bread and Breadmaking." Light and Stearns, Boston.

GRANDE, F. (1967). *American Journal of Clinical Nutrition* **20**, 176.

HAY, W. H. (1935). "A New Health Era." Harrap, London.
HEATON, K. W. (1972). "Bile Salts in Health and Disease." Churchill Livingstone, Edinburgh.
HIMSWORTH, H. P. (1949). *Proceedings of the Royal Society of Medicine* **42**, 323.
HIPSLEY, E. H. (1953). *British Medical Journal* **2**, 420.
JERMYN, M. A. and ISHERWOOD, F. A. (1956). *Biochemical Journal* **64**, 123.
KENT, N. L. (1970). "The Technology of Cereals." Pergamon Press, Oxford. (a) pp. 115–134; (b) p. 37.
KENT-JONES, D. W. and AMOS, A. J. (1967). "Modern Cereal Chemistry", 6th edition, p. 564. Food Trade Press, London.
KEYS, A. (1971). *Atherosclerosis* **14**, 193.
McCANCE, R. A. and LAWRENCE, R. D. (1929). "The Carbohydrate Content of Foods." Special Report Series, Medical Research Council, London, No. 135. Her Majesty's Stationery Office, London.
McCANCE, R. A. and WIDDOWSON, E. M. (1956). "Breads, White and Brown." Pitman Press, London.
McCANCE, R. A. and WIDDOWSON, E. M. (1960). "The Composition of Foods." Special Report Series, Medical Research Council, London, No. 297. Her Majesty's Stationery Office, London.
McCANCE, R. A., WIDDOWSON, E. M., MORGAN, T., PRINGLE, W. J. S. and MACRAE, T. F. (1945). *Biochemical Journal* **39**, 213.
McCARRISON, R. (1921). "Studies in Deficiency Disease." Hodder and Stoughton, Oxford.
McCARRISON, R. (1943). "Nutrition and Health." Faber and Faber, London.
MACDONALD, I. (1972). *In* "Sugar" (J. Yudkin, J. Edelman and L. Hough, eds), p. 198. Butterworth, London.
PAINTER, N. S. (1964). *Annals of the Royal College of Surgeons of England* **34**, 98.
PLATT, B. S. (1971). "Tables of Representative Values of Foods Commonly Used in Tropical Countries", p. 2. Special Report Series, Medical Research Council, London, No. 302. Her Majesty's Stationery Office, London.
RUBNER, M. (1885). *Zeitschrift Biologie* **21**, 250.
RUBNER, M. (1901). *Ibid.* **42**, 261.
SOUTHGATE, D. A. T. (1969). *Journal of the Science of Food and Agriculture* **20**, (a) 326; (b) 331.
SOUTHGATE, D. A. T. (1973). *Plant Foods for Man* **1**, 45.
SOUTHGATE, D. A. T. and DURNIN, J. V. G. A. (1970). *British Journal of Nutrition* **24**, 517.
STOCKS, P. (1944). *Journal of Hygiene, Cambridge* **43**, 242.
THORNBER, J. P. and NORTHCOTE, D. M. (1961). *Biochemical Journal* **81**, (a) 449; (b) 455.
TOVEY, F. (1962). Ch.M. Thesis, University of Liverpool.
TROWELL, H. (1960). "Non-infective Disease in Africa." Edward Arnold, London.
TROWELL, H. (1972a). *Atherosclerosis* **16**, 138.
TROWELL, H. (1972b). *American Journal of Clinical Nutrition* **25**, 926.
TULLOCH, J. A. (1962). "Diabetes Mellitus in the Tropics", p. 1. Livingstone, Edinburgh.

VAN SOEST, P. J. and McQUEEN, R. W. (1973). *Proceedings of the Nutrition Society* **32**, 123.

WALKER, A. R. P. (1947). *South African Medical Journal* **21**, 590.

WALKER, A. R. P. (1949). *Nature* **164**, 825.

WALKER, A. R. P. (1961). *South African Medical Journal* **35**, 114.

WALKER, A. R. P. (1966). *Ibid.* **40**, 814.

WALKER, A. R. P. (1971). *Atherosclerosis* **14**, 137.

WILLIAMS, R. D. and OLMSTED, W. H. (1935). *Journal of Biological Chemistry* **108**, 653.

WILLIAMS, R. D. and OLMSTED, W. H. (1936). *Journal of Nutrition* **11**, 433.

WRIGHT, S. (1962). "Applied Physiology" (C. A. Keele and E. Neil, eds), 10th edition, p. 448. Oxford University Press, London.

YUDKIN, J. (1957). *Lancet* **2**, 155.

YUDKIN, J. (1972). *In* "Sugar" (J. Yudkin, J. Edelman and L. Hough, eds), pp. 14–17. Butterworth, London.

Chapter 4

Some historical aspects of milling cereals and refining sugar

HUGH TROWELL

I. Ancient history 43
II. Milling wheat 43
III. Milling other cereals 44
    A. Rye 44
    B. Oats 45
    C. Maize (corn) 45
    D. Rice 45
IV. Refining sugar 45
References 46

I. Ancient history

The history of man's attempt to refine carbohydrate foods is as long as the history of man, or even longer. His primate ancestors ate starch in seeds, nuts and buds; they sucked sugar in the sweet tropical fruits, spitting out coarse pith. The molar teeth of paleolithic man and the excavation of their habitation sites have demonstrated that they munched seeds, dug up starchy roots and gathered fruit. Possibly they obtained over half their daily energy from vegetable sources, as do African Bushmen at the present day.

II. Milling wheat

About 10,000 years ago in the lands of the Middle East, notably Iran, wild wheat and barley were first cultivated as crops, and wild sheep and goats were domesticated. Stored cereals became the basis of city life of the first civilizations (Trowell, 1973). Paleolithic man had gathered seeds and ground them between stones, but the first sieves to sift the coarse bran from the ground meal were those of Egypt. There, grain was ground by hand on stone slabs.

Some bran was sifted from the flour to make the off-white bread as eaten by the upper classes of Greece and Rome. The Romans introduced circular mill-stones, while later in Britain water-power from the rivers drove the stone-ground mills. Sieves, however, still remained primitive, being made of wool and linen threads, until fine silk sieves were introduced in the eighteenth century. The first sieving removed the coarse horse bran, the second the fine bran (McCance and Widdowson, 1956). In that century mills too were altered. The upper mill-stone was raised to inaugurate the "high-grinding" system which provided for the first time flours of diverse qualities; some contained less bran (Kent, 1970a), were expensive and prized by the rich.

The agricultural revolution of the eighteenth century, coupled with the enclosure of the common fields, prevented small-holders from cultivating their own barley and rye, so that wheat, which had been gaining in popularity for a long time, became the farm crop of the new system. The flour for the common man was changing; thus in 1775 there was a complaint that "bakers do not make as they formerly did, bread of unsifted flour" (Hammond and Hammond, 1911). At that time dispossessed labourers drifted to the new industrial towns. Authorities have stated that even there "the best quality 'white flour' prior to the middle of the nineteenth century was a wholemeal flour, produced by stone grinding, from which coarse particles of bran were removed by bolting through fine linen and woollen cloths. It contained a great deal of finely ground bran and most of the germ" (Drummond and Wilbrandon, 1957).

The new fine silk bolting cloths (sieves) introduced in the middle of the nineteenth century probably did even more to reduce the bran than the new steel roller mills introduced from the Continent in 1878 (Jones, 1958). By 1910 almost all the old stone-ground mills had been pulled down or converted.

The pressure in the roller mills can be adjusted, so that gentle pressure is exerted in order to fracture the starchy endosperm along its cell-boundaries. It is important to note that only 9% of the starch granules are damaged. This is called "available starch" by the miller: it can be attacked by β-amylase of the flour; if too much is "available", it will not bake a good loaf (Kent, 1970b).

III. Milling other cereals

A. Rye

Until the seventeenth century rye, taken with barley and wheat as maslin bread, was commonly eaten in Britain. Rye is still an important bread grain in Scandinavia and Eastern European countries, and is often eaten as fibre-rich wholemeal or coarsely ground flour.

B. Oats

Oats, taken as fibre-rich oatmeal or oat cakes, used to be widely eaten in Scotland and Wales, primitive milling techniques then being employed.

C. Maize (corn)

As long ago as 5000 B.C. maize was the cereal of the ancient civilizations of Mexico and Central America (Trowell, 1973). It was pounded in mortars or ground by hand between stones. In the last century the American negro relied on coarsely ground maize meal (hominy). American Indians were hunter food-gatherer tribes, until restricted by the white man; they too were introduced to hominy. The Spaniards took maize to Africa and Asia, where it competed with, and partially supplanted, traditional cereals such as millet. Irish potatoes, sweet potatoes and manioc (cassava) also spread from America to other continents, but remained unprocessed starchy carbohydrate foods.

Eventually simple milling techniques, based on those employed in wheat milling, were used to produce coarse maize meal. It was seldom a high extraction flour. Maize is deficient in tryptophan and niacin and there have been outbreaks of pellagra wherever it has been the main item of diet.

D. Rice

Rice became the dominant crop of Eastern civilizations of India and China. It was and still is prepared for cooking by simple techniques described in Chapter 3.

IV. Refining sugar

The cultivation of sugar spread slowly from the South Pacific Islands where it is indigenous, to reach India about 300 B.C. (Deerr, 1949). A small amount was cultivated in Persia by the Arabs in the first millennium A.D., but sugar remained an expensive rare luxury in Europe during the Middle Ages until the West Indies started production about A.D. 1600. Primitive mills for crushing the cane and refineries for removing the impurities were built at about the same time and provided a small amount of sugar, which in the eighteenth century was drunk in chocolate, tea and coffee by the upper classes. The vacuum pan method of manufacturing refined sugar started in 1813; this and other improvements allowed production to increase rapidly, and large modern refineries were built to refine the crude products. The whole process of refinement consists of removing impurities and colouring matter from the crude liquid. Even unrefined products contain only negligible traces of fibre and no vitamins or protein, and there are no known nutrients present in unrefined sugar which are absent in refined sugar. There are, however, certain slight changes in chemical composition; for instance, pyrophosphates are not the same in refined and unrefined sugar. Sucrose is a palatable food, a cheap source of calories and stores well. The main question for nutritionalists is whether large amounts can be consumed with impunity throughout life. About 60% of sugar comes from sugar cane, 40% from sugar beet. Sugar is the same chemically in the sugar cane, in unrefined sugar and in refined sugar.

References

DEERR, N. (1949). "The History of Sugar", p. 14. Chapman and Hall, London.

DRUMMOND, J. C. and WILBRANDON, A. (1957). "The Englishman's Food: a History of Five Centuries of English Diet", p. 43. Jonathan Cape, London.

HAMMOND, J. L. and HAMMOND, B. (1911). "The Village Labourer, 1760–1832", p. 124. Longmans Green, London.

JONES, C. R. (1958). *Proceedings of the Nutrition Society* **17**, 7.

KENT, N. L. (1970). "Technology of Cereals." Pergamon Press, Oxford. (a) p. 115; (b) p. 175.

McCANCE, R. A. and WIDDOWSON, M. (1956). "Breads, White and Brown: Their Place in Thought and Social History", pp. 31–46. Pitman Press, London.

TROWELL, H. (1973) *Plant Foods for Man* **1**, 11.

Chapter 5

Dietary changes in modern times

HUGH TROWELL

I. The complexity of the dietary problem	. . . . .	47
II. Wheat and flour	. . . .	48
A. The structure of wheat grain .	. . . .	48
B. Flours of different extraction rates .	. . . .	49
III. Dietary changes in England and Wales	. . . .	50
A. Starch	. . . .	50
B. Sugar	. . . .	52
C. Fat	. . . .	53
D. Energy (calories)	. . . .	53
IV. Dietary changes in developing countries	. . . .	54
A. Food-gatherers and hunters .	. . . .	54
B. Wheat eaters and maize eaters	. . . .	55
C. Rice eaters	. . . .	55
References	. . . .	56

I. The complexity of the dietary problem

This book is concerned primarily with the consumption of highly processed starchy food and sugar in relation to disease. It is, however, unwise to study only one facet of diet. If fats and sugar increase, bread consumption and the intake of cereal fibre will decrease. If certain diseases, such as ischaemic heart disease, diabetes and diverticular disease, then increase in frequency, it will prove difficult to assess which factor, or factors, were responsible: too much fat, or too much sugar, or too little starch and too little fibre. It is important to recognize that the consumption of fat, all of it processed in various ways, has increased in the past hundred years. Protein consumption has also increased in western society and vitamin and mineral intakes have usually been plentiful. Infant feeding has also altered in western society. Few infants are breast-fed for many months before they are offered processed powdered cow's milk mixtures, often supplemented with sugar, and they grow faster and mature more rapidly than those who have been fed in a traditional manner. Perhaps this, too, is not wholly beneficial: menarche occurs at an age of lower psychological maturity.

II. Wheat and flour

A. The structure of wheat grain

Chaff is removed during threshing to reveal the oval grain of wheat, with an infolded crease running from one end to another. A cross-section (Fig. 5.1) discloses (1) the covering layers of pericarp, seed coat and

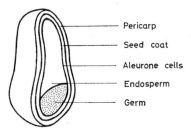

FIG. 5.1. Cross-section of wheat grain, showing: covering layers of pericarp, seed coat and aleurone cells; starchy endosperm; germ.

aleurone cells, (2) the main mass of starchy endosperm cells and (3) the germ towards one end. The starch is in the form of granules embedded in a protein matrix, which contains a small quantity of hemicelluloses and only a trace of cellulose. The covering layers consist of a tough pericarp and seed coats, the inner layer of which is called the aleurone cells. These outer layers are especially rich in the B-complex vitamins and dietary fibre. The germ is rich in protein, fat, mineral salts and dietary fibre. The bran, removed in milling, consists of the pericarp, seed coat and aleurone layer (Table 5.1).

TABLE 5.1. Percentage of the total constituents of wheat (after Kent, 1970a)

Part	Weight	Constituents				
		Starch	Crude fibre	Protein	Fat	Ash
Endosperm (flour)	82	100	8	72	50	23
Pericarp, seed coat and aleurone (bran)	15	0	70	20	30	67
Embryo (germ)	3	0	3	8	20	10

Note: only 81% of the crude fibre has been reported but methods of estimation are unsatisfactory.

B. *Flours of different extraction rates*

Milling fractions do not correspond exactly with the particular parts of
the grain. Nevertheless, in the case of wheat, modern milling methods are
designed to remove all the germ and to separate the bran as completely
as possible from the starchy flour of the endosperm. The weight of flour
produced per 100 parts of wheat milled is known as the percentage
extraction rate. Any flour below 80% is often spoken of as a low-extraction
flour, because at this point of extraction there is a sudden change from the

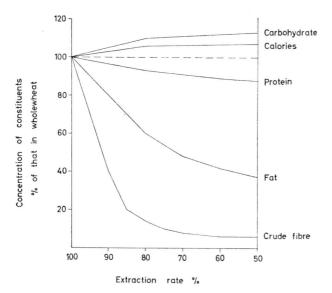

FIG. 5.2. Nutrient composition of flours of various extraction rates compared with
that of whole wheat (after Kent, 1970b; constructed from data of McCance *et al.*,
1945).

very high content of various nutrients in high-extraction flours (80–100%)
to a low content of all these nutrients in low-extraction flours (70–80%)
(Fig. 5.2). This is especially true of fibre, which is proportionally reduced
more than any other nutrient in low-extraction flours.

Table 5.2, derived from various sources (McCance and Widdowson,
1969; Kent, 1970c), shows that the components of wheat vary. Manitoba
wheat has more protein than English wheat. White flour, 70% extraction
from any variety of wheat, has slightly more calories, slightly less protein,
and much less fat than wholemeal flour of 100% extraction. All B group
vitamins (thiamin, niacin, riboflavin) are reduced to about one-fifth, and
the crude fibre content is decreased to about one-twentieth. Bran and the
germ are correspondingly rich in B vitamins and fibre. Associated with the

fibre of cereal grains is a substance called phytic acid (inositol hexa-phosphate) which decreases the absorption of calcium and iron in the flour. Probably some 60% of phytic acid is hydrolysed in breadmaking (Kent, 1970d), but those communities who take much unleavened bread may develop rickets. The risk is believed to be greater in children who grow up in industrial areas of the north, where there is little sunshine because of the smoky atmosphere. Rickets may be prevented by liberal supplements of vitamin D. In 1942 it was feared that the British high

TABLE 5.2. Composition of wheat flour, Manitoba and English (g/100 g and mg/100 g) (McCance and Widdowson, 1969; Kent, 1970c)

Flour	Extraction rate %	Calories	Protein g	Fat g	Carbo-hydrate g	Fibre g	Calcium mg	Iron mg	Thian mg
MANITOBA									
Wholemeal	100	339	13·6	2·5	69	2·2	28	3·8	0·4
National	85	350	13·6	1·7	74	0·4	19	2·7	0·3
White	70	352	12·8	1·2	77	0·1	13	2·2	0·0?
ENGLISH									
Wholemeal	100	333	8·9	2·2	73	2·0	36	3·0	0·4
National	85	346	8·6	1·5	79	0·4	25	2·2	0·3
White	70	349	7·9	1·0	82	0·1	19	1·4	0·0?
Bran	—	—	12·0	4·0	—	10–13	—	—	0·5

extraction war-time National flour, coupled possibly with a decreased supply of milk, might lead to negative calcium balance, so that the supplementation of flour with added chalk was recommended. Actually during the war milk consumption rose 25%. Experience in sunny South Africa has demon-strated that Bantu who take whole cereals, little milk, and no supplements of calcium, remain healthy and have a low incidence of rickets. They have a lower blood calcium and fewer renal calculi. Results of research in that country cast doubt on the advisability of adding chalk to bread (Walker et al., 1970). Osteoporosis is ten times commoner in South African Whites than in South African Bantu (Solomon, 1968); the latter eat much fibre-rich maize meal, and are also more active physically.

III. Dietary changes in England and Wales

A. Starch

Since 1770 the amount of starch and sugar consumed in England and Wales has altered profoundly (Hollingsworth and Greaves, 1967; Board of Trade, 1968) (Fig. 5.3). The amount of starchy carbohydrate food in the diet, especially wheat, has declined considerably and the wheat crude fibre intake has decreased even more so (Fig. 5.4c). In 1770 wheat flour consumption was approximately 500 g/day. This was usually stone-ground, lightly sifted wholemeal, with its crude fibre content varying probably from 0·5 to 2 g/100 g, so that the cereal crude fibre intake was 2·5–10 g/day,

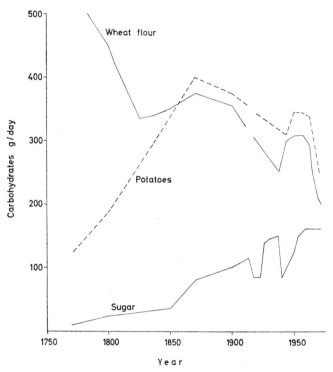

FIG. 5.3. Trends in the consumption of wheat flour, potatoes and sugar in England and Wales 1770–1970. No detailed records during 1914–18 War for wheat flour and potatoes. (Hollingsworth and Greaves, 1967; Board of Trade, 1968.)

an approximate mean of 6·25 g/day. By 1870 wheat flour consumption had fallen to approximately 375 g/day and its crude fibre content to 0·2– 0·5 g/100 g (Robertson, 1972), so that the approximate mean wheat flour crude fibre intake was 1·3 g/day. By 1970 wheat flour consumption had fallen to 200 g/day and the crude fibre content of white 70–72% extraction flour to 0·1 g/100 g (Kent, 1970e), which means that the average wheat flour crude fibre intake was about 0·2 g/day. This figure applies to those who habitually eat white bread and white flour, such as is consumed by nearly 95% of the population. Other cereal products also contributed fibre, but modern breakfast foods are usually low in fibre compared with oatmeal porridge. Thus in the two centuries from 1770 to 1970 wheat flour daily crude fibre intakes had decreased in the majority of people to between one-twelfth and one-fifteenth of the 1770 amount; in the last century, 1870–1970, it had decreased to about one-sixth of the 1870 amount. Meanwhile the consumption of potatoes had risen from a low level in 1770 to a peak level of 400 g/day by 1870 and provided 1·6 g/day of crude

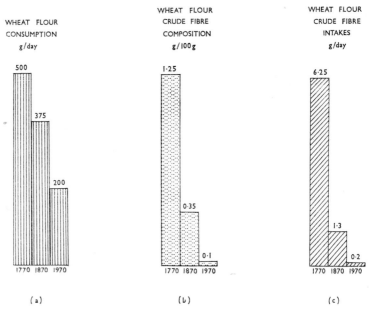

FIG. 5.4. Wheat flour and wheat flour crude fibre consumption England and Wales 1770–1970.

1770   stone-ground lightly sifted wholemeal.
1870   stone-ground moderately sifted "white" flour.
1970   roller milled, white 70–72% extraction flour.
(a) Wheat flour consumption, approximate mean.
(b) Crude fibre composition, approximate mean.
(c) Wheat flour crude fibre intakes, approximate mean.

fibre. By 1970 consumption had fallen to the level of 285 g/day, which provided 1·2 g/day of crude fibre. Fibre from other non-starchy plant foods, leafy vegetables and fruit, has probably increased during the last century 1870–1970, but there are no data concerning supplies prior to 1909 (Robertson, 1972).

B. Sugar

During the period 1700–1850 sugar consumption had been minimal (Fig. 5.3); it rose steeply only after 1850 and closed the energy gap produced by decreasing consumption of wheat flour and potatoes. Sugar consumption rose from 80 g/day in 1870 to 100 g/day in 1900, and continued to rise except for the periods of rationing during the two World Wars. It has been almost stationary since about 1958 at 164 g/day, providing 17% of the daily calories (Board of Trade, 1968). The consumption of sugar, which contains neither protein, minerals nor vitamins, doubled in the century 1870–1970; during the same period of time the wheat white flour crude fibre intake had decreased to one-sixth. Sugar has no fibre and its inclusion in diet will usually cause a reduction of the consumption of starchy foodstuffs which do contain fibre.

C. Fat

Fat consumption increased markedly in Britain during the period 1770–1970. In 1770, before the Agricultural Revolution resulted in the production of milk and butter throughout the year, fat consumption was low, probably about 25 g/day; it rose to about 75 g/day by 1870 and to 145 g/day by 1970, when it contributed nearly 40% of the daily calories. Fat consumption therefore doubled in the century 1870–1970. The consumption of milk and cheese, which contain among other nutrients fat, protein and vitamins, has also risen, more particularly in the present century. There has been about a 25% increase in these foods during the last 30 years.

D. Energy (calories)

Concern must be expressed, however, at the rising intake of calories not only in Britain but in all advanced western nations. There has been a concomitant reduction in physical activity due to the use of transport and machinery in factory, field and home, and this should be offset by a reduction in energy intake to prevent obesity. The matter will be reviewed more fully in Chapter 16. Suggestive lessons may be drawn from the British war-time rationing which began in 1939 and was progressively relaxed during 1945–1954. The pre-war average daily calorie intake has been assessed as 3050 kcal/day and it fell some 5% as soon as rationing of fat and sugar started in 1940. Energy intakes remained below the pre-war level until total fat intakes rose to 93% of their pre-war level in 1944. As soon as fat intakes exceeded their pre-war level, as in 1950 and again from 1954 onwards, assessed calorie intakes exceeded by 3–5% the pre-war level of 3050 kcal/day (Board of Trade, 1968; Table 16.1).

During the period of rationing sugar consumption did not correlate so closely with fluctuations in the average daily energy intakes. The latter exceeded the pre-war level in 1944, 1945 and from 1949 onwards, but sugar consumption did not reach and exceed its pre-war level until 1954. The daily average energy intakes exceeded the pre-war level by 5% only once, namely in 1954, the first complete year in which the high-fibre National bread ceased to be compulsory and gave way to low-fibre white bread. In that year the consumption of white bread and items made from white flour actually fell 10% and have decreased almost every year since that date, likewise the cereal fibre intakes, while energy intakes have persisted at 3–5% above the pre-war level, due largely to more fat and more sugar (Board of Trade, 1968).

IV. Dietary changes in developing countries

A. Food-gatherers and hunters

Communities who have relied on hunting and food-gathering have difficulty in adapting to western diets. For example Red Indians, African Bushmen and Australian Aborigines had previously obtained the majority of their energy in fibre-rich starchy foods, gathered or dug up. In the Arctic, fat and flesh provided most of the calories and the Eskimos ate a little vegetable fibre such as lichen, moss, the contents of the paunch of the caribou and of the intestines of fish (Sinclair, 1953): these contain fibre from plants or plankton. When western foods such as sugar and white flour became available they easily displaced traditional foods and consequently dental caries became common. Diabetes is probably still rare among traditionally living Eskimos, but serum cholesterol levels can be as high as in the U.S.A., even if ischaemic heart disease is said to be still uncommon (Bang et al., 1971).

Red Indian groups who lived in the southern states of the U.S.A. had adapted to maize (corn), until this was supplanted by white flour and sugar. Diabetes and gross obesity then became common (Carpenter and Steggarda, 1939). More than 50% of Pima Indians over 35 years of age have diabetes (Bennett et al., 1971).

In Africa most Bushmen still eat their traditional diet and like Paleolithic man take no salt, which was first mined only in Neolithic times (Brothwell and Brothwell, 1969). Many tribes in Africa used vegetable potash in place of salt until modern times. In certain African tribes including the Bushmen blood-pressure declined with advancing years. The hypothesis that hypertension is due partly to man's poor adaptation to a high intake of salt, coupled with the strain of living in modern technological society, the disease affecting only susceptible genotypes, deserves serious investigation.

B. Wheat eaters and maize eaters

Only a few isolated groups, such as the Bedouin and Yemenite Jews (Groen *et al.*, 1966) and other rural folk in the Lebanon and Iran still consume large amounts of stone-ground unsifted wheat wholemeal and take a negligible amount of sugar. In other countries of the Middle East and in Europe, beginning with the most affluent, milling techniques were altered during the eighteenth and nineteenth centuries and refined white flour was first produced there. At about the same time sugar consumption started to rise, at first only in the upper classes, and more milk products and fats were consumed.

As long as the rural life of Africa remained unchanged, traditional methods of grinding cereals and preparing other starchy foods were not altered. In rural areas starchy carbohydrates, which have been only lightly processed, may still provide 70–85% of the calories; fat intakes are low (15–25% of the calories), protein intakes are moderate (10–15% of the calories). If there is enough food most adults fare well, but many infants and children are apt to suffer from undernutrition or kwashiorkor (protein-energy malnutrition—PEM).

The first dietary change in developing countries is usually the addition of sugar which stores well and is a cheap source of calories. Consumption has risen rapidly within a decade or two to 60–70 g/day in rural areas and to 70–80 g/day, as in lower classes of South African Whites (Walker *et al.*, 1971). In many urban areas of southern and eastern Africa lightly milled maize (corn) meal provides the bulk of the calories, but meal decreases when fat consumption rises from 30 g/day (10% of calories) to 75 g/day (25% of calories). Better-off Africans tend to consume polished rice and white bread, less of their traditional unprocessed foods and far less fibre.

Similar dietary changes have occurred in the tropical countries of Asia, Central and South America, the islands of the Pacific and among the Maoris of New Zealand.

C. Rice eaters

For many centuries, if not millennia, rice has been milled and polished to varying degrees in the ancient civilizations of the East. It was mainly in the poorer rural areas of India that dehusked rice was consumed as paddy rice, without milling or polishing. Milled, lightly polished rice, with the vitamins and fibre reduced to about a quarter, has been the staple food of the cities and upper classes of eastern countries for decades, if not centuries. Fat consumption remains low and animal protein may be very low in the poorer social groups. In most eastern countries sugar intakes of 20–60 g/day are less than half those taken in advanced western nations.

Energy intakes although low maintain a steady, if light, body-weight throughout adult life in short people.

White wheat flour is eaten increasingly in industrial areas in India, and in the cities of Japan. In urban areas the consumption of white bread, sugar, fat and protein has increased, while that of carbohydrate has fallen; the latter is more highly processed, so that total fibre intakes, derived from starchy foods, are markedly reduced.

Comparable changes of diet and disease have occurred in the islands of the Pacific, such as Hawaii, where diets are now intermediate between those traditional of Asia and the new processed foods of America.

These dietary changes have been reflected in altering patterns of disease.

References

BANG, H. O., DYERBURG, J. and NIELSEN, A. (1971). *Lancet* 1, 1143.

BENNETT, P. H., BURCH, T. A. and MILLER, M. (1971). *Lancet* 2, 125.

Board of Trade Journal (1968). **194**, 753.

BROTHWELL, D. and BROTHWELL, P. (1969). "Food in Antiquity", p. 162. Thames and Hudson, London.

CARPENTER, T. M. and STEGGARDA, M. (1939). *Journal of Nutrition* 18, 297.

GROEN, J. J., BALOGH, M. and YARRON, E. (1966). *Israel Journal of Medical Sciences* 2, 202.

HOLLINGSWORTH, D. F. and GREAVES, J. P. (1967). *American Journal of Clinical Nutrition* 20, 65.

KENT, N. L. (1970). "Technology of Cereals." Pergamon Press, Oxford. (a) p. 39; (b) p. 162; (c) pp. 159–170; (d) p. 165; (e) p. 163.

McCANCE, R. A., WIDDOWSON, E. M., MORAN, T., PRINGLE, J. S. and MACRAE, T. F. (1945). *Biochemical Journal* 39, 213.

McCANCE, R. A. and WIDDOWSON, E. M. (1969). "The Composition of Foods." Special Report Series, Medical Research Council, London, No. 297. Her Majesty's Stationery Office, London.

ROBERTSON, J. (1972). *Nature* 238, 290.

SINCLAIR, H. M. (1953). *Proceedings of the Nutrition Society* 12, 69.

SOLOMON, L. (1968). *Journal of Bone and Joint Surgery* 50B, 2.

WALKER, A. R. P., HOLDSWORTH, C. M. and WALKER, E. J. (1971). *South African Medical Journal* 45, 516.

WALKER, A. R. P., WALKER, B. F., RICHARDSON, B. D. and CHRIST, H. H. (1970). *American Journal of Clinical Nutrition* 23, 244.

Part III

Refined carbohydrate foods in the gastrointestinal tract

Chapter 6

The effects of carbohydrate refining on food ingestion, digestion and absorption

KENNETH HEATON

I. Ingestion. 60
II. Digestion and absorption 61
    A. Gastroduodenal function 61
    B. Enzymic digestion 62
    C. Small intestinal function 63
    D. Bile salt absorption and metabolism 64
References 66

The manufacture of refined carbohydrate foods involves major changes in the physical state and chemical composition of man's diet. The part of man's body most directly concerned with his food is the gastrointestinal tract. It is only reasonable, therefore, to expect its function to be affected when the diet is changed to include refined carbohydrate. Surprisingly, the behaviour of the digestive tract with different foods is a barely explored field. However, the limited observations that are available, together with everyday experience and logical reasoning, do allow certain generalizations to be made.

Reduced to the bare essentials, the three functions of the digestive tract are ingestion, digestion and absorption (excretion may be regarded as an after-function and is not further considered in this chapter). As a generalization, it may be said that ingestion, digestion and absorption are all easier with refined than with unrefined foods. They therefore proceed more quickly or more completely. This gain in efficiency may seem an advantage at first sight, but closer inspection suggests that the price paid may be excessive.

I. Ingestion

Plant fibre is a hindrance to ingestion. This can be seen on comparing the rates of ingestion of refined and unrefined foods. When six normal volunteers were asked to eat, on separate occasions, a 300 g meal of wholemeal bread and an equivalent meal of white bread, they all took longer to eat the wholemeal bread (McCance et al., 1953). The average eating times were 34 min for white bread and 45 min for wholemeal (Fig. 6.1). In this experiment, satiety was not assessed, but it is common experience that white bread is less satisfying than wholemeal. Since white bread is eaten more quickly and is less satisfying, it is probable that at bread-containing meals more food will be ingested with white than with wholemeal bread. The overall effect on nutritional status cannot be deduced without knowing how long the satiety from the two breads lasts, and data on this point are lacking, but it seems likely that total food intake will tend to be higher on a white bread diet (Heaton, 1973).

Fibre-depleted bread is quick to eat because it requires less chewing. Chewing stimulates the secretion of saliva. The volume of saliva entering the stomach is likely to be less during a refined meal than an unrefined one. Chewing also stimulates the secretion of gastric juice (Davenport, 1966). After eating refined food, therefore, the stomach will contain less saliva and less gastric juice and so will be less distended. In their bread experiment, McCance et al. (1953) did in fact note that after white bread the stomach was smaller and its contents were more concentrated (as judged by the greater density of barium given with the bread). Distension of the stomach evokes the sensation of satiety. White bread is less satisfying than wholemeal partly, no doubt, because it distends the stomach less. It is literally less filling.

With sugar, these effects of fibre-depletion are much greater. No direct comparisons of refined and unrefined sugar have been reported, but common sense can predict the results. Whereas flour-refining produces a material which requires less chewing, the refining of sugar cane and sugar beet goes a stage further and produces a substance which requires no chewing at all: refined sugar is soluble in water and so can be drunk, merely passing through the mouth. The time required to ingest a given amount of carbohydrate is dramatically reduced when it can be taken in liquid form. Thirty-eight grams of sucrose can be swallowed in a single $11\frac{1}{2}$ oz can of cola drink, in say 1 or 2 min. For the same 38 g of sugar to be ingested in unrefined form, that is as fruit, the teeth will have to chew 330 g of say apples (equivalent to four medium-sized apples). This will take at least 10 min and induce a far greater feeling of satiety than the cola drink. Sucrose can also be added to flour, as in cake, biscuits and pastry, without increasing the amount of chewing required.

It is clear, therefore, that the availability of refined sucrose greatly increases the rate at which man can ingest sugars. Man's inborn desire for sweetness ensures that he *wants* to ingest sugars fast, but it is only since the sugar-producing and refining industries have made refined sucrose widely available and cheap, that man has been *able* to ingest sugars fast. In recent years, the average Englishman has had no difficulty in slipping past his decaying or false teeth about 140 g of refined sugar per day, and it is not unusual for intakes to exceed 300 g. The "normal" intake of 140 g is equivalent to 1·25 kg (or nearly 3 lb) of apples, which is far more than most people would wish or be able to eat in one day. Because of its extreme "ingestibility", sucrose has a unique place in human nutrition. It has been blamed by Cleave as the main cause of overnutrition and hence as the chief culprit in the diseases associated with overnutrition, notably diabetes and coronary heart disease (Cleave *et al.*, 1969).

In summary, carbohydrate refining makes the consumption of starch and sugar quicker, easier and less satisfying. As a natural obstacle to food ingestion, fibre adds effort to eating. Nutritionally, the role of fibre may be to act as a natural preventive of overnutrition.

II. Digestion and absorption

A. Gastroduodenal function

Little is known of the effects of different diets on gastric function, but it is likely that the stomach behaves differently with refined and unrefined foods. As noted above, McCance *et al.* (1953) found that a white bread meal results in stomach contents which are smaller and more concentrated than after a wholemeal bread meal. In addition, the stomach emptied more slowly after white bread in all their six volunteers, the average delay being 1·1 h (Fig. 6.1). This may have been because the less distended stomach received less stimulus to contract. Distension of the gastric antrum provokes the release of the hormone gastrin from the antral mucosa (Davenport, 1966). Gastrin has many actions. In particular, it stimulates gastric motility and acid-pepsin secretion, and also contraction of the lower oesophageal sphincter. If, as seems possible, gastrin secretion is reduced with a refined diet, any or all of these functions may be altered. Inefficient contraction of the lower oesophageal sphincter is currently regarded as the major factor leading to gastro-oesophageal reflux, and hence to dyspeptic symptoms such as heartburn and regurgitation (Cohen and Harris, 1972). There is a crying need for research in this area.

The capacity of food to buffer acid depends on its protein content. Cleave (1962) has pointed out that in carbohydrate refining, protein is removed, and in a study comparing whole maize meal with refined maize flour Lennard-Jones *et al.* (1968) showed that intragastric pH is significantly lower during digestion of the refined meal. Much more work is needed along these lines, but meanwhile it may be noted that saliva has some buffering capacity and salivary secretion is reduced with fibre-depleted, non-masticatory foods.

Because all sugars (mono- and di-saccharides) are soluble in water, any ingested sugar confers high osmotic activity on the stomach contents, unlike the insoluble starches and proteins. As we have seen, the rate of sugar ingestion is artificially increased by the availability of refined sucrose. The use of sucrose must therefore raise the osmolality of gastric contents to unphysiological levels. Fordtran and Locklear (1966) found that after a

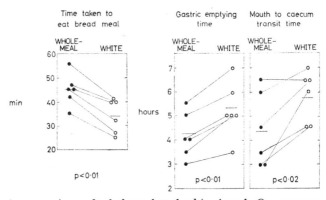

FIG. 6.1. A comparison of wholemeal and white bread. On separate occasions, six healthy volunteers each ate a large meal of white bread and one of wholemeal bread. Each meal contained a little barium, so that its progress through the alimentary tract could be followed by serial X-rays. The lines join the results in each individual after eating wholemeal bread (closed circles) and white bread (open circles). Drawn from the data of McCance *et al.* (1953).

steak meal the osmolality of stomach contents was 240–250 mOsm which is slightly hypotonic, whereas after a milk and doughnut meal it was about 450 mOsm, which is extremely hypertonic. Experimentally, hypertonic solutions are toxic to cells and work is needed on the effect of hypertonic sugar solutions on the gastric and duodenal mucosa. One effect of very hypertonic solutions (700 mOsm) is to delay gastric emptying (Hunt *et al.*, 1951), probably through the stimulation of osmoreceptors in the duodenum.

B. Enzymic digestion

Indigestible cell-wall material acts as a mechanical barrier between the contents of plant cells and their environment. Since a proportion of the

cell-walls are ruptured or removed in the refining process, refined carbohydrate foods may be more accessible to digestive enzymes. With sugars
this is of no consequence since sugars are not digested in the intestinal
lumen. However, the fine milling and sifting of flour may increase the rate
of digestion of starch to glucose by pancreatic amylase, and of protein to
peptides and amino acids by trypsin and chymotrypsin. This in turn would
increase the availability of glucose for absorption. Faster digestion of
refined starch may, however, be counteracted by its slower emptying from
the stomach. In ten normal volunteers, we have found no significant
difference in the blood sugar curves after equivalent meals of white and
wholemeal bread (Pomare, Heaton and Hartog, 1972, unpublished
data).

C. Small intestinal function

Radiologically, the contents of the small intestine are more bulky and
dilute after wholemeal bread than after white bread (McCance *et al.*,
1953). The same is presumably true after eating four apples as compared
with drinking a can of sweetened mineral water. The increased bulk is
unlikely to be due solely to the actual mass of fibre, but also to an increased
volume of digestive secretions. Saliva and gastric juice secretion are
increased by chewing. Furthermore, bulkier stomach contents may, on
entry into the duodenum, be more powerful stimulators of the digestive
hormones, secretin and cholecystokinin, which promote the secretion of
bile and pancreatic juice. Another possible factor is the formation by fibre
of a polysaccharide mesh or gel in which osmotically active substances are
trapped and water with them. Whatever their cause, changes in the bulk
and dilution of small bowel contents probably explain why the small bowel
behaves differently on full-fibre and fibre-depleted diets.

The careful experiments of Southgate and Durnin (1970) established the
important fact that the small bowel performs less efficiently as the fibre
content of the diet is increased. This was most clearly brought out in
young women who, on three diets of increasing fibre content, excreted
faeces containing progressively more energy, fat and nitrogen (Fig. 6.2).
On a high-fibre diet, containing 89 g of fat per day, these healthy subjects
excreted on average 6·24 g of fat daily; technically, they had steatorrhoea.
The calorific value of stools was markedly raised on the higher fibre diets.
The availability of energy in the diet was reduced by 0·16% for each 1 g
increase in the intake of fibre (as cellulose and hemicelluloses). Subjects
with ileostomies excrete more water and dry matter in their ileostomy
effluent when they eat cabbage or baked beans (Kramer *et al.*, 1962). This
supports the idea that dietary fibre reduces small bowel efficiency (perhaps

to the physiological level), but much work needs to be done on small bowel function with different diets.

How does fibre hinder the absorption of nutrients? There are probably two factors at play. Firstly, by diluting the small bowel contents and simply by acting as an inert obstacle, fibre may physically prevent contact between nutrient and mucosa. Secondly, fibre accelerates the rate of passage of small bowel contents. McCance *et al.* (1953) found that the residue of a whole-meal bread meal reached the caecum in 4·4 h, that of a white bread meal in 5·8 h (Fig. 6.1). Experimentally, increasing the transit rate of the small bowel reduces its absorptive capacity (Kendall, 1973; Manninen *et al.*, 1973).

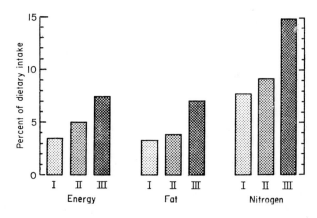

Fig. 6.2. Faecal excretion of energy, fat and nitrogen in young women on diets of low (I), medium (II) and high (III) fibre content. The data are expressed as percentages of the dietary intake. Diet I contained 6·2 g, Diet II 16·2 g and Diet III 31·9 g of cellulose and pentosans. Drawn from the data of Southgate and Durnin (1970).

It seems reasonable to conclude that on fibre-depleted food the small bowel contents are concentrated and slow moving, and there is over-efficient absorption of nutrients. This may be relevant to the aetiology of small bowel diseases which are mediated by toxic materials in the small bowel lumen, especially Crohn's disease, and also to the aetiology of obesity and other diseases of overnutrition.

D. *Bile salt absorption and metabolism*

Bile salts are the major breakdown products of cholesterol. They are also potentially toxic materials especially when degraded by intestinal bacteria. Consequently there has been considerable interest in the effect of diet upon bile salts. This subject has been fully reviewed elsewhere (Heaton, 1972), and it was concluded that dietary fat and dietary cholesterol seem to exert little if any effect on bile salt metabolism.

There is good evidence, mainly from animal experiments, that a refined or fibre-depleted diet causes marked changes in bile salt metabolism. When rats or rabbits are given a semi-synthetic diet, containing refined sugar or starch, they show a marked fall in the rate of bile salt synthesis (Portman and Murphy, 1958; Gustafsson and Norman, 1969). The rate of synthesis must in the steady state equal the rate of excretion in the faeces, and bile salt excretion does tend to be depressed. It is not at present clear which comes first, decreased excretion from the gut or decreased synthesis by the liver. Experimental evidence suggests that fibre-depleted diets are capable of producing both abnormalities.

Decreased excretion of bile salts could result from abnormally efficient intestinal reabsorption or conservation. As noted above, fibre-depleted diets do seem to permit over-efficient absorption of nutrients from the small intestine, and it is plausible that the same should apply to the reabsorption of bile salts from the terminal ileum. In this case the restoration of fibre to the diet should increase the excretion of bile salts. Experimentally, feeding large amounts of purified cellulose (to 20% of the total food intake) has been shown to increase faecal bile salt output in rats fed a semi-synthetic diet (Portman and Murphy, 1958) and in young Indian girls fed a hypercholesterolaemic diet (Shurpalekar et al., 1971). Feeding the more realistic amount of 15 g per day of cellulose to adult volunteers, Stanley et al. (1972) showed a 25% increase in the excretion rate of radioactive cholate. In experiments on South African prisoners, Antonis and Bersohn (1962) showed faecal bile acids to be 24–43% higher on a low-fat diet containing about 15 g crude fibre than on a similar diet containing 4 g crude fibre. On the other hand, Eastwood et al. (1972) have reported that adding 16 g of cellulose or bran daily to the diet of normal volunteers made no difference to total faecal bile acids. Similarly, Pomare et al. (1974) noted no change in the half-lives of radioactive bile salts when 57 g daily of bran were added to the diet, which simplies that even this large amount of bran did not impair bile salt reabsorption significantly. The question of whether or not fibre promotes bile salt excretion must therefore remain sub judice, regardless of the fact that, in vitro, fibre absorbs bile salts (Eastwood and Hamilton, 1968).

Recent studies in the author's laboratory have shown that feeding bran alters the metabolism of bile salts (Pomare and Heaton, 1973; Pomare et al., 1974). The primary effect of bran seems to be to reduce the absorption from the colon of deoxycholate, which is a bacterial metabolite of cholate. At the same time, there is increased synthesis by the liver of chenodeoxycholate, but not of cholate. The possible significance of these findings in relation to gallstone formation are discussed in Chapter 14. More work is needed to determine whether bran and other fibrous materials reduce the bacterial degradation of bile salts in the colon, or whether they simply hinder the absorption of the degradation products from the colonic lumen.

References

ANTONIS, A. and BERSOHN, I. (1962). *American Journal of Clinical Nutrition* **11**, 142.

CLEAVE, T. L. (1962). "Peptic Ulcer." John Wright, Bristol.

CLEAVE, T. L., CAMPBELL, G. D. and PAINTER, N. S. (1969). "Diabetes, Coronary Thrombosis and the Saccharine Disease", 2nd edition. John Wright, Bristol.

COHEN, S. and HARRIS, L. D. (1972). *Gastroenterology* **63**, 1066.

DAVENPORT, H. W. (1966). "Physiology of the Digestive Tract", 2nd edition. Year Book Medical Publishers, Chicago.

EASTWOOD, M. A. and HAMILTON, D. (1968). *Biochimica et biophysica Acta* **152**, 165.

EASTWOOD, M. A., HAMILTON, T., KIRKPATRICK, J. R. and MITCHELL, W. D. (1972). *Proceedings of the Nutrition Society* **32**, 22A (abstract).

FORDTRAN, J. S. and LOCKLEAR, T. W. (1966). *American Journal of Digestive Diseases* **11**, 503.

GUSTAFSSON, B. E. and NORMAN, A. (1969). *British Journal of Nutrition* **23**, 429.

HEATON, K. W. (1972). "Bile Salts in Health and Disease." Churchill Livingstone, Edinburgh.

HEATON, K. W. (1973). *Lancet* **2**, 1418.

HUNT, J. N., MACDONALD, I. and SPURRELL, W. R. (1951). *Journal of Physiology* **115**, 185.

KENDALL, M. J. (1973). *British Medical Journal* **2**, 179 (letter).

KRAMER, P., KEARNEY, M. M. and INGELFINGER, F. J. (1962). *Gastroenterology* **42**, 535.

LENNARD-JONES, J. E., FLETCHER, J. and SHAW, D. G. (1968). *Gut* **9**, 177.

McCANCE, R. A., PRIOR, K. M. and WIDDOWSON, E. M. (1953). *British Journal of Nutrition* **7**, 98.

MANNINEN, V., APAJALAHTI, A., MELIN, J. and KARESOJA, M. (1973). *Lancet* **1**, 398.

POMARE, E. W. and HEATON, K. W. (1973). *British Medical Journal* **4**, 262.

POMARE, E. W., HEATON, K. W., LOW-BEER, T. S., and WHITE, C., (1974). *Gut* **15**, 824 (abstract).

PORTMAN, O. W. and MURPHY, P. (1958). *Archives of Biochemistry and Biophysics* **76**, 367.

SHURPALEKAR, K. S., DORAISWAMY, T. R., SUNDARAVALLI, O. E. and NARAYANA RAO, M. (1971). *Nature* **232**, 554.
SOUTHGATE, D. A. T. and DURNIN, J. V. G. A. (1970). *British Journal of Nutrition* **24**, 517.
STANLEY, M., PAUL, D., GACKE, D. and MURPHY, J. (1972). *Gastroenterology* **62**, 816 (abstract).

Chapter 7

Gastrointestinal transit times; stool weights and consistency; intraluminal pressures

DENIS BURKITT and NEIL PAINTER

I. Historical aspects	69
II. Recent studies	70
A. Methods used	70
B. Results	71
C. General considerations	78
III. Intraluminal pressures	79
A. Some methods used to measure intracolonic pressures . .	79
B. Segmentation and colonic physiology	81
C. Factors that influence intracolonic pressures	82
References	83

I. Historical aspects

The laxative effects of the unabsorbable fibre content of food has long been recognized. Hippocrates observed that "To the human body it makes a great difference whether the bread be made of fine flour or coarse, whether of wheat with the bran, or without the bran".

Hakim, a Persian physician, wrote in the ninth century A.D., "Wheat is a beneficial cereal. Chupatties are made from wheat flour. The chupatties containing more bran come out of the digestive tract quicker but are less nutritious. Chupatties containing a little bran take a long time to be excreted."

Cogan wrote in the sixteenth century, "Such as have been costive, by eating browne bread and butter have been made soluble" (McCance *et al.*, 1953).

In the present century the American workers Cowgill and Anderson (1932) and Fantus *et al.* (1940) drew attention to the effect of bran on bowel behaviour and content. In Britain, Dimock (1936) emphasized the role of cellulose fibre in maintaining normal colon activity. He found the commercial breakfast cereal "All Bran" to be highly successful in the treatment of constipation. He drew on the previous experience of Gallant (1912) who treated mucous colitis with bran, of Hurst (1919) who attributed the rarity of constipation in German troops to the coarse bread in their diet, and of Austin (1919) who considered bran the best remedy for constipation. Hurst *et al.* (1934) subsequently recommended a high-residue diet for the treatment of both mucous colitis and constipation. During his 30 years in the Royal Navy as a consultant physician, Cleave successfully treated constipation with bran and experienced no complications (Cleave, 1941; p.c. 1971).

II. Recent studies

Recent epidemiological studies throughout the world have confirmed this relationship between reduced dietary fibre and constipation. The time taken for markers of various types to pass through the gastrointestinal canal has been recorded by many workers.

A. Methods used

1. Millet seeds

Burnett (1923) used swallowed millet seeds to measure transit times, and related stool consistency to the time taken for the seeds to be evacuated.

2. Melon seeds

Abdel A'al Osman (p.c., 1970), a Sudanese surgeon, recognizing that swallowed melon seeds were passed unaltered in the stools, gave seeds of different colours with the morning, midday and evening meals of volunteers. The seeds were recovered by washing the stools with water through a wire mesh and the colour of the seeds indicated which meal was represented by the stool examined.

3. Carmine capsules

Carmine is swallowed in gelatine capsules and the time that elapses before red coloration appears in the stool is measured. This method was used in children as early as 1909 by Triboulet and in adults by Strauss in 1914. Later results by this method are shown in Table 7.1.

4. Barium meal studies

Eve (1966), studying British volunteers, found that in 28 out of 52 (53·8%) the head of the column of barium had not been evacuated after 48 h, and in 14 (26·9%) not even after 72 h. The average daily weight of stools was 131 g. Manousos *et al.* (1967) found that it took over 5 days for all barium to leave the bowel in a third of their normal subjects. Cleave and Campbell (1968) observed that in six tribal Zulus all barium had left the bowel within 48 h, but in another six subjects on a more westernized diet some barium still remained in three of the colons after the same period.

5. Radiography of stools following ingestion of radio-opaque plastic pellets

This method was first advocated by Hinton *et al.* (1969). It is much more accurate than other methods, does not depend on subjective impressions such as stool coloration, and does not expose the volunteer to radiation. Pellets about the size of grains of rice are cut from plastic impregnated with barium. It has been customary to give 25 pellets at one time, and since a few of these will move up and down the colon long after the majority have been excreted, the transit time is usually calculated as the number of hours that elapse between swallowing the "shapes" and the recovery of 20 of the 25 (80%) in the stools.

Each volunteer is given five or more plastic bags into which he is instructed to pass his stools. The bags are labelled so as to identify the volunteer and the order in which the stools are passed. The time when each bag is used is recorded, and the bags are subsequently weighed and X-rayed so that the number of "shapes" in each can be counted. In some trials the volume of stools has been estimated by measuring the water displaced when a bag of faeces, with air removed, has been immersed in a vessel full of water. This is a somewhat inaccurate measurement, and the relation between stool weight and volume is sufficiently close to rely on stool weights and transit times when assessing the bowel behaviour.

6. Ingestion of plastic pellets followed by sieving of stools

Walker *et al.* (1970), when estimating intestinal transit times in situations where radiography was not available, collected the stools in cartons and subsequently forced them through a copper wire sieve with the aid of a wooden spoon and water. The pellets, held back by the wire mesh, can then be counted.

B. Results

The results obtained by using carmine as a marker are shown in Table 7.1 and those obtained by radio-opaque markers in Table 7.2. Since it is not possible to relate results by different methods, discussion will mostly be limited to results obtained by the second, more accurate method. A point which clearly emerges is the inverse relationship between intestinal transit times and stool weights, as depicted in Fig. 7.1a, b, c and d and Fig. 7.2. Each mark indicates one volunteer and is positioned according to his or her transit time, measured vertically, and average daily stool weight,

TABLE 7.1. Transit time of digesta as reflected by first appearance of ingested carmine

Population	Reference	Mean time of first appearance (h)
Whites, U.K., adults	Rothman and Katz (1964)	40–48
Whites, U.K., adults	Mulinos (1935)	28
Whites, South African students	Walker (p.c., 1972)	28
Whites, U.K., adults	Wolman (1957)	20
Whites, U.K., children	Mulinos (1935)	28
Whites, U.K., children	Dimson (1970)	26
Whites, U.K., children	Wolman (1957)	20
Africans, Rhodesia, medical students	Holmgren and Mynors (1972)	28
Africans, South Africa, urban children, Johannesburg	Walker (p.c., 1972)	23
Africans, Rhodesia, high-school teachers	Holmgren and Mynors (1972)	20
Africans, Rhodesia, miners (unrefined diet)	Holmgren and Mynors (1972)	14
Africans, South Africa, rural children, Johannesburg	Walker (p.c., 1972)	12

measured horizontally. This inverse relationship between transit time and stool weight has been measured in many ethnic groups in different environmental circumstances. Although it has only been possible to measure stool consistency in terms such as firm and soft, formed and unformed, this consistency has also been shown to relate to transit time and weight, small slowly passing stools being firm, formed and often faceted, and large more rapidly passing faeces being soft and often unformed. The latter are voided with minimal straining.

TABLE 7.2. Transit times as shown by Hinton's method

Subjects	Country	Race	Type of diet	No. of subjects	Time of appearance of first pellets (h)		Transit time (h)		Weight of stools passed per day (g)		Comments
					Range	Mean	Range	Mean	Range	Mean	
Naval ratings and wives	U.K.	White	Refined	15	22–110	45.7	44–144	83.4	39–223	104	Shore-based personnel (cf. Wozasek and Steigman, 1942)
Teenage boarding-school pupils	U.K.	White	Refined	9	18–103	57.4	35–120	76.1	71–142	110	Institutional diet together with cakes, sweets, and so on from school shop
Teenage boarding-school pupils	U.K.	White	Refined	19	15–54	31.0	22–157	64.5	39–244	135	Institutional diet together with cakes, sweets, and so on from school shop
Naval ratings	U.K.	White	Refined	30	7–99	33.0	17–115	59.0	65–261	144	Very good, varied meals
Students	South Africa	White	Refined	100	13–54	30.5	28–60	48.0	120–195	173	These ate more fruit than is usual in the U.K.
Nurses	South Indian	Indian	Intermediate	13	9–34	27.6	23–64	44.0		155	Less refined diet than that of western world
Urban school-children	South African	African	Intermediate	500	9–40	28.5	24–59	45.2	120–260	165	Partly Europeanized diet
Manor House Hospital patients	U.K.	White	Intermediate	6	15–24	22.0	27–48	41.0	128–248	175	U.K. diet plus wholemeal bread and added bran
Senior boarding school pupils	Uganda	African	Intermediate	27	4–54	27.6	22–118	47.0	48–348	185	Traditional Ugandan diet plus refined sugar, white bread, jam, butter
Vegetarians	U.K.	White	Intermediate	24	8–49	22.0	18–97	42.4	71–488	225	Note similarity of values to those of African groups
Rural school-children	South Africa	African	Unrefined	500	5–28	12.8	20–48	33.5	150–350	275	Traditional diet
Rural villagers	Uganda	African	Unrefined	15	4–32	19.8	19–68	35.7	178–980	470	Villagers not yet supplementing their diet with processed food of western type

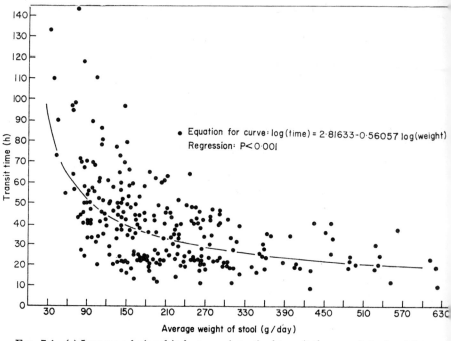

FIG. 7.1. (a) Inverse relationship between intestinal transit times and stool weights. This includes groups on different diets.

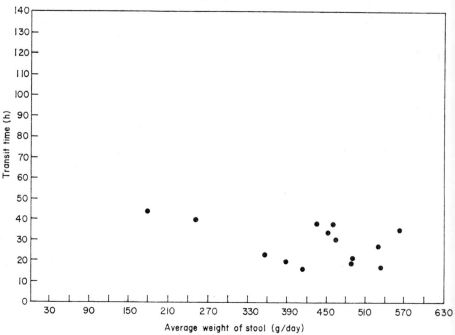

FIG. 7.1. (b) Transit times and stool weights in African villagers (high-fibre diet).

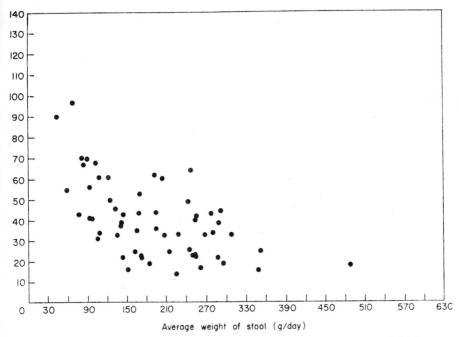

FIG. 7.1. (c) Transit times and stool weights in English vegetarians and African boarding school (intermediate diet).

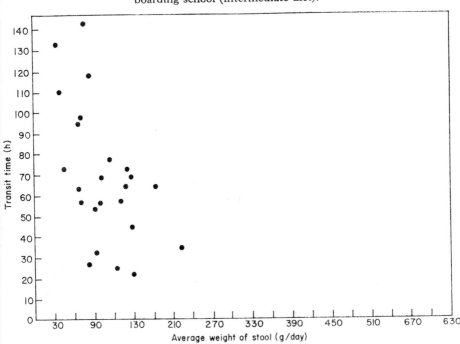

FIG 7.1. (d) Transit times and stool weights in English boarding school and British Navy (refined diet).

Many studies were done on individuals, or groups too small for reliable comparisons. It will therefore be best to compare groups large enough to represent different and relatively distinct communities and each having a fairly constant dietary pattern.

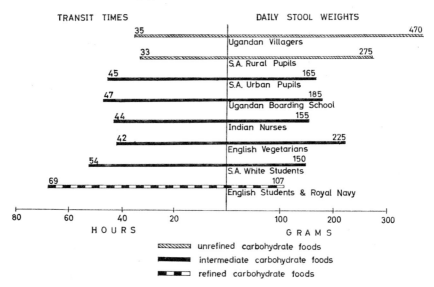

FIG. 7.2. Average intestinal transit times and stool weights in communities on different diets.

1. Refined carbohydrate diets

The average time taken for 15 shore-based naval ratings and their wives to pass 80% of swallowed markers was 83 h, and the average of their daily stool weights was only 104 g.

Nine senior students in an English boarding-school who supplemented their institutional diet with cakes and confectionery from the tuck shop took, on average, 76 h to pass 20 (80%) of their swallowed markers and their average daily weight of stool was 110 g (Burkitt *et al.*, 1972) (Table 7·2).

At another English boarding-school intestinal transit times in 19 students and two members of staff were found to average 64·5 h and average daily stool weights were 135·5 g on normal school diet (Payler, 1973) (Table 7.2).

Transit times of 59 h and average daily stool weights of 144 g were recorded for 30 naval personnel at sea on a very substantial diet (G. Milton-Thompson, p.c. 1972) (Table 7.2).

One hundred white South African students, eating considerably more fruit than is customary in the United Kingdom, had mean transit times of 48 h and average daily stool weights of 173 g (Burkitt *et al.*, 1972) (Table 7.2).

All except the last of these accord with average daily stool weights of 115 g in North America (Wozasek and Steigmann, 1942) and transit times exceeding 72 h in over 50% of volunteers recorded by Kopstein (1940). Brocklehurst and Khan (1969), who used this method to estimate transit times in sedentary geriatric patients, found that in five out of eight patients some markers still remained in the bowel after 2 weeks.

2. Intermediate diets

J. Iswariah (p.c., 1971), recorded transit times of 44 h and average daily stool weights of 155 g in nurses in a mission hospital in South India (Fig. 7.2; Table 7.2). In a much larger group of nurses in India F. Tovey (p.c., 1972) recorded average daily stool weights of 215 g, but did not estimate transit times.

Walker *et al.* (1970) studied 500 urban African pupils on an intermediate diet; their intestinal transit times averaged 45 h and they passed an average of 165 g of stool per day (Fig. 7.2; Table 7.2).

Twenty-seven senior students at an African boarding-school in Uganda, eating traditional carbohydrate food supplemented by sugar, white bread, butter, meat and preserves, had transit times and stool weights intermediate between African villagers and westerners. They took on average 47 h to pass their markers and had stool weights averaging 185 g daily (Fig. 7.2; Table 7.2). The academic curriculum and sporting activities of these boys were similar to those in the English boarding-school (Burkitt *et al.*, 1972).

Painter *et al.* (1972) observed mean transit times of 41 h and average daily stool weights of 175 g in six British subjects whose diet was supplemented by wholemeal bread and bran (Table 7.2).

The average daily weight of stool passed by 24 English vegetarians and vegans was 225 g and their average transit time was 42 h (Fig. 7.2; Table 7.2). Both these figures are comparable with those recorded for more educated Africans on an intermediate diet.

3. Unrefined carbohydrate diets

Burkitt *et al.* (1972) reported that 500 rural African pupils on an unrefined carbohydrate diet passed 80% of swallowed markers in an average of 33·5 h and evacuated 275 g (Fig. 7.2; Table 7.2). Similar findings were recorded for 15 African villagers in Uganda living on a traditional high-fibre diet. They showed transit times averaging 35 h, and passed on average 470 g of stool daily.

4. Fibre-free diet

A diet with the least possible residue was supplied to astronauts, with the specific purpose of minimizing bowel action. On this fibre-free diet 5–6 days can elapse without stools being passed (Winitz et al., 1965).

5. Small bowel transit time

Little information on the effect of different diets on small bowel transit time is available. McCance et al. (1953) recorded stomach to caecum time of 4·4 h in volunteers on wholemeal bread, as compared with 5·8 h in those on white bread (Fig. 6.1). Possible implications of this in regard to absorption of bile salts and other intestinal constituents will be discussed in Chapters 14, 15 and 16.

C. General considerations

These illustrative groups of people with diets containing variable amounts of unabsorbed fibre show that reduction in fibre content prolongs intestinal transit times, reduces the bulk and hardens the consistency of stools. Diets rich in fibre have the reverse effect. The replacement of fibre in the diet can restore normal bowel activity, and its laxative effect has been repeatedly reported (Avery Jones, 1972).

In the English school boys, reported by Payler (1973) above, the average transit time was reduced from 64·5 to 45·9 h and average daily stool weights increased from 135 to 163 g following the replacement of white by wholemeal bread, and the addition of two heaped dessertspoonsful of bran to the daily diet. Harvey et al. (1973) have shown that replacing white with wholemeal bread or adding about 30 g of bran a day reduced the longest transit times by about 3 days and actually lengthened the transit times in those with a tendency to diarrhoea. McCance et al. (1953) found that intestinal transit times were on average 24 h longer in those eating white bread compared to those eating brown bread.

Holmgren and Mynors (1972), using carmine as a marker, confirmed these findings. They showed that in African miners in Rhodesia, eating unrefined carbohydrate foods, ingested carmine first appeared in the stools in 14 h. In school teachers on an intermediate diet the dye took 20 h to appear, and in university medical students on more refined carbohydrate foods 28 h (Table 7.1).

A. Osman (p.c., 1970), using different coloured melon seeds, found that transit times in Sudanese nomads living largely on milk were similar to those of villagers eating a mainly vegetarian diet. The average time elapsing before the first appearance of markers in both groups was under 24 h. Average daily weight of stool was 155 g for the nomads and 220 g for the villagers. This apparently satisfactory intestinal behaviour observed in those traditionally subsisting on a low-residue diet may reflect an adaptation, over many generations, to a particular environment, similar to the way the Masai have adapted to a diet of blood and milk and maintain low serum cholesterol levels by metabolizing their cholesterol in a different way from other tribal groups (Mann et al., 1972).

No instance is known where prolonged transit times, reduced stool weights and altered stool consistency have not followed the replacement of a high-fibre diet for a low-fibre diet. Many students and doctors coming to the U.K. from Africa and India have testified to the constipation that has followed their adoption of normal English food.

As a historical footnote it is significant that in the second half of the eighteenth century Stark studied his own intestinal transit times in Britain using mustard and caraway seeds and found that "*during periods of constipation* it took 36–40 h for the passage but normally he could recover the seeds the morning after swallowing them" (McCay, 1973). A far cry from what is now regarded as normal.

III. Intraluminal pressures

Before discussing the effect of refined carbohydrate foods on intraluminal pressures in the colon it is necessary to appreciate the normal mechanisms of colonic behaviour. It is only within the past 20 years that techniques and apparatus capable of providing reliable measurements of intraluminal pressures have become available.

A. Some methods used to measure intracolonic pressures

1. Balloons

These have been inserted into the bowel lumen and filled to varying extents with air or water. The pressures within them have been recorded without appreciating that these do not equate with pressures in the bowel outside the balloon (Quigley and Brody, 1952). This is clearly illustrated in Fig. 7.3.

The upper longitudinal section of the colon (Fig. 7.3a) shows three balloons A, B, C; A and B are of the same size but bear a different relation to haustra of the colon; C is small. Movements of the colonic wall will distort balloons A and B differently (Fig. 7.3b), particularly when the colon contracts (Fig. 7.3c). In these circumstances balloons A and B will record different changes in pressure, neither of which will correspond to pressure changes in the lumen of the bowel. Although balloon C will respond to pressure changes, elasticity and resistance of its skin may result in the pressure within it differing from that in the colonic lumen. If the colon contracts so that its lumen is occluded (Fig. 7.3c), then balloon A will be distorted differently from balloon B, which will in fact act as a foreign body if its contents cannot escape. Balloon C, being smaller, will be less liable to act as a foreign body and be less distorted by the colonic wall. Theoretically the ideal balloon would merely be a membrane across the mouth of the recording tube. Even then the elasticity of the membrane might affect the accuracy of pressure recording.

It is thus evident that intraluminal balloons are an unreliable means of measuring intracolonic pressures.

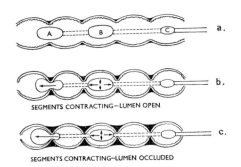

FIG. 7.3. Showing why balloons do not accurately record intraluminal pressures. Balloons of different sizes in different situations will be affected differently by colonic contractions. (From Painter, 1968a. Reprinted by kind permission of the editor of the *American Journal of Digestive Diseases*.)

2. Open-ended tubes

These water-filled tubes accurately measure the intraluminal pressures in the region of their tips. When used singly, however, they fail to show why or how pressure changes occur, nor do they distinguish between pressures generated near their tips and those created at some distance away. The mechanism whereby the colon can localize pressures to the region of the tip of a measuring tube can only be shown with the addition of cineradiography.

3. Simultaneous cineradiography with intraluminal pressure recording

If simultaneous cineradiographic films are taken while intraluminal pressures are recorded, the behaviour of the colon and the configuration of its lumen can be correlated with intracolonic pressures. The appearance of the bowel in the vicinity of the tips of the tubes can thus be correlated with the pressures recorded by these tubes. This technique has shown that very high pressures can be produced within a localized portion of the sigmoid colon (Painter, 1962, 1964, 1968a, b; Painter *et al.*, 1965).

B. Segmentation and colonic physiology

Combined cineradiography and pressure recording has shown that segmentation is involved in the generation and localization of intracolonic pressures (Painter, 1962). This is depicted diagrammatically in Fig. 7.4a, b and c. After segments of circular muscle contract to form rings in the

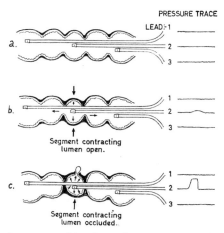

FIG. 7.4. Showing how a combination of pressure recording from open-ended tubes and cineradiography can detect pressure changes in portions of the bowel localized by segmentation.

bowel, the whole wall of a segment, localized between two contracting rings, contracts and consequently builds up pressure between the closed inlet and outlet of the occluded segment (Painter, 1962, 1964; Painter *et al.*, 1965).

Normal segmentation is essential for both the transportation and halting of the contents of the colon (Fig. 7.5b and c). Figure 7.5a shows how pressure is produced within a segment between contracting rings. Figure 7.5b shows how relaxation of one contracting ring allows the content to move to the next segment wherein the pressure is lower. This is the normal mechanism by which contents are moved. Figure 7.5c shows how contents are halted. Segmentation is seen in the sigmoid as faeces are shunted back and forth. This process aids absorption of water from the faeces and renders them more concentrated and viscous.

It is thus obvious that a wide colon is less liable to contract its lumen by segmentation than is a narrow one which may segment sufficiently to occlude its lumen intermittently. The greater the degree of segmentation, the greater the intracolonic pressures.

A consideration of Figs 7.4 and 7.5 makes it obvious that changes in the viscosity of the faeces must affect the work of the sigmoid. The harder the contents of the colon, the greater the pressure that will be required to move them. This will necessitate more vigorous segmentation, and more powerful contraction of colonic muscles. Consequently intrasigmoid pressures must be influenced by any dietary changes that affect the consistency of the faeces, and it has been shown above that reduction in dietary fibre results in increased firmness of stools.

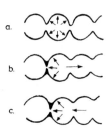

FIG. 7.5. Showing how segmentation of the colon is an essential element in both propelling and halting the contents of the colon. (From Painter, 1964. Reprinted from *Annals of the Royal College of Surgeons of England* with kind permission.)

C. Factors that influence intracolonic pressures

Under resting conditions intracolonic pressures differ little from that of the atmosphere and can be altered by a variety of influences, including the ingestion of food or emotional stimulus.

Drugs like morphine and Prostigmin also increase both the number and amplitude of contraction waves, with corresponding changes in intraluminal pressure. These drugs increase segmentation and narrow the colonic lumen. By contrast, pethidine (Demerol) lessens segmentation and diminishes the response of the bowel to mechanical stimuli, thus decreasing intracolonic pressure. Pro-Banthine paralyses colonic muscles, with resultant widening of its lumen and abolition of pressure changes, including those induced by morphine (Painter and Truelove, 1964; Painter *et al.*, 1965).

Heaton (1973) has aptly summarized the effect of dietary fibre on intestinal physiology in the phrase "Hard in—soft out; soft in—hard out" (Fig. 7.6).

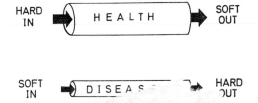

FIG. 7.6. Reciprocal relationship... ...ncy of food and of stools.

References

AUSTIN, R. F. E. (1919). *Indian Medical Gazette* **54**, 56.
AVERY JONES, F. (1972). Management of Constipation in Adults. *In* "Management of Constipation" (F. Avery Jones and E. W. Godding, eds), p. 97. Blackwell Scientific Publications, Oxford.
BROCKLEHURST, J. C. and KHAN, M. Y. (1969). *Gerontologia Clinica* **11**, 293.
BURKITT, D. P., WALKER, A. R. P. and PAINTER, N. S. (1972). *Lancet* **2**, 1408.
BURNETT, F. L. (1923). *American Journal of Roentgenology and Radium Therapy* **10**, 599.
CLEAVE, T. L. (1941). *British Medical Journal* **1**, 461.
CLEAVE, T. L. and CAMPBELL, G. D. (1968). *British Medical Journal* **1**, 579.
COWGILL, G. R. and ANDERSON, W. E. (1932). *Journal of the American Medical Association* **98**, 1866.
DIMOCK, E. (1936). "The treatment of habitual constipation by the bran method." M.D. Thesis, University of Cambridge.
DIMSON, S. B. (1970). *Archives of Diseases in Childhood* **45**, 232.
EVE, I. S. (1966). *Health Physics* **12**, 131.
FANTUS, B., KOPSTEIN, G. and SCHMIDT, H. R. (1940). *Journal of the American Medical Association* **114**, 404.
GALLANT, A. E. (1912). *New York Medical Journal* **96**, 414.
HARVEY, R. F., POMARE, E. W. and HEATON, K. W. (1973). *Lancet* **1**, 1278.
HEATON, K. W. (1973). *Nutrition* **27**, 170.
HINTON, J. M., LENNARD-JONES, J. E. and YOUNG, A. C. (1969). *Gut* **10**, 842.
HOLMGREN, G. O. R. and MYNORS, J. M. (1972). *South African Medical Journal* **46**, 918.
HURST, A. F. (1919). "Constipation and Allied Intestinal Disorders", 2nd edition, p. 335. Oxford University Press, Oxford.
HURST, A. F., HOLMES, G., BURNFORD, J., SPRIGGS, E. I., RUSSELL, K. and BATTEN, G. B. (1934). *Proceedings of the Royal Society of Medicine* **27**, 677.
KOPSTEIN, G. G. (1940). *Radiology* **35**, 39.
McCANCE, R. A., PRIOR, K. M. and WIDDOWSON, E. M. (1953). *British Journal of Nutrition* **7**, 98.
McCAY, C. M. (1973). "Notes on the History of Nutrition Research" (F. Verzár, ed.). Hans Huber, Bern.
MANN, G. V., SPOERRY, A., GRAY, M. and JARASHOW, D. (1972). *American Journal of Epidemiology* **95**, 26.

MANOUSOS, O. N., TRUELOVE, S. C. and LUMSDEN, K. (1967). *British Medical Journal* **3**, 760.

MULINOS, M. G. (1935). *Review of Gastroenterology* **2**, 292.

PAINTER, N. S. (1962). Master of Surgery Thesis, University of London.

PAINTER, N. S. (1964). *Annals of the Royal College of Surgeons of England* **34**, 98.

PAINTER, N. S. (1968a). *American Journal of Digestive Diseases* **13**, 468.

PAINTER, N. S. (1968b). *British Medical Journal* **3**, 475.

PAINTER, N. S. and TRUELOVE, S. C. (1964). *Gut* **5**, 201.

PAINTER, N. S., TRUELOVE, S. C., ARDRAN, G. M. and TUCKEY, M. (1965). *Gastroenterology* **49**, 169.

PAINTER, N. S., ALMEIDA, A. Z. and COLEBOURNE, K. W. (1972). *British Medical Journal* **2**, 137.

PAYLER, D. K. (1973). *Lancet* **1**, 1394.

QUIGLEY, J. P. and BRODY, D. A. (1952). *American Journal of Medicine* **13**, 73.

ROTHMAN, M. M. and KATZ, A. B. (1964). *In* "Gastroenterology" (H. L. Bockus, ed.), Vol. II, p. 695. Saunders, Philadelphia.

STRAUSS, H. (1914). *Archiv für Verdauungskrankheiten, mit Einschluss der Stoffwechselpathologie und der Diätetik* **20**, 299.

TRIBOULET, H. (1909). *Bulletins de la Société de Pédiatrie de Paris* **11**, 512.

WALKER, A. R. P., WALKER, B. F. and RICHARDSON, B. D. (1970). *British Medical Journal* **3**, 48.

WINITZ, M., GRAFF, J., GALLAGHER, N., NARKIN, A. and SEEDMAN, D. A. (1965). *Nature* **205**, 741.

WOLMAN, I. J. (1957). "Laboratory Application in Clinical Pediatrics", p. 696. McGraw-Hill, New York.

WOZASEK, O. and STEIGMANN, F. (1942). *American Journal of Digestive Diseases* **9**, 423.

Part IV

Diseases of the large intestine

Chapter 8

Appendicitis

DENIS BURKITT

I. Geographical and socio-economic distribution 87
   A. Countries largely populated by Caucasians 87
   B. Africa 87
   C. Indian sub-continent 90
   D. West Malaysia and Haiti 90
II. Emergence in the western world 91
III. Changes in incidence following westernization, urbanization or dietary change 91
IV. Changes in incidence following emigration 92
V. Dietetic factors possibly responsible for differences and changes in incidence. 92
VI. Possible causative mechanisms 95
References 96

I. Geographical and socio-economic distribution

A. Countries largely populated by Caucasians

Appendicitis has its highest prevalence in Europe, North America and countries such as Australia, New Zealand and South Africa to which people from western countries have emigrated. In the United States nearly a quarter of a million appendices are removed annually and in England many large provincial hospitals admit about one case of appendicitis every 12 h. Both in the U.S.A. and England appendicectomy is the most frequent emergency abdominal operation.

B. Africa

Appendicitis is still very rare in rural Africa. It was uncommon even in urban Africans 30–40 years ago, but the incidence is rising, sometimes rapidly, in urbanized communities and among those most affected by western customs (Burkitt, 1971).

1. Ghana

Badoe (1967) stated that in the 1940s there were only 6–10 appendicectomies annually at Korle Bu Hospital, Accra. By 1954–60 this figure had risen to 70, and by 1965–6 to 145, with a further 65 treated conservatively. Bowesman (1960) drew attention to the higher incidence in urban areas in Ghana.

2. Kenya

The situation has been similar here. In Nairobi the absence of a single case in Vint's 1937 series of 1000 autopsies on Africans contrasts with the present situation in which over 150 African patients are admitted annually to the Kenyatta Hospital suffering from appendicitis (J. R. Miller, p.c. 1972).

3. Natal

Two large mission hospitals in Natal saw approximately one case per 1000 admissions, and most of these were students and nurses (A. Barker, p.c. 1971). At least two Africans with acute appendicitis were admitted weekly to the King Edward VI Hospital in Durban (L. Baker, p.c. 1970).

4. Nigeria

In 1964 and 1965, 158 African patients with acute appendicitis were admitted to the teaching hospital in Lagos, accounting for nearly one-third of all abdominal emergencies. It is interesting that 90% were city dwellers and approximately three-quarters were students, clerks, professional men, and their wives (Omo-Dare and Thomas, 1966). At University College Hospital, Ibadan, 67 African patients had appendicectomies during 1959 and 1960 (Udeh, 1962). Between 1965 and 1972 over 400 cases were seen (T. E. Solanke, p.c. 1973).

5. Rhodesia

Between 1940 and 1945 only eight cases of appendicitis were recorded in a series of 2000 autopsies on Africans in Salisbury (Gelfand, 1957). By 1970 an average of 75 African patients were being operated on annually (J. Mynors, p.c. 1971).

6. South Africa

Thirty years ago appendicitis was rare in the Bantu. Erasmus (1939) stated that it was eight times more common in the white than in the black population. All of the 38 African patients he reported were or had been in close contact with western civilization and were city dwellers. Eighteen were and the others had been domestic servants in European households, three were mine labourers, two were nurses and one was the daughter of a clergyman. Bremner (1971) reported that in the Baragwanath Hospital, Johannesburg, "histologically proven appendicitis increased seven-fold between the years 1956–69". The increased frequency of appendicitis far exceeds the overall increase in other abdominal emergencies.

7. Sudan

In the years 1928–31 appendicectomy accounted for less than 1% of major surgical operations in Khartoum. In the period 1938–41 the figure had risen to 3·7%, in 1948–51 to 5·7%, and in 1958–61 to 13·4% (A. Osman, p.c. 1972).

8. Uganda

In Kampala some 20 years ago, only four out of 300 emergency abdominal operations on Africans during a 2 year period were for appendicitis, while in an English hospital there 74% of a series of 300 abdominal emergencies were for appendicitis (Burkitt, 1952). In 1969 appendicectomy was performed on 47 African patients (P. Bewes, p.c. 1972).

9. Zaire

Janssens and De Muynck (1966) discussed the prevalence of appendicitis in the Congo before that country became independent in 1962, and quoted figures from many rural hospitals to emphasize the rarity of appendicitis in Africans in comparison with its frequency in Europeans. One surgeon could remember no African case prior to 1940. Africans who did develop this disease were almost exclusively clerks, domestic servants, or in some of their customs partly westernized. Fronville (1931) did not find a single case among 2500 autopsies on Africans. S. G. Browne (p.c., 1971) saw one case in 28 years in Central Zaire.

10. Rural hospitals throughout Africa

Replies to questionnaires sent to doctors in 96 rural hospitals in 15 countries in Africa indicated that 74 admitted less than one case of appendicitis a year. Only one saw more than four confirmed cases. Monthly returns completed with varying degrees of regularity by doctors in 63 hospitals in seven countries in East and Central Africa over a period of 1 year indicated that each hospital was admitting an average of one case of appendicitis per year. Even in West Africa, which is considerably more westernized, on average only five cases were admitted annually to rural hospitals in four countries.

All available evidence indicates that this disease is becoming increasingly common amongst urban Africans, but throughout rural Africa it is still very rare.

C. Indian sub-continent

In 1924 Hallilay wrote "During the whole of my time at Lyallpur (five years), a populous district of over a million inhabitants containing some 30 dispensaries, and for the whole of the statistical reports of which I was responsible, I never encountered or saw reported a single case of appendicitis". Neither did he encounter a single case during two years' tenure as surgeon at Kangra in the Himalayan Hills, nor during a year at Ambala as surgeon responsible for 10,000 Indian troops. He saw this condition commonly among the much smaller numbers of British troops. As surgical specialist in Poona he saw no appendicitis amongst the thousands of Indian troops, although "gangrenous appendicitis was not uncommon at the Sassoon Hospital, but all that I saw were in Indians of the well-to-do and professional classes".

Bradfield (1924) reported that of 29 appendicectomies in 1 year in Madras, ten were Europeans, nine Anglo-Indians, three Indian Christians and one was a Parsee. Appendicitis is becoming increasingly common in urban and more westernized Indians.

Replies to a questionnaire completed by doctors in 15 rural hospitals in India, Pakistan, Bangladesh and Nepal showed that eight admitted less than one case of appendicitis a year and only one admitted more than three.

In 89 monthly returns from 11 rural hospitals in India 111 cases of appendicitis were reported, an annual average of 1·4 cases per hospital.

In contrast, two mission hospitals serving urban communities in Assam, visited by the author, admitted two to four cases monthly, largely from the upper socio-economic class. In city communities appendicitis has become very common. At the Irvine Hospital in Delhi, S. Nair (p.c., 1973) estimates an admission rate of five cases of acute appendicitis a week, and M. J. Joshi (p.c., 1973) reports a similar experience in Poona.

D. West Malaysia and Haiti

Salleh and Balasegaram (1972) reported that in West Malaysia the lowest prevalence of appendicitis was found amongst the least affluent groups living largely on plant and vegetable products.

Only 51 patients with acute appendicitis were admitted to the 400-bed Albert Schweitzer Hospital in Haiti in just over 5 years (F. G. Lepreau, p.c. 1970). The staple foods were rice, corn, sweet potatoes and beans.

II. Emergence in the western world

Between 1820 and 1840, 33 cases of abscesses in the right iliac fossa were reported, and between 1840 and 1860, 102 cases; these were widely distributed in Europe and North America (Short, 1920). Although Melier (1827) suggested that such abscesses were derived from perforation of the appendix, the term "perityphlitis" was generally retained. The name "appendicitis" was adopted following what Short termed "the epoch-making treatise" of Fitz in 1886.

Between 1901 and 1918 deaths from appendicitis doubled in England and Wales (Short, 1920). Elliot-Smith (1971) studied the rise in incidence of appendicitis over the last 100 years, from the records at the Radcliffe Infirmary, Oxford. He found that in the last 70 years the incidence of appendicitis had risen from five to ten annually to the present incidence of 500 cases a year.

The incidence of appendicitis rose in the United States at an earlier stage than in most European countries, but it is significant that this rise in incidence was considerably slower in American negroes than in the white community. In 1896 Matas remarked on the relative rarity of appendicitis in negroes, and even in 1942 Boland made the same observation. Short (1920) stated "many doctors practising in the 'black belt' of Alabama can scarcely recall a case in a negro". In the early 1930s appendicitis in New Orleans had been four times more common in the white than in the negro community, but by 1950 this difference had fallen to 2-fold (Boyce, 1951). Maes and McFetridge (1936) commented on the negro's relative immunity to appendicitis.

This racial disparity in the United States has now almost disappeared, and where both races live in an identical environment, as in the armed forces, appendicitis is equally common.

III. Changes in incidence following westernization, urbanization or dietary change

In Africa the manner in which the incidence of appendicitis rises following urbanization is well illustrated in the geographical distribution and chronological emergence described above.

Another example of an increased prevalence following the impact of modern western customs is demonstrated in the results which followed the provision of European food to African troops in the Second World War. Appendicitis first became prevalent amongst a detachment of Sudanese soldiers after they had received British Army rations in North Africa (A. Elliot-Smith, p.c. 1971). A similar experience was reported from Singapore after West African troops were supplied with standard British rations.

IV. Changes in incidence following emigration

Appendicitis is considerably more prevalent amongst the Japanese in Hawaii than it is in Japan (G. N. Stemmermann, p.c. 1972). De Muynck and his colleagues (1965) reported that 3% of 200 African students going to Antwerp each year from Zaire for further training developed appendicitis while in Belgium. Appendicitis is the only non-infective disease of the bowel which increases in incidence within a few months of entering a new environment.

V. Dietetic factors possibly responsible for differences and changes in incidence

The epidemiological observations outlined above indicate that appendicitis must be due primarily to environmental rather than genetic factors. The factor that most determines the environment of the mucosa of the large bowel, including the appendix, is the nature of the faecal content, which in turn is dependent on the food eaten. In any search for the cause of appendicitis it would therefore seem reasonable to consider dietary differences between communities with a high and a low incidence of the disease, and changes in eating habits which have preceded a rise in incidence in different situations. Over 50 years ago Short (1920) was impressed by the observation that appendicitis was nearly ten times more prevalent in well-to-do boys at an English boarding-school who were eating a refined diet, than it was in a large orphanage where the fare was much coarser. He contrasted the rarity of appendicitis in Rumanian city dwellers, i.e. 1 in 221 patients, with that of rural peasants on a mainly vegetarian diet, 1 in 22,000 patients. Information which Short collected on the geographical distribution and time of emergence of this disease led him to the conclusion that "by far the most probable explanation is that the rise in incidence of appendicitis is due to some changes in the food habits of the people". Consequently he looked for changes in western diet that occurred concurrently with the rise in incidence of appendicitis. After dismissing many other items of food he came to the conclusion that the cause lay in the replacement of foods with a high cellulose content by those with only a little. He blamed the popularization of white flour in particular, and contrasted its low cellulose content with that of unrefined wheat, rice, and a wide variety of fruits and vegetables.

Epidemiological evidence shows indisputably that appendicitis is most prevalent in communities consuming a refined diet and that it is rare or unknown in communities on a high-residue and low-sugar diet. Moreover, the disease can increase in frequency shortly after a change from a high to a much lower fibre diet, as illustrated by its appearance among African soldiers following the provision of western rations.

The relationship between appendicitis and diet has long been recognized, though widely differing opinions as to the items of diet responsible have been expressed. Bowesman (1960), recognizing that the disease was commoner in urban communities, blamed the increased consumption of meat. McCarrison (1922) incriminated the removal of vitamins and other ingredients in the processing of food. Erasmus (1939) thought that the addition of meat and fine flour to the diet was responsible. Janssens and de Muynck (1966) blamed bacterial, protozoal or helminthic infections. Nuttall (1947) was, it would seem, nearer the truth in endeavouring to account for the greater incidence of appendicitis among Anglo-Saxons when he observed that their diet contained less cellulose and more protein, with consequent changes in bowel behaviour. Similarly Omo-Dare and Thomas (1966) attributed the higher urban incidence to their patients having "forsaken the simple village diet, rich in cellulose, for the more sophisticated diet, rich in proteins". Cleave et al. (1969) in the light of epidemiological evidence, blamed a refined diet but put more emphasis on the increase in sugar consumption than on the reduction in fibre, though they recognized the importance of each.

J. R. Miller (p.c., 1970) studied the dramatic rise in appendicitis in Africans in Nairobi, Kenya, and considered the most influential factor was the replacement of home-ground cereals by machine-refined flour. He found that approximately one-third of all out-patients attending the Kenyatta Hospital in Nairobi ate white bread daily and that probably all took sugar.

As mentioned above, all the 38 African patients with appendicitis reported from Johannesburg by Erasmus in 1939 had had access to European-type food, as had the students from Zaire temporarily living in Belgium. It is significant that in Port Sudan appendicitis is said to be commoner in dockers fed with European-type food from the ships than in other low-income groups.

The increased prevalence of appendicitis in higher income groups in Africa seems most likely to be related to dietary changes. The rarity in rural Rumania before the First World War, in contrast to the prevalence of the condition in cities, was attributed by Wilkie (1914) to the fact that "the Rumanian peasants subsist on a diet almost wholly vegetarian, whereas in the cities an animal diet is the rule".

R. M. Clark (p.c., 1971) records that appendicitis "arrived" in the part of China where he worked in 1940 following the instalment of a roller mill, the cases all occurring in government employees and students who obtained their flour from the roller mill, while those living on stone-ground flour remained free of the disease. Sugar was almost unavailable to either group.

It is of interest that Battle (1913) attributed the rising incidence of appendicitis to the replacement of stone-grinding by roller mills. His reasoning was, however, wide of the mark, since he thought that the damage was done by fragments of metal from the rollers.

P. Harrison (p.c., 1972), who worked in southern Arabia between the wars, stated that appendicitis suddenly became common after coarsely milled wheat bread was replaced by highly milled imported white flour and imported sweet jams became popular.

Walker and his associates (1973) questioned over 15,000 16–20-year-old South African pupils of all races in both rural and urban situations, to ascertain the prevalence of appendicectomy and to relate it to dietary customs. They also obtained from sections of these groups data on their crude fibre intake, frequency of defaecation and intestinal transit times. Appendicectomy was very uncommon in rural Bantu (0·5%) and in peri-urban Bantu (0·9%), slightly more common in urban Bantu (1·4%) and very common in Caucasians (16·5%). In Indian and coloured groups the prevalence was 2·9% and 1·7% respectively. In the rural Bantu population there was a much larger fibre intake and frequency of defaecation, with shorter transit times. Data on these variables were similar in all ethnic groups in urban areas despite the difference in appendicectomy pre-valence, suggesting other possible aetiological factors, bacteriological or chemical.

Not only has an increase of appendicitis been observed to follow changes from high to lower fibre diets, but the reverse has also been noted. Examples are cited of a decreased incidence during war time when there was, in many countries, a return to less sophisticated foods (Fleisch, 1946).

Van Ouwerkerk (1951) reported on the fall in incidence of appendicitis in the Netherlands during the Second World War and emphasized that it was almost unknown amongst Dutch prisoners of war in Japanese intern-ment camps who were fed on "coarse vegetables and almost no meats or fats".

Walker et al. (1973) found that white South Africans in prison, living on a higher fibre diet, were significantly less prone to appendicitis than those consuming less fibre as free men. This is consistent with the rarity of the disease in an English prison referred to by Short (1920).

VI. Possible causative mechanisms

The effect of dietary fibre on both intestinal content and behaviour has been described in preceding sections of this chapter. The fibre content of food is the only constituent known to affect the consistency, bulk and speed of transit of the faeces. The prolonged hold-up of intestinal content in the large bowel associated with fibre-depleted carbohydrate foods is likely to allow proliferation of any organisms whose presence in the faeces is the result of changes in other dietary constituents. The amount of dietary fibre present in unrefined cereals is known to influence the electrolyte composition and also the microbial flora of the large bowel and probably of the lower ileum. Changes in bowel function, content and bacteria may all play a causative role in appendicitis.

Clinical and pathological evidence suggests that the initial change is a pressure phenomenon leading to devitalization of mucosa, bacterial invasion being secondary. This increased pressure can be explained on the basis of altered muscular behaviour and the presence of faecaliths. The bacterial invasion may be enhanced by changes in faecal bacterial flora. Raines and Capper (1971) wrote: "When an acutely inflamed appendix has been removed some form of obstruction to its lumen can be demonstrated in a large percentage of cases".

The following evidence suggests that the factor initiating appendicitis is likely to be an increase in intraluminal pressure:

1. The inflammatory change in the mucosa affects the whole circumference of the appendix-lumen distal to a line of demarcation. This indicates some uniform change throughout the whole area of mucosa, distal and never proximal to a line of demarcation.

2. The frequency with which a faecalith obstructs the lumen. Faecaliths rarely if ever form in the soft faeces associated with a high-fibre diet.

3. In view of the fact that the small faecal volume associated with a low-fibre diet can result in contractions of the circular muscles of the colon sufficient to obstruct its lumen, it seems highly probable that the smaller lumen of the appendix could more easily be obstructed.

4. Inflammatory changes rarely if ever extend beyond the base of the appendix into the wall of the caecum.

5. Inflammatory changes in the mucosa are more or less generalized beyond the line of demarcation between normal and inflamed mucosa. A localized ulcer is rarely if ever encountered other than pressure necrosis at the site of faecalith impaction.

6. The epigastric colic present in the early stages of the disease indicates muscular contraction rather than initial inflammation.

7. It is significant that barium meal studies have shown that the addition of bran to the diet increases emptying of the appendix (Fantus et al., 1940).

8. There is evidence that raised intraluminal pressure can result in devitalization of the mucosa.

In 1904 Van Zwalenburg showed how the viability of the bowel mucosa could be impaired by increased pressures, and postulated that subsequent inflammation could result from bacterial invasion. He believed that faecal concretions could exert a valve-like action and thus lead to raised intraluminal pressures (Van Zwalenburg, 1905). Subsequently Wilkie (1914) endorsed these conclusions and Wangensteen and Bowers in 1937 wrote, "Obstruction and infection are the two causative factors important in bringing about a picture of acute appendicitis". These workers showed experimentally that intraluminal pressures from 5 to 15 cm of water maintained for 6–18 h are followed invariably by changes in the appendix wall.

Any changes in the bacterial flora of the faeces, either as a result of arrest in the colon or directly due to dietary changes as suggested by Cleave *et al.* (1969), could well modify the results of bacterial invasion following initial mucosal devitalization.

All available evidence thus suggests that refined carbohydrate foods may be an important factor in the pathogenesis of appendicitis.

References

BADOE, E. A. (1967). *Ghana Medical Journal* 6, 69.

BATTLE, W. H. (1913). *Lancet* 2, 135.

BOLAND, F. K. (1942). *Annals of Surgery* 115, 939.

BOWESMAN, C. (1960). "Surgery and Clinical Pathology in the Tropics." Livingstone, Edinburgh.

BOYCE, F. F. (1951). *Annals of Surgery* 133, 631.

BRADFIELD, E. W. C. (1924), *Indian Medical Gazette* 59, 515.

BREMNER, C. G. (1971). *South African Journal of Surgery* 9, 127.

BURKITT, D. P. (1952). *East African Medical Journal* 29, 190.

BURKITT, D. P. (1971). *British Journal of Surgery* 58, 695.

CLEAVE, T. L., CAMPBELL, G. D. and PAINTER, N. S. (1969). "Diabetes, Coronary Thrombosis and the Saccharine Disease", 2nd edition. John Wright, Bristol.

ELLIOT-SMITH, A. (1971). Changing Patterns of Disease. *In* "Just Consequences" (R. Waller, ed.), p. 143. Knight, London.

ERASMUS, J. F. P. (1939). *South African Medical Journal* 13, 601.

FANTUS, B., KOPSTEIN, G. and SCHMIDT, H. R. (1940). *Journal of the American Medical Association* 114, 404.

FITZ, R. H. (1886). *American Journal of Medical Sciences* 92, 321.

FLEISCH, A. (1946). *Schweizerische Medizinische Wochenschrift* 76, 889.

FRONVILLE, G. (1931). *Annales des Sociétés belges de Médecine tropicale de Parasitologie et de Mycologie humaine et animale* 11, 445.

GELFAND, M. (1957). "The Sick African", 3rd edition, p. 720. Juta, Cape Town.

HALLILAY, H. (1924). *Indian Medical Gazette* 59, 403.

JANSSENS, P. G. and DE MUYNCK, A. (1966). *Tropical and Geographical Medicine* **18**, 81.

MAES, U. and MCFETRIDGE, E. M. (1936). *American Journal of Surgery* **33**, 5.

MATAS, R. (1896). *Transactions of the American Surgical Association* **14**, 483.

MCCARRISON, R. (1922). *Journal of the American Medical Association* **78**, 1.

MELIER, F. (1827). *Journal général de Médecine, de Chirurgie et de Pharmacie, françaises et étrangères* **100**, 317.

DE MUYNCK, A., LIMBOS, P. and JANSSENS, P. G. (1965). *Annales des Sociétés belges de Médecine tropicale de Parasitologie et de Mycologie humaine et animale* **45**, 111.

NUTTALL, H. C. W. (1947). *In* "British Surgical Practice" (E. Rock Carling and J. Paterson Ross, eds), Vol. 1, p. 293. Butterworth, London.

OMO-DARE, P. and THOMAS, H. O. (1966). *West African Medical Journal* **15**, 217.

RAINES, A. J. H. and CAPPER, W. M. (1971). *In* Bailey and Love's "Short Practice of Surgery", 15th edition, p. 974. H. K. Lewis, London.

SALLEH, H. BIN D. and BALASEGARAM, M. (1972). *Medical Journal of Malaysia* **27**, 43.

SHORT, A. R. (1920). *British Journal of Surgery* **8**, 171.

UDEH, F. N. (1962). *British Journal of Surgery* **50**, 39.

VAN OUWERKERK, L. W. (1951). *Archivum chirurgicum neerlandicum* **3**, 164.

VAN ZWALENBURG, C. (1904). *Journal of the American Medical Association* **42**, 820.

VAN ZWALENBURG, C. (1905). *Annals of Surgery* **41**, 437.

VINT, F. W. (1937). *East African Medical Journal* **13**, 332.

WALKER, A. R. P., WALKER, B. F., RICHARDSON, B. D. and WOOLFORD, A. (1973). *Postgraduate Medical Journal* **49**, 243.

WANGENSTEEN, O. H. and BOWERS, W. F. (1937). *Archives of Surgery* **34**, 496.

WILKIE, D. P. D. (1914). *British Medical Journal* **2**, 959.

Chapter 9

Diverticular disease of the colon

NEIL PAINTER and DENIS BURKITT

I. Present geographical and socio-economic distribution . . . 99
   A. Western countries and other Caucasian communities . . 99
   B. Africa 102
   C. The Indian sub-continent and the Middle East . . . 104
   D. Other areas 105
II. Emergence as a clinical problem in the western world . . . 105
III. Changes in incidence following the adoption of western customs
   either within a country or on emigration 107
IV. Dietetic factors that may explain variations and alterations in
   incidence 107
   A. The relation of dietary fibre to the pathogenesis of diverticular
   disease 108
   B. Origin of the low-fibre diet in the treatment of diverticular
   disease 110
   C. The treatment of uncomplicated diverticular disease of the colon
   by a high-fibre diet 110
V. Effect of bran on intracolonic pressures 111
VI. Animal experiments that bear on the pathogenesis of diverticular
   disease 112
VII. Intraluminal pressures, colonic pain and diverticular disease. . 112
VIII. Conclusion 114
References 114

I. Present geographical and socio-economic distribution

A. Western countries and other Caucasian communities

The emergence of diverticular disease as a clinical problem was first recognized from the rising incidence of diverticulitis, a condition which could be clinically diagnosed.

The advent of contrast radiology confirmed that diverticulosis was a common condition and prompted attempts to discover its true prevalence.

TABLE 9.1. Incidence of colonic diverticula: necropsy series

Country and author	Incidence of diverticula		No. in series	Comments
	%	No.		
United Kingdom:				
Drummond (1917)	4·4	22	500	
Fifield (1927)	2·1	—	10,167	London Hospital, 55% of subjects were under age 30, so incidence over 40 would probably have been 5%
Parks (1968)	37	111	300	Northern Ireland, 50% in ninth decade
United States:				
Hartwell and Cecil (1910)	5	—	81	New York, 1909–10
Rankin and Brown (1930)	5·6	111	1925	All but one subject aged over 40
Oschner and Bargen (1935)	6·9	—	447	All necropsies in one year
Kocour (1937)	3·58	—	7000	Over age 40
	15·2	—		White women over age 70
	7·1	—		White men over age 70
	2·0	—		Coloured men over age 70
	3·0	—		Coloured women over age 70
Morton (1946)	6·3	—	8500	Rochester, N.Y.
Australia:				
Cleland (1968)	2·6	78	3000	Refers to 1940–8. Incidence rose with age
	6·2	36	589	Over age 70 in this period
Hughes (1969)	45	90	200	43% if caecal diverticula excluded

Country and author	Incidence of diverticula		No. in series	Comments
	%	No.		
United Kingdom:				
Sriggs (1920)	0·6	6	1000	
Sriggs and Marxer (1925)	10	100	1000	Mainly adult patients. Importance of postevacuation film had been realized
Edwards (1934a)	10·8	—	507	Period 1925–31, King's College Hospital. Patients aged over 40
Grout (1949)	8	—	2179	Relates to previous 13½ years and all patients over age 35
Edwards (1953)	16	25	1623	
Manousos et al. (1967)	7·6	—	} 109	7·6% below age 60 } Deliberate study by Ba meal and follow-through in normal people
	34·9	—		34·9% over age 60 }
Sweden:				
Lunding (1935)	4·2	87	2090	
France:				
Debray et al. (1961)	40	—	500	40% over age 70. All patients had gastrointestinal symptoms
United States:				
Enfield (1924)	1·2	—	—	Found incidentally on barium studies
Mayo (1930)	5·71	1819	31,838	Mayo Clinic
Rankin and Brown (1930)	5·67	1398	24,620	Mayo Clinic
Oschner and Bargen (1935)	7	—	2747	Enemas given for intestinal symptoms
Willard and Bockus (1936)	8·2	38	463	Consecutive enemas in private practice
Eggers (1941)	7·5	—	647	Barium meal followed through colon
Allen (1953)	44·5	—	428	Barium enemas
	30	—	2000	Enemas given for symptoms. No diverticula under age 35, 5% at 45, 66% in older age-groups
Welch et al. (1953)	8·5	—	47,000	Collected series; 66% incidence over age 80
Smith and Christensen (1959)	22	—	1016	Consecutive enemas. Years 1954–8; incidence doubled at 80 years

(From Painter and Burkitt, 1971)

Necropsy studies showed that diverticula were rare before the age of 40, thus confirming that they are an acquired abnormality. Necropsy and barium enema estimates of the prevalence of diverticula are given in Tables 9.1 and 9.2. Both methods have their limitations: autopsies are performed more on elderly subjects than on young ones and barium enemas are usually undertaken because of symptoms of illness. Radiological series exaggerate the prevalence while necropsy findings vary with pathologist's personal interest in diverticulosis. The present true incidence of the disease could be established only by subjecting a sample of the population to annual barium enemas, a method which would not be practicable.

B. Africa

The rarity of diverticular disease in centres where ample autopsy and radiological evidence is available is, as might be expected, abundantly substantiated by experience in rural hospitals. Although uncomplicated diverticulosis would pass undetected in these circumstances diverticulitis, if it occurred, could not be consistently missed by successive doctors in many large hospitals. Repeated questionnaires distributed personally or by post to doctors in over 130 mission and other rural hospitals in Africa have indicated that diverticular disease is virtually unknown in their African patients (Trowell et al., 1974).

Some specific information gleaned both from writings and personal contact, given below, adds further evidence of the rarity of diverticular disease in rural Africa and its increase with the adoption of western customs.

1. Ethiopia

Goulston (1967) states that diverticulosis is infrequent and diverticulitis unknown.

2. Ghana—Accra

E. Badoe (p.c., 1971) saw only one case of diverticulitis in 16 years in the medical school hospital.

3. Liberia—Monrovia

J. Diggs (p.c., 1974) found two patients with diverticular disease in approximately 300 barium enema examinations, both in the highest socio-economic group.

4. Sierra Leone—Freetown

O. Williams (p.c., 1974) saw seven patients with diverticular disease in over 20 years' surgical practice in the General Hospital. All were in the upper socio-economic group.

5. Nigeria—Lagos

Kyle *et al.* (1967) recorded that only two cases of diverticulitis were observed in the University Hospital over a period of 3 years.

6. Rhodesia—Salisbury

Wapnick and Levin (1971) reported what they believed to be the only recorded case of diverticular disease in a Rhodesian African.

7. South Africa—Johannesburg

In the 2000 bed Baragwanath Hospital, which serves the most urbanized Africans, Keeley (1958) found no diverticula in a series of 2367 autopsies between 1954 and 1956. At the same hospital A. Solomon (p.c., 1971) found six cases in approximately 1000 barium enemas done in a 3 year period on Bantu patients. J. I. Levy (p.c., 1972) who was carrying out 100–150 barium enema examinations annually at the non-European Hospital, which also cares for the most urbanized Africans, saw no cases in 13 years.

Higginson and Simson (1958) found only one case with diverticula in over 2000 consecutive autopsies.

Bremner and Ackerman (1970) stated that the Bantu practically never develop diverticulosis.

—Pretoria

I. Simson (p.c., 1972) found only five cases in 3000 Bantu autopsies which had been done with meticulous care.

—Durban

D. Chapman (p.c., 1971) saw only one African case in 14 years in the Department of Surgery at the King Edward VII teaching hospital.

8. Kenya—Nairobi

J. R. Miller (p.c., 1971) saw only one case of diverticular disease in an African in 11 years in the Department of Surgery at the Kenyatta Hospital.

9. Uganda—Kampala

Davies (quoted by Trowell, 1960) found only two diverticula in 4000 autopsies in a 15-year period.

A. C. Templeton (p.c., 1970) made a detailed study of over 300 autopsies on subjects over the age of 30 years, specifically searching for evidence of diverticulosis, and found only one case of diverticular disease in an African. This involved the sigmoid colon in a woman aged over 80 years. Three caecal diverticula were observed, but these are considered to be aetiologically distinct.

10. Zaire—Kinshasa

A. Jain (p.c., 1971) saw one case only in 9 years in a medical school hospital.

C. The Indian sub-continent and the Middle East

Even in the urban communities in these regions diverticular disease is still very rare, as will be seen from the evidence given below.

1. India—Delhi

O. P. Bhardwaj (p.c., 1973) found only nine cases in over 9000 barium enema examinations. In 15 years S. Bhargava (p.c., 1973) has seen only 12 cases, all in more "westernized" Indians, in a series of several thousand barium enemas.

—Calcutta

N. M. Bannerjee (p.c., 1973) diagnosed less than one case a year in a department carrying out over 300 barium enema examinations annually.

—Assam

G. G. Ahmed (p.c., 1973) saw no case in 3 years in the Department of Radiology at Gauhati Medical College.

2. Iran—Shiraz

R. Zarabi and A. Farpour (p.c., 1971) saw only five cases in 8 years in two university hospitals totalling 700 beds.

3. *Iraq—Baghdad*

Mohammed Abu-Tabikh (p.c., 1973) reported that approximately 1000 barium enema examinations were done annually in the University Radiological Department and not more than three cases of diverticulosis were detected.

D. *Other areas*

In Japan diverticular disease has until recently been very rare (Sato *et al.*, 1970). In Singapore, Kyle *et al.* (1967) saw three cases of diverticulitis in 15,000 Europeans, but only 10 in 1,500,000 Chinese, Indian and Malay inhabitants over a period of 5 years. They saw only a single case among 137,000 native Fijians but two in 7000 Europeans. M. K. Kutty (p.c., 1970) found no case at autopsy during a 3 year period at Kuala Lumpur (Malaysia), and Kim (1964) found no diverticula in 500 barium meal examinations in Korea. V. Plengvanit (p.c., 1972) commented on the rarity of this disease in Bangkok (Thailand) where he had detected two cases in 91 barium enemas.

II. Emergence as a clinical problem in the western world

Diverticular disease of the colon was unknown to clinicians at the turn of this century.

The term "divertikel" was used by Fleischman in 1815 (quoted by Spriggs and Marxer, 1925). Gross (1845), Cruveilhier (1849), Rokitansky (1849), Haberschon (1857) and Klebs (1869) all realized that colonic diverticula were acquired and thought these were caused by constipation. However, they regarded diverticula only as interesting phenomena, except for Cruveilhier, who pointed out that they might become infected and perforate. In 1859, Sidney Jones described vesicocolic fistula due to diverticulitis, but when Cripps (1888) collected 63 examples of entero-vesical fistula he believed that they were often caused by ingested foreign bodies. He took pains to emphasize that they were usually the result of "inflammatory mischief" and not of cancer, but he blamed diverticulitis only in the case reported by Jones.

Virchow in 1853 described perisigmoiditis while Loomis (1870) recorded peritonitis resulting from diverticulitis. Since this complication was still regarded as a surgical rarity 30 years later, it seems very unlikely that perforated diverticulitis was common at that time.

Our nineteenth-century predecessors accurately described diverticula and their complications, but regarded them as curiosities.

In 1899, Graser stressed that if diverticula became infected, perisig-moiditis and perforation with peritonitis would follow and his warning proved timely within a decade. Five years later, Beer (1904) described 18 infected diverticula and the complications of peritonitis, adhesions, fistula and stenosis, but he still believed that diverticula seldom caused symptoms. "Diagnoses" such as pericolitis sinistra, perisigmoiditis, torsion and inflammation of appendices epiploica lingered on, being still considered respectable by Bland-Sutton (1903), d'Arcy Power (1906), Donaldson (1907) and Roberts (1908). Even as late as 1910, Taylor and Lakin were reluctant to attribute peritonitis to diverticulitis but they did so when they saw two examples of this complication within a few months. The ability of diverticulitis to mimic cancer was still thought newsworthy at this time, both in Britain and America, Mayo, et al., 1907; Moynihan 1907.

Diverticulitis changed from a rare to a relatively common disease within two decades. Dr Telling of Leeds first saw the disease in 1899 when none of his colleagues was familiar with it, but by 1908 he could describe all its complications and in 1917 he published his classic paper on diverticulosis and diverticulitis. Even so, the condition was still not mentioned in text-books in 1920 (Telling, 1908, 1920; Telling and Gruner, 1917).

The appearance of diverticulitis early in this century surprised even surgeons of repute but, by 1920, Sir John Bland-Sutton remarked that "in the last ten years, acute diverticulitis is recognized with the same certainty as appendicitis and is a newly discovered bane of elders".

By 1930 Mayo estimated that 5% of patients over the age of 40 years bore diverticula. At about the same time barium enema studies were indicating a prevalence of 4–10%. Morton (1946), reviewing American autopsies and Edwards (1953) quoting English barium enema studies, recorded similar figures.

The incidence of diverticulosis has obviously risen dramatically in the United Kingdom, the U.S.A., Australia and France in the last 20 years. About one-twentieth of those over the age of 40 and more than one-third of those over 60 have diverticula. The incidence rises to two-thirds at 80 years (Parks, 1968; Hughes, 1969). The disease must have become commoner in Australia, as it was much less frequent there in the 1940s (Cleland, 1968).

All available evidence thus suggests that diverticular disease of the colon was almost unknown at the beginning of this century, but that it has become increasingly common and is now the commonest disease of the colon.

This evidence could be almost endlessly multiplied. It leaves no possible doubt that diverticular disease of the colon, almost unknown at the beginning of this century, is now exceedingly common amongst those most influenced by the environment associated with modern economic develop-ment, but is, in striking contrast, still almost unknown in communities who have until recently been little affected by customs characteristic of modern western civilization.

III. Changes in incidence following the adoption of western customs either within a country or on emigration

Some 40 years ago diverticular disease was significantly less prevalent in American negroes than in whites (Kocour, 1937), but this difference has now almost disappeared (Cleave *et al.*, 1969).

It was until recently almost unknown in Japan but Dr Chikai Yazana reported to the International Conference of University Colon and Rectal Surgeons at their Meeting in Rhodes, 1972, that in the Tokyo Women's Hospital from December 1967 to August 1971, 1987 barium enemas had demonstrated diverticula in 131 patients, a rate of 6·6%, and this was in the ratio of three males to one female; the incidence increased with age to 22% over the age of 70. The disease is more prevalent in Japanese who have been born and bred in Hawaii and who have been reared on a western-type diet (G. N. Stemmermann, p.c. 1970).

The few cases recorded in India and Iran have for the most part been in the upper socio-economic group.

IV. Dietetic factors that may explain variations and alterations in incidence

The dramatic increase in incidence of diverticular disease in the western world occurred within some 70 years and, theoretically, can only be explained in three ways. First, it might be due to a genetic change in the whole population, but this idea is too ridiculous to contemplate seriously. Second, this change may be due to observer error and hence be more apparent than real, but the quality of their writings shows that the clinicians and pathologists of the last century were just as capable of recognizing diverticulitis as those of today. A third possibility remains: namely, that the colon's environment has been changed and that diverticula are caused by our modern diet, in particular by changes in the composition of that fraction of diet which reaches the colon.

The changes which have occurred in the fibre content of western diet have been described in Chapter 5 and the relationship between dietary fibre and intestinal transit times, and stool weights and consistency have been outlined in Chapter 7, together with the results of studies of intra-luminal pressure relative to diet.

Since the epidemiology of diverticular disease is consistent with the hypothesis that it is causally related to a low residue diet it must now be considered by what mechanisms these changes may be brought about.

Only when cineradiography and pressure recording became available were diverticula shown to be the result of functional obstruction due to segmèntation dividing the colon into "little bladders" (Fig. 7.4). These become "trabeculated" so that the colonic wall is distorted with its muscle thrown into ridges of varying thickness before the herniation of the mucosa takes place (Edwards, 1934a, b; Painter, 1962, 1963, 1964; Arfwiddson, 1964).

Modern workers, who are not limited to the study of dead tissues, have confirmed the opinion of Gross (1845) that diverticula are caused by obstruction "by which the muscular fibres are separated from each other so as to permit the mucous membranes to protrude. . .". Haberschon (1857) blamed constipation for thickening of the muscle and for diverticula, while Lane (1885) realized that diverticula were not caused by distension behind some obstruction but that they were produced by a mechanism similar to that which causes bladder diverticula and which involves muscular contraction. Bristowe (1854) also believed that colonic diverticula were caused in a manner which resembled that operating in the sacculated bladder and that costiveness might mimic the effects of obstruction.

Around 1880 the British diet became so depleted of cereal fibre as to damage the colon. The evidence suggests that the refining of flour and other cereals is the primary cause of diverticulosis, while the increased consumption of refined sugar at the expense of bread further decreases the intake of dietary fibre. Although much bran had been removed from flour before this date, it would appear that the colon failed to adapt to this further reduction of dietary fibre.

It is significant that only during the Second World War was the rising incidence of this disease halted—during a time when the manufacture of higher extraction national flour was mandatory and refined sugar was in short supply (Painter and Burkitt, 1971).

Although dietary changes are taking place rapidly in Africa south of the Sahara a low-fibre diet has not yet been eaten for long enough to cause diverticulosis. Close observation of these dietary changes and the altering incidence of disease in this part of the world may well reveal the causation of these and other diseases.

A. The relation of dietary fibre to the pathogenesis of diverticular disease

If a deficiency of dietary fibre causes diverticulosis, this must be related to colonic segmentation which is the mechanism responsible for the mucosal herniation. The role of segmentation in colonic physiology is summarized in Fig. 7.5. Its postulated role in the causation of diverticular disease is depicted in Fig. 9.1 (Painter, 1962, 1964; Painter et al., 1965).

The protrusion of diverticula between the muscle fibres of the colonic wall can well be likened to the manner in which mud held in a closed fist extrudes between the fingers when the fist is clenched (Fig. 9.2).

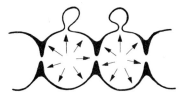

FIG. 9.1. Diagrammatic representation of the manner in which excessive segmentation can convert the lumen of the colon into "little bladders" in which pressure can build up and force diverticula out between fibres in the colon wall.

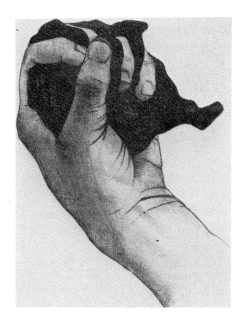

FIG. 9.2. Diverticula represented as mud extruding between the fingers of a clenched fist.

It is suggested that an unrefined diet containing adequate fibre may prevent diverticulosis for the following reasons:

1. The colon that copes with a large volume of faeces is of a wider diameter and does not develop diverticula. This is true in man (Wells, 1949) and experimental animals such as rats (Carlson and Hoelzel, 1949) and rabbits (Hodgson, 1972a). Such a colon having a wide bore *ab initio* segments less efficiently than does a narrow colon (Chapter 7) and is consequently less prone to diverticulosis (Painter, 1964).

2. Studies of transit times and stool weights are described in Chapter 7. In most instances, the food residue passes through the African gut within 40 h, whereas in an Englishman this may take twice as long (Burkitt *et al.*, 1972). The African's colon thus absorbs water for a shorter time, and propels a less viscous faecal stream. Water is retained in the faeces also by the hydrophilic celluloses and hemicelluloses of the dietary fibre. Consequently, his colon has to do less work and produces less pressure by segmentation. His colon is therefore unlikely to become "trabeculated" and to bear diverticula than is a colon that has to struggle for many years with the viscous contents which result from a low-fibre diet.

3. In western countries custom often demands the suppression of the call to stool which favours the drying of faeces and increased pressure generation. On the other hand, the South African Bantu can pass large motions on demand without straining (Walker *et al.*, 1970).

In short, the swiftly passed soft stool subjects the sigmoid to less strain and does not favour the development of diverticula.

B. Origin of the low-fibre diet in the treatment of diverticular disease

The low-fibre diet which was the mainstay of the medical management of diverticulosis for nearly 50 years was founded on a misunderstanding of the cause of this condition. Spriggs and Marxer (1927) believed that constipation and the stagnation of faeces in the sigmoid led to infection and so they gave paraffin to cleanse the colon. Undigested fragments of food and bone had been found close to diverticula and were reported by Cripps (1888), Bland-Sutton (1903) and Brewer (1907) who believed that these were connected with the perforation. Hence, a low-fibre diet, in which fruit and vegetables were made into a purée, and stalks and pips were eliminated, was advocated by authorities such as Slesinger (1930), Oschner and Bargen (1935), Willard and Bockus (1936), Brown and Marcley (1937) and by Edwards (1939).

Despite the profession's adoption of this diet, there is no evidence to show that it is of any benefit. It is now known that a diet low in fibre is contraindicated in the treatment of diverticular disease because it is believed to be the cause of the condition.

C. The treatment of uncomplicated diverticular disease of the colon by a high-fibre diet

If a diet that is deficient in fibre causes diverticulosis, then it is logical to ask whether the replacement of fibre in the diet in the form of miller's bran would alleviate the symptoms of the uncomplicated disease. The restoration of dietary fibre in this form was shown to be effective in 88·6% of 70 patients thus treated by Painter *et al.* (1972). These authors asked patients to restrict their intake of refined sugar, whether brown or white, by not adding it to their food or drinks, and persuaded them to eat wholemeal instead of white bread and to add miller's bran to their diet in such a quantity as was necessary to enable them to pass one or two soft stools a day. The correct amount of bran was established by trial and error; an average of two teaspoonsful three times a day was found to be sufficient in the majority of patients, but some had to increase this to several tablespoonsful. This regimen of treatment not only relieved the abdominal aching, heaviness and distension that is often associated with diverticular disease, but even the colic which was sometimes so severe that it had been mis-diagnosed as left renal colic.

It is not yet known whether this "bran diet" will lessen the liability of patients with the disease to suffer attacks of acute diverticulitis, but certainly it is highly effective in diminishing or abolishing the symptoms of painful diverticular disease. It is of great interest to note that taking bran often improved the appetite and no patient reported that bran had diminished appetite. Patients who ate little because of post-prandial abdominal discomfort and distension were usually able to eat normally once the bran diet had taken effect. This shows that the old belief that "roughage irritates the gut" is merely a myth; bran becomes "softage" when wet (Painter, 1971; Painter *et al.*, 1972).

The ability of bran to afford much effective relief of symptoms even when the disease is well established adds to the evidence that fibre affects intestinal behaviour and is consistent with the view that fibre-deficiency causes diverticulosis. No one would claim, however, that this evidence in itself proves that a deficiency of fibre is a causative factor.

V. Effect of bran on intracolonic pressures

A. N. Smith (p.c., 1973) has provided evidence of a connection between dietary fibre and intracolonic pressures. Reilly's operation of sigmoid myotomy has been shown to reduce intracolonic pressures and widen the lumen of the colon, thus relieving symptoms (Smith *et al.*, 1969; Smith *et al.*, 1971), but these pressures rise again after about 2 years in patients who remain on their previous diet. Smith persuaded patients who had undergone myotomy to add bran to their diet and found that after nearly 4 years the reduction in intracolonic pressures achieved by this operation had been maintained. These observations suggest that the correction of a deficiency of dietary fibre had resulted in the removal of the cause of the high pressures that would have recurred had his patients continued to eat a fibre-deficient diet.

Hodgson (1972b) has recently shown that methyl-cellulose given to six patients with diverticular disease reduced intracolonic pressures and relieved symptoms in every case. This small series supports the view that the colon does not generate high pressures in the presence of a soft faecal stream. Moreover it seems unnecessary to use methyl-cellulose (Celivac), which has been known to clump and cause obstruction, when bran, which is natural and safe, is available at but a fraction of the cost.

VI. Animal experiments that bear on the pathogenesis of diverticular disease

Rats fed on a high-fibre diet by Carlson and Hoelzel (1949) did not develop diverticula while others fed on a low-fibre diet had contracted colons which bore diverticula. These authors suggested that the rat colons, which narrow as a result of eating a low-fibre diet, were more prone to become obstructed at the acute angle where the rat's colon joins the rectum and that this caused the diverticula to develop. Painter (1964) and Painter et al. (1965) suggested another explanation, namely, that the narrow colon could segment more efficiently and so produce higher localized intracolonic pressures which resulted in the appearance of diverticula.

Hodgson (1972a) fed six New Zealand white rabbits on white bread, butter, milk and sugar supplemented by vitamins. He measured their intracolonic pressures before and after Prostigmin, prior to giving this "refined" diet and again afterwards. The diet caused the rabbits to gain weight while their general condition deteriorated and they became constipated. Their colons became narrower and the administration of prostigmine caused scattered wide-necked reducible diverticula to appear. The total pressure produced within their colons had been altered by this low-fibre diet. Hodgson's findings were essentially similar to those reported in humans by Painter (1962, 1964) and Painter et al. (1965).

These experiments lend support to the view that low-fibre diets are the primary cause of diverticulosis, but they must be interpreted with caution if only because of the different life-span of the species investigated.

VII. Intraluminal pressures, colonic pain and diverticular disease

Pain, usually of a colicky nature felt in the left iliac fossa, and associated with the presence of diverticula, was once thought to be due to diverticulitis, but when Morson (1963) studied sigmoid colons which had been resected for "diverticulitis" he found in only one-third histological evidence of sufficient inflammation to account for the symptoms which had led to operation. In some of his specimens, *thickening of the colonic muscle was the only abnormality, and no diverticula were present.* These observations, coupled with those of Arfwiddson (1964), who showed that high pressures were present in the colon even in the "pre-diverticular state", led Painter (1964) to suggest that the pain of so-called diverticulitis was often the colic of intermittent functional obstruction brought about by excessive colonic segmentation. He called this "painful diverticular disease" (Painter, 1964). Later it was shown that this pain could be relieved by replacing in the form of bran the cereal fibre that is deficient in our modern diet (Painter *et al.*, 1972).

These observations leave no reasonable doubt that thickening or "trabeculation" of the colonic muscle, segmentation and abnormally high intracolonic pressures are closely related to diet. The colic that is usually attributed to "diverticulitis" or to a "spastic" or "irritable" colon is in the majority of cases due to abnormal activity of the colonic muscle. Consideration of the diagram illustrating segmentation (Fig. 7.5) will make it obvious that the sigmoid which has to cope with a viscous faecal content will have to work harder, becomes hypertrophied and will be more likely to produce high pressure and colic due to functional obstruction than will a wide-bore colon that has only to propel soft stools (Painter, 1964; Painter and Burkitt, 1971). This would explain how a high-fibre diet relieves the colic of painful diverticular disease. Painter *et al.* (1972) have suggested that, if a low-fibre diet can so damage the colon that it eventually "ruptures" itself producing diverticula, then it is very unlikely that such a diet would harm the colon (and usually only the sigmoid colon) exclusively. They believe that a low-fibre diet probably adversely affects the rest of the gut and may be responsible for some of the "upper intestinal" symptoms attributed to diverticulosis or to the "irritable bowel syndrome".

Some evidence to support this contention was obtained by Holdstock *et al.* (1969), who investigated nine patients with severe abdominal pain for which no organic cause had been found. In two of these patients the attacks of pain coincided with bouts of raised intraluminal "pressure" measured by balloons, in the small intestine, and in five, lower abdominal colic was associated with similar episodes of exaggerated colonic activity. Pro-Banthine, given in a dosage that paralyses the intestinal muscle, stopped both the generation of pressure and the pain. Their observations show beyond any doubt that the contraction of intestinal muscle can cause abdominal pain in the absence of any structural abnormality.

VIII. Conclusion

The theory that diverticular disease of the colon is a deficiency disease due to a lack of dietary fibre is consistent with what is known of the pathogenesis of colonic diverticula and with the few studies which have been made concerning the effect of diet on the pressures in the human colon. Moreover, the pain and colic once attributed to inflammatory diverticulitis is now known to be caused by abnormal intestinal behaviour which is almost certainly the result of the bowel's having to struggle with contents of an abnormal consistency due to an unnatural diet.

At the time of writing, diverticular disease of the colon has the unique distinction, with the exception of constipation, of being the only common disease whose symptoms have been relieved by the replacement of the cereal fibre that is missing from our modern diet. Consequently there is every reason to believe that the disease, like scurvy, need not occur. It is contended that if we retraced our dietary footsteps and consumed a less refined diet, the prevalence of this disease would be greatly reduced in succeeding generations.

References

ALLEN, A. W. (1953). *American Journal of Surgery* **86**, 545.

ARFWIDDSON, S. (1964). *Acta chirurgica scandinavica* Suppl. No. 342.

BEER, E. (1904). *American Journal of Medical Science* **128**, 135.

BLAND-SUTTON, J. (1903). *Lancet* 1148.

BLAND-SUTTON, J. (1920). *Proceedings of the Royal Society of Medicine, Section of Surgery* **13**, 64.

BREMNER, C. G. and ACKERMAN, L. V. (1970). *Cancer* **26**, 991.

BREWER, G. E. (1907). *American Journal of the Medical Sciences* **134**, 483.

BRISTOWE, J. S. (1854). *Transactions of the Pathological Society of London* **6**, 191.

BROWN, P. W. and MARCLEY, D. M. (1937). *Journal of the American Medical Association* **109**, 1328.

BURKITT, D. P., WALKER, A. R. P. and PAINTER, N. S. (1972). *Lancet* **2**, 1408.

CARLSON, A. J. and HOELZEL, F. (1949). *Gastroenterology* **12**, 108.

CLEAVE, T. L., CAMPBELL, G. D. and PAINTER, N. S. (1969). "Diabetes, Coronary Thrombosis and the Saccharine Disease", 2nd edition. John Wright, Bristol.

CLELAND, J. B. (1968). *British Medical Journal* **1**, 579.

CRIPPS, H. (1888). "The Passage of Air and Faeces from the Bladder", p. 98. Churchill, London.

CRUVEILHIER, J. (1849). "Traité d'Anatomie pathologique générale", Vol. 1, p. 59. Baillière, Paris.

DEBRAY, C., HARDOUIN, J. P., BESANCON, F. and RAIMBAULT, J. (1961). *Semaine des Hôpitaux de Paris* **37**, 1743.

DONALDSON, R. (1907). *British Medical Journal* **2**, 1705.

DRUMMOND, H. (1917). *British Journal of Surgery* **4**, 407.

EDWARDS, H. C. (1934a). *Lancet* 1, 221.
EDWARDS, H. C. (1934b). *British Journal of Surgery* 22, 88.
EDWARDS, H. C. (1939). "Diverticula and Diverticulitis of the Intestine." John Wright, Bristol.
EDWARDS, H. C. (1953). *Postgraduate Medical Journal* 29, 20.
EGGERS, C. (1941). *Annals of Surgery* 113, 15.
ENFIELD, C. D. (1924). *American Journal of Roentgenology* 12, 242.
FIFIELD, L. R. (1927). *Lancet* 1, 277.
GOULSTON, E. (1967). *British Medical Journal* 2, 378.
GRASER, E. (1899). *Münchener medizinische Wochenschrift* 46, 721.
GROSS, S. (1845). "Elements of Pathological Anatomy", p. 554. Blanchard and Lea, Philadelphia.
GROUT, J. L. A. (1949). *British Journal of Radiology* 22, 442.
HABERSCHON, S. O. (1857). "Observations on the Alimentary Canal." Churchill, London.
HARTWELL, J. A. and CECIL, R. L. (1910). *American Journal of the Medical Sciences* 140, 174.
HIGGINSON, J. and SIMSON, I. (1958). *Schweizerisch zeitschrift für Allgemeine Pathologie und Bakteriologie* 21, 577.
HODGSON, J. (1972a). *British Journal of Surgery* 59, 315.
HODGSON, J. (1972b). *British Medical Journal* 3, 729.
HOLDSTOCK, D. J., MISCIEWICZ, J. J. and WALLER, S. (1969). *Gut* 10, 19.
HUGHES, L. E. (1969). *Gut* 10, 336.
JONES, S. (1859). *Transactions of the Pathological Society of London* 10, 131.
KEELEY, K. J. (1958). *Medical Proceedings* 4, 281.
KIM, E. H. (1964). *New England Journal of Medicine* 271, 764.
KLEBS, E. (1869). "Handbuch der pathologischen Anatomie", p. 271. Hirschwald, Berlin.
KOCOUR, E. J. (1937). *American Journal of Surgery* 37, 433.
KYLE, J., ADESOLA, A. O., TINCKLER, L. F. and DE BEAUX, J. (1967). *Scandinavian Journal of Gastroenterology* 2, 77.
LANE, A. (1885). *Guy's Hospital Reports* 43, 48.
LOOMIS, A. L. (1870). *New York Medical Record* 4, 497.
LUNDING, K. (1935). *Acta medica scandinavica* Suppl. No. 72.
MANOUSOS, O. N., TRUELOVE, S. C. and LUMSDEN, K. (1967). *British Medical Journal* 3, 760.
MAYO, W. J. (1930). *Annals of Surgery* 92, 739.
MAYO, W. J., WILSON, L. B. and GIFFIN, H. Z. (1907). *Surgery, Gynecology and Obstetrics* 5, 8.
MORSON, B. C. (1963). *British Journal of Radiology* 36, 385.
MORTON, J. J. (1946). *Annals of Surgery* 124, 725.
MOYNIHAN, B. G. A. (1907). *British Medical Journal* 2, 1381.
OSCHNER, H. C. and BARGEN, J. A. (1935). *Annals of Internal Medicine* 9, 282.
PAINTER, N. S. (1962). M.S. Thesis, University of London.
PAINTER, N. S. (1963). *British Medical Journal* 1, 309.
PAINTER, N. S. (1964). *Annals of the Royal College of Surgeons of England* 34, 98.
PAINTER, N. S. (1971). *British Medical Journal* 2, 156.

PAINTER, N. S. and BURKITT, D. P. (1971). *British Medical Journal* 2, 450.
PAINTER, N. S., ALMEIDA, A. Z. and COLEBOURNE, K. W. (1972). *British Medical Journal* 2, 137.
PAINTER, N. S., TRUELOVE, S. C., ARDRAN, G. M. and TUCKEY, M. (1965). *Gastroenterology* 49, 165.
PARKS, T. G. (1968). *Proceedings of the Royal Society of Medicine* 61, 932.
POWER, D'ARCY (1906). *British Medical Journal* 2, 1171.
RANKIN, F. W. and BROWN, P. W. (1930). *Surgery, Gynecology and Obstetrics* 50, 836.
ROBERTS, L. J. (1908). *British Medical Journal* 1, 1174.
ROKITANSKY, C. (1849). "A Manual of Pathological Anatomy", Vol. 2, p. 48. The Sydenham Society, London.
SATO, T., MATSUZAKI, S., FUJIWARA, Y., TAKAHASHI, J. and SUGURO, T. (1970). *Naika* 25, 563.
SLESINGER, E. G. (1930). *Lancet* 1, 1325.
SMITH, A. N., ATTISHA, R. P. and BALFOUR, T. (1969). *British Journal of Surgery* 56, 895.
SMITH, A. N., GIANNAKOS, V. and CLARKE, S. (1971). *Journal of the Royal College of Surgeons of Edinburgh* 16, 276.
SMITH, C. C. and CHRISTENSEN, W. R. (1959). *American Journal of Roentgenology* 82, 996.
SPRIGGS, E. I. (1920). *Proceedings of the Royal Society of Medicine, Section of Surgery* 13, 65.
SPRIGGS, E. I. and MARXER, O. A. (1925). *Quarterly Journal of Medicine* 19, 1.
SPRIGGS, E. I. and MARXER, O. A. (1927). *Lancet* 1, 1067.
TAYLOR, G. and LAKIN, C. E. (1910). *Lancet* 1, 495.
TELLING, W. H. M. (1908). *Lancet* 1, 843.
TELLING, W. H. M. (1920). *Proceedings of the Royal Society of Medicine, Section of Surgery* 13, 5.
TELLING, W. H. M. and GRUNER, O. C. (1917). *British Journal of Surgery* 4, 468.
TROWELL, H. C. (1960). "Non-infective Disease in Africa", p. 218. Edward Arnold, London.
TROWELL, H. C., PAINTER, N. S. and BURKITT, D.P. (1974). *American Journal of Digestive Diseases* 19, 864.
VIRCHOW, R. (1853). *Virchows Archiv für pathologische Anatomie und Physiologie und für klinische Medizin* 5, 335.
WALKER, A. R. P., WALKER, B. F. and RICHARDSON, B. D. (1970). *British Medical Journal* 3, 48.
WAPNICK, S. and LEVIN, L. (1971). *British Medical Journal* 4, 115.
WELCH, C. E., ALLEN, A. W. and DONALDSON, G. A. (1953). *Annals of Surgery* 138, 33.
WELLS, C. (1949). *British Journal of Radiology* 22, 449.
WILLARD, J. H. and BOCKUS, H. (1936) *American Journal of Digestive Diseases and Nutrition* 3, 580.

Chapter 10

Benign and malignant tumours of large bowel

DENIS BURKITT

I. Anatomical classification 119
II. Geographical distribution 119
    A. Cancer 119
    B. Adenomatous polyps 122
III. Emergence in western countries 123
IV. Influence of urbanization and western civilization 123
    A. Urbanization 123
    B. Western civilization 124
V. Rising incidence following emigration 125
VI. Dietetic factors 125
    A. Changes in food 126
    B. Faecal bacterial flora 126
    C. Postulated roles of dietary fibre and fat 129
    D. Factors altering incidence 129
    E. Possible significance of the anatomic distribution . . . 130
References 131

The association between benign and malignant tumours of the large bowel is so close that they might be considered as but different effects of common causes (Oettle, 1967; Morson and Bussey, 1970; Burkitt, 1971). The anatomical (Fig. 10.1), geographical and age distribution are almost identical for both conditions. Moreover, they tend to occur together in the same patients (Figs 10.2 and 10.3) (Rider *et al.*, 1954, 1959; Bockus *et al.*, 1961; Burkitt, 1971) and can both be induced experimentally by the same means (Spjut and Spratt, 1965; Cleveland *et al.*, 1967; Navarrete and Spjut, 1967). Rider *et al.* (1954) concluded that the relationship between cancer and polyps in the same patient suggests that the whole mucosal surface has an increased tendency to develop both benign and malignant neoplasms. Cancer and adenomatous polyps will therefore be discussed together in considering their epidemiological aspects and possible causative factors.

Hyperplastic polyps have been excluded.

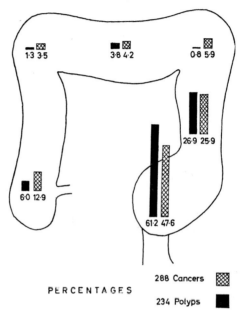

FIG. 10.1. Distribution of adenomatous polyps and cancer in the large bowel.

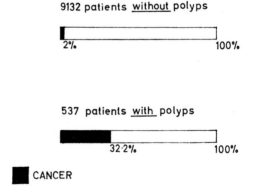

FIG. 10.2. Showing that the presence of polyps increases the likelihood of coexisting cancer.

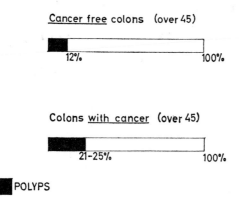

FIG. 10.3. Showing that the presence of cancer increased the likelihood of coexisting polyps.

I. Anatomical classification

From an epidemiological standpoint tumours of the colon and rectum should be considered together. Both have their maximum and minimum frequencies in the same communities. The variations between the relative proportions of colonic and rectal tumours in different communities are small compared to the very great variations in frequency of cancer of the large bowel, as a whole, in different parts of the world. Colon/rectum ratios seldom vary more than 3-fold, whereas the age-adjusted incidence of large bowel cancer varies 15-fold (Fig. 10.4), which strongly suggests major environmental factors common to tumours of the whole of the large bowel. Additional local aetiological factors must, however, operate in varying degrees to account for the different colon/rectum ratios in communities.

A further reason for considering tumours of the colon and rectum together is that tumours are frequently found at or near the pelvi-rectal junction, making classification by bowel segment difficult.

II. Geographical distribution

A. Cancer

No other form of cancer is so closely related to economic development and modern western civilization as cancer of the colon and rectum (Higginson, 1967; Burkitt, 1971). In North America and many countries in Europe, it is responsible for more deaths than any other form of cancer, with the exception of bronchial carcinoma (Doll, 1969; Doll *et al.*, 1966). In the United States alone over 70,000 new cases are reported annually and some two-thirds of these prove fatal (Silverberg and Holleb, 1972). In Britain the Registrar-General's figure for deaths from cancer of the colon and rectum for 1962 was 14,543.

In striking contrast these tumours are rare in developing countries, especially in rural communities.

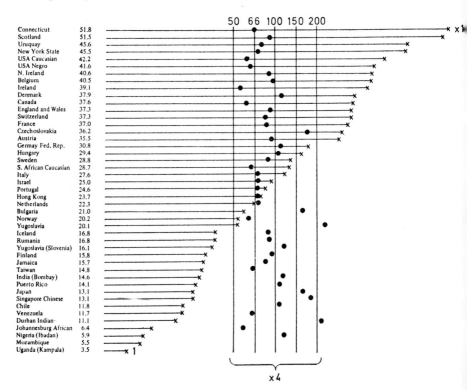

FIG. 10.4. Age-standardized rates for cancer of the colon and rectum in men 35–64 years of age arranged in order of incidence (modified from Doll, 1969). The variations in the ratio of rectal/colon tumours are shown by black dots on the same scale. 100 = parity. (Reprinted from "Modern Trends in Oncology". Butterworth, London, 1973.)

Information available from cancer registries indicates that as areas become more westernized and industrialized, so incidence rates increasingly rise. The rates for cancer of the colon and rectum in men per 100,000, standardized for 35–64 years of age (Doll, 1969), arranged in order of incidence, clearly indicate the relationship to economic development (Fig. 10.4). Kampala (Uganda), which serves a largely rural community in Africa, is at the bottom of the list.

For most of Africa incidence rates are not available but the general rarity of large bowel cancer can be judged from its ratio to the total cancer cases recorded. Information collected from reports published in some African countries is summarized in Table 10.1. Figures from 57 rural hospitals,

TABLE 10.1. Proportion of cancer of the colon and rectum to total cancer in different parts in Africa. (From "Modern Trends in Oncology". Butterworth, London, 1973.)

	Reported series		Percentage of total cancer of colon and rectum	Reference
	Period	Total series		
Johannesburg (S. Africa)	1952–54	1076	2·6	Robertson (1969)
Johannesburg (S. Africa)	1962–64	2407	2·4	Robertson (1969)
Durban (S. Africa)	1964–66	1040	2·1	Schonland and Bradshaw (1968)
Lourenço Marques (Mozambique)	1956–60	603	1·3	Prates and Torres (1965)
Sudan	1954–61	2234	2·8	Lynch et al. (1963)
Accra (Ghana)	1942–55	1192	1·8	Edington (1956)
Kampala (Uganda)	1954–60	615	2·8	Davies et al. (1965)
Nairobi (Kenya)	1957–63	4206	2·5	Linsell (1967)
Dakar (Senegal)	1955–64	1838	2·5	Camain and Lambert (1964)
Salisbury (Rhodesia)	1963–65	1415	1·6	Skinner (1967)
Ilesha (Nigeria)	1954–67	465	5·8	Mulligan (1969)
Stanleyville (Congo Kinshasa)	1939–55	2536	1·1	Thijs (1957)

M.R.C. survey of up-country hospitals

	Hospitals			
Kenya	5	934	1·5	
Uganda	7	613	2·1	
Tanzania	23	1743	2·3	
Malawi	22	827	1·7	

from which regular reports of all cases of cancer have been received, are given for comparison.

Doll and his colleagues (1970) emphasized the importance of environmental rather than genetic factors in their observation that in Israel the incidence of cancer of the colon and rectum is considerably higher in immigrants from Europe than in those born in Asia or Africa. The difference between the two groups is much more marked for bowel tumours than for other forms of cancer.

Four other small series from Uganda (Buckley, 1967), Tanzania (Eshleman, 1966), Acornhoek, South Africa (Sutherland, 1968) and Lambarene, Gabon (Denues and Munz, 1967) each with a total of less than 300 cases, reported relative frequencies of large bowel cancer varying from 0·2% to 4·4% of the total.

The most remarkable feature is that in all the larger series, with the sole exception of Ilesha, Nigeria, where 5·8% of over 400 cancers were in the colon or rectum (Mulligan, 1969), there is in sub-Saharal Africa a uniform and low figure of about 2%. This corresponds to the lowest figure given in the list in Fig. 10.4 and would appear to represent a basic minimum rate of cancer of the large bowel in the absence of those environmental factors which probably increase with industrialization. Templeton (1973) suggested that colon cancer relative to total cancer might be inadequately recorded in areas distant from major centres.

Although small bowel tumours are rare, there is a close correlation throughout the world between the incidence of cancer of the large and small bowel, which suggests some causative factor common to each (Lowenfels, 1973).

B. Adenomatous polyps

Since benign tumours of the large bowel are not recorded in cancer registries, information on their geographical distribution is less easily obtainable than that of malignant tumours. There is, however, ample evidence that adenomatous polyps are very common in the western world and virtually unknown in developing countries. In Europe and North America the incidence rises markedly with age, and in 1000 autopsy examinations Arminski and McLean (1964) gave an incidence as high as 25% in all patients over the age of 20 years. Spjut and Spratt (1965) considered that adenomatous polyps are "almost ubiquitous in older Americans". Spiro (1970) stated that if the bowel mucosa is examined with a magnifying glass small polyps can be found in nearly 70% of autopsies.

In contrast, polyps are so rare in Africa that Bremner and Ackerman (1970) found only six in a review of surgical specimens received over a 12-year period in a 2000-bed hospital for Bantu patients in South Africa. In a series of 14,000 autopsies at the same hospital no polyps were found, although the bowel was opened and inspected in each case. Parker and Skinner (quoted by Bremner and Ackerman, 1970) found no polyps in over 13,000 autopsies in Rhodesia. During a 5 year period in Kampala, Uganda, Templeton (1973) found only one adenomatous polyp of the large bowel in over 40,000 surgical specimens from Africans. Six were found in operation and post mortem specimens and two of these were from patients educated in England who had adopted a "rather western way of life". In a further two cases carcinoma had developed in colons bearing multiple polyps. No adenomas were found in the colon in 2000 autopsies performed on adults during this 5 year period. A particularly careful search was made for polyps in a series of 343 autopsies performed by Templeton in patients over 25 years, but none was found.

In 1960 Trowell stated that there was no known report of this condition in an African.

In Shiraz, Iran, P. Haghighi (p.c., 1972) found only eight polyps in 370 autopsies.

In Japan, S. Yamagata and T. Takebe (p.c., 1972) found 294 cases with large bowel polyps in over 81,000 autopsies, giving a frequency of 0·36%, which, like the colon cancer incidence in Japan, is a figure intermediate between those of African countries and those of North America.

V. Ramalingaswami (p.c., 1973), Director of the All-India Institute of Medical Sciences, has commented on the great rarity of adenomatous polyps of the large bowel in India.

Both polyps and cancer of the large bowel are rare in rural communities in Peru, and at autopsy more cancers than polyps are seen (J. Berrios, p.c. 1974).

Experience of Brazil is similar. H. Miziara (p.c., 1974) sees only one or two polyps a year in over 1000 autopsies in Brasilia.

III. Emergence in western countries

Unlike appendicitis and diverticular disease there is no available evidence concerning the date at which bowel cancer became common in the western world. Experience in other countries and in American negroes would suggest that the appearance of colonic cancer as a common disease may have been a relatively recent phenomenon probably preceding the emergence of diverticular disease as an important clinical problem.

IV. Influence of urbanization and western civilization

A. Urbanization

Large bowel cancer has, in several countries, been shown to be consistently more prevalent in urban than in rural communities, as has been demonstrated in Norway, Sweden, Finland and Denmark (Ringertz, 1967;

Fig. 10.5) and in Poland, figures for which are given below for 1965–66, in city and urban groups, all ages (Doll *et al.*, 1970) (Table 10.2):

TABLE 10.2. Incidence of large bowel cancer in Poland.

	Warsaw city	Four rural areas
MEN		
Colon	6·2	2·7
Rectum	5·5	3·1
WOMEN		
Colon	10·2	3·6
Rectum	5·6	3·6

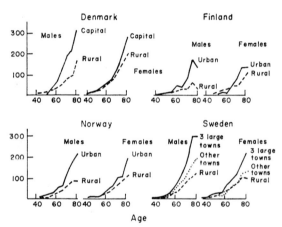

FIG. 10.5. A comparison of the incidence of large bowel cancer in rural and urban communities (adapted from Ringertz, 1967).

In the United States the highest incidence is in the more industrialized areas (Haenszel and Dawson, 1965).

In Japan the incidence of colonic and rectal cancer is steadily increasing and is commoner in upper-income groups (Wynder and Shigematsu, 1967).

B. *Western civilization*

Formerly cancer of the large bowel was considerably less frequent in negroes than in whites in the United States (Quinland and Cuff, 1940; Steiner, 1954) and intestinal polyps were also much less common in negroes (Helwig, 1947). However, as they have increasingly adopted the white man's way of life this disparity has, in respect of colon cancer, totally disappeared (Doll *et al.*, 1966). From discussions with many

American gastroenterologists it is clear that there is now no great disparity between the prevalence of adenomatous polyps in the white and the black communities.

In 1924 Dolbey and Mooro reported 671 cases of all forms of cancer from Egypt, wherein they found it to be "very rare" in the colon and only seven cases in the rectum, suggesting that these tumours accounted for a low proportion of total cancer. In 1967 Nasr gave a figure of nearly 6%.

American influence has rapidly been changing the way of life in Puerto Rico. The proportion of cancer represented by tumours of the lung and large bowel, both of which are universally associated with western civilization, has been steadily increasing (Martinez, 1968).

V. Rising incidence following emigration

Cancer of the large bowel has been notably uncommon in Japan (Doll et al., 1966) but, as mentioned previously, the incidence has been rising, particularly in urban areas. In second generation immigrants to California and Hawaii the incidence has now almost reached that of their Caucasian compatriots (Wynder and Shigematsu, 1967; Stemmermann, 1970). Adenomatous polyps are three times more common in Japanese living in Hawaii than in those living in Japan (G. N. Stemmermann, p.c. 1972).

VI. Dietetic factors

The epidemiological features previously mentioned indicate that these tumours are dependent almost exclusively on environmental rather than on genetic influences.

The fact that multiple primary tumours are found more commonly in the large bowel mucosa than in any other organ or structure, except the skin, suggests some environmental factor affecting the large bowel mucosa as a whole (Moertel et al., 1961). The faecal content, the nature of which is determined mainly by the food and fluid ingested, is the most important factor influencing the environment of the colonic and rectal mucosa. The part played by direct contact between the faecal stream and the mucosal lining of the bowel is illustrated by the fact that whenever neoplasms have been induced experimentally these tumours do not appear in bowel loops detached from the faecal stream (Spjut and Spratt, 1965). The rarity of bowel cancer in communities whose traditional way of life has changed little, and also in wild animals, suggests that the customary diet to which man or animal has been for long adapted is not highly carcinogenic.

The total mucosal surface of the small intestine has been estimated to be over 100 times that of the large bowel. Epithelial tumours are over 100 times more prevalent in the large bowel than in the small bowel.

Relative to surface area, therefore, tumours are more than 10,000 times more likely to develop in the large than in the small bowel mucosa. This might be explained either by differences in susceptibility to certain carcinogenic agents exhibited by the large and small bowel mucosa, which has some experimental support, or by the formation or activation of the responsible carcinogens within the large bowel. Carcinogens ingested in an active form might be expected more often to induce tumours in the enormous area of small bowel mucosa.

A. Changes in food

From the evidence presented previously it seems probable that an increased incidence of bowel tumours is most likely to be caused by changes of diet. The particular change responsible must be that which several decades ago preceded their rise in incidence in the western world, and more recently preceded an increase in developing countries. Any dietary change that has also been associated with an increasing prevalence of other diseases of the large bowel which are epidemiologically associated with bowel cancer must be particularly suspect.

As outlined above, the major dietary changes preceding the increased incidence of other non-infective bowel diseases have been a reduction in the content of the fibre, and particularly of cereal fibre, in the diet and an increase in fat, protein, refined starchy food and sugar consumption. In this connection it is significant that when the diet of American negroes had a higher cereal fibre content and less fat and protein than that of white Americans the incidence of both benign and malignant bowel tumours was much lower in the former than in the latter, whereas today, when the diet of the black community is very similar to that of the white community, the incidence of bowel cancer and polyps is closely comparable in the two ethnic groups. It has already been shown that changes in dietary fibre have profound effects on the behaviour of the bowel and on the nature of the stools and that all dietary factors probably affect the nature of faecal bacteria.

Seventh Day Adventists, who are vegetarians, and usually consume more fibre than non-vegetarians, have a lower risk of developing bowel cancer (Wynder and Shigematsu, 1967).

From all the evidence a possible relationship between bowel tumours and dietary fibre is suggested and must therefore be further considered.

B. Faecal bacterial flora

It appears likely that faecal bacteria play an important role in the causation of bowel tumours. Rats kept in a sterile environment developed no bowel tumours after being given chemicals which had induced tumours in animals living normally (Cole, quoted by Wynder *et al.*, 1969). Lagueur (1964) reported that oral cycasin produced bowel tumours in normal but not in germ-free animals. The faeces of the latter lacked the enzyme which splits the cycasin meal to produce the carcinogen.

Consistent with this is the evidence presented by Aries *et al.* (1969), Hill and Aries (1971), Hill *et al.* (1971), and Drasar and Hill (1972), which suggests that differing incidence rates of cancer of the colon and rectum in different countries may be related to the concentration of carcinogens in the faeces deriving possibly from bacterial action on bile acids in the large bowel. The bacterial flora of stools from three areas where bowel cancer is low—Uganda, South India and Japan—was compared with that of stools from three high-risk areas—England, Scotland and the U.S.A. (Table 10.3). It was found that the stools of Britons and Americans contained more Gram-negative non-sporing anaerobes, and in particular more bacteroides, whereas those from people in countries with a low cancer incidence contained more aerobic bacteria (*Enterococci* and *Enterobacteria*). Faecal bacteria were found to be essentially the same in white and coloured Americans, and British residents in Uganda had the same bacterial pattern as that found in the United Kingdom.

In the light of this evidence several workers suggested that the increased fat content of western diets might be responsible for an increase in faecal carcinogens. They pointed out that stools from high-risk countries had a greater concentration of steroids and bile acids than that found in stools from low-risk areas (Table 10.3) and that the bacteria which predominated in the western stools had the property of degrading bile acids to deoxycholic acid, a potential carcinogen.

These observations suggested that diet rather than race or climate was the determining factor.

Table 10.3 records the incidence of cancer of the colon and rectum (Doll, 1969), the faecal bacterial flora, steroid metabolism, the fat and the animal protein of the average diet (Drasar and Hill, 1972), together with estimates of the crude fibre consumption in England and Wales (Robertson, 1972), the U.S.A. (Tecumseh heart study, J. R. K. Robson, p.c. 1974) and Uganda (H. Trowell, p.c. 1974). Kampala Africans eat liberal amounts of unprocessed carbohydrate foods: beans, groundnuts and plantains. Plantains contain much more hemicellulose than would be suggested from their low crude fibre content (Southgate, 1969). No reliable data has been obtained concerning the crude fibre content of the average national diet of Japan or South India.

The evidence that the additional fat in western diets alters both the bacteria and the substrate requires confirmation. Such changes could enhance carcinogen formation. The observation that cholestyramine, which increases the amount of bile acids reaching the colon, can raise the incidence of experimentally induced bowel cancer (Nigro et al., 1973) is consistent with this hypothesis, likewise the fact that removal of fat from the diet results in a fall in the faecal concentration of bile acids.

TABLE 10.3. Incidence of cancer of the colon and rectum, bacterial flora, steroid metabolism and diet in six countries

	U.S.A.	Scotland	England	Japan	South India	Uga
Cancer of colon and rectum/100,000 population	41·6	51·5	38·1	13·1	14	
Selected bacteria (log 10/g faeces)						
Bacteriodes	9·8	9·8	9·8	9·4	9·2	
Streptococci	5·9	5·3	5·8	8·1	7·3	
Faecal steroids (mg/g dry weight)						
Neutral steroids	10·7	10·1	10·8	4·5	1·5	
% degraded	64	77	69	43	62	5!
Acid steroids	6·0	6·2	6·2	0·9	0·5	
% degraded	46	49	51	13	21	3:
Diet (g/person/day) assessment only						
Fat	96	—	76	32	15	1(
Animal protein	68	—	54	28	5	1(
Crude fibre	3–4	—	4·2	?	?	8–1

Constructed from data of incidence of cancer of colon and rectum (Doll, 1969), faecal bacterial flora and steroids, also estimates of the fat and protein of the average diet (Drasar and Hill, 1972); together with estimates of the crude fibre content of the diet in England (Robertson, 1972), U.S.A. (Tecumseh heart study, J. R. K. Robson, p.c. 1974) and Uganda (H. Trowell, p.c. 1974).

Lacassagne et al. (1961) demonstrated that apocholic acid, a product of the mild degradation of cholic acid (one of the two main bile acids), could be carcinogenic, and later (1966) they reported the sarcomagenic property of a product of the degradation of bile acids.

Low-Beer (1974) has drawn attention to the fact that although the liver, biliary tree and small intestine are daily in contact with deoxycholate in quantities and concentrations far greater than in the colon, cancer in these structures is much less common than in the colon. This does not suggest that deoxycholate is a primary factor in large bowel cancer. It might well be, however, that it serves as an index to bacterial activity in the colon and that some other product of bacterial activity may be the carcinogenic agent.

C. *Postulated roles of dietary fibre and fat*

Diets in western countries, where there is a high incidence of large bowel cancer, contain less fibre and more fat than do diets in communities with a low cancer incidence. An increased fat content is associated with a higher proportion of bacteria capable of degrading bile acids. A diminished fibre content leads to concentrated faeces and prolongation of intestinal transit time (Chapter 7). The possible relative roles of these two factors must be considered, for it has frequently been suggested that faecal stasis may enhance tumour formation by concentrating carcinogens and by ensuring their prolonged contact with the bowel mucosa (Oettle, 1967; Wynder and Shigematsu, 1967; Edington and Gilles, 1969; Burkitt, 1971).

D. *Factors altering incidence*

It has been postulated that a number of interacting factors may alter the incidence of large bowel cancer. These include:

1. The amount of carcinogen formed, which, if not an exogenous carcinogen, might depend on:

(a) Bacteria
   (i) Variety: this will depend on the quality of available nutrients, mineral salts and pH.
   (ii) Number: this will depend on the quantity and quality of nutrients and on the time available. This has been shown to relate to dietary fibre.

(b) Bile Acids
   (i) Metabolism. Pomare and Heaton (1973) showed that feeding with cereal fibre in the form of bran reduced dehydroxylation of bile salts.
   (ii) Time. The time available for bacterial degradation of bile acids will depend on the extent of faecal stasis.

2. The retention of carcinogen in the large bowel, which will be influenced by

   (a) Prolonged transit times
   (b) Frequency of bowel evacuation
   (c) Inhibitions against immediate evacuation when the desire is felt.

3. Concentration of carcinogens.

Celluloses and hemicelluloses have a bulk-forming property partly due to
their ability to retain water. In addition there is, with more rapidly
progressing faeces, less time for water absorption by the colon.

E. Possible significance of the anatomic distribution

Epithelial tumours are very rare in the small bowel in spite of the fact
that the area of its mucosal surface greatly exceeds that of the colon and
rectum. This suggests that in spite of the more rapid small bowel transit
times the carcinogenic agents responsible for large bowel tumours are not
ingested, at least in an active form, but are produced, concentrated or
activated, or their effects otherwise enhanced in the lumen of the colon.

The carcinogenic potential might be expected to be greater in the distal
colon since more bile acid degradation will probably have taken place by
the time the faeces reach this region. Moreover, there will be increased
concentration of potential carcinogens through water absorption as the
faeces proceed through the large bowel. The higher incidence in the caecum
and ascending colon relative to the transverse colon and splenic flexure
calls for explanation, as does the varying ratio between tumours of the
rectum and pelvic colon in different communities.

In African countries the apparently high incidence of tumours in the
ascending colon is no longer believed to be a true picture but merely
reflects the rarity of tumours of the distal colon. Likewise cancer of the
male breast was once thought to be unduly common among Africans, but
this merely reflected the rarity of tumours in the female breast.

Recent studies (K. Heaton, p.c. 1972; A. Connell, p.c. 1972) suggest
that the faecal stream is much more delayed in the ascending and the
pelvic portions than in the transverse portion of the colon, and this may
well relate to tumour distribution. One of the factors responsible for the
accumulation of faeces in the first and last stages of the colon may be
gravity, which, in the erect position, would tend to localize the faeces in
these more dependent sites. Halls (1965) has shown that the previously held
conception that the rectum is normally empty is no longer tenable; the
rectal mucosa is apparently in contact with contained faeces for much
longer periods than had previously been believed.

An additional factor predisposing to the retention of faeces in more
westernized communities is the social custom that requires the suppression
of the desire to defaecate when it is experienced at inconvenient times.

Rose et al. (1974) have shown a correlation between deaths due to
ischaemic heart disease and cancer of the colon in different countries
(Fig. 10.6) which is consistent with the hypothesis set forward in this book

that a deficiency of dietary fibre might be an aetiological factor common to both diseases.

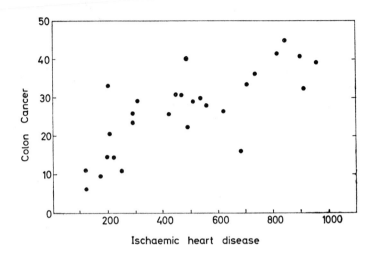

(Rose et al. 1974, Lancet)

FIG. 10.6. Deaths per 100,000 for ischaemic heart disease and colon cancer in different countries (from Rose *et al.*, 1974).

References

ARIES, V., CROWTHER, J. S., DRASAR, B. S., HILL, M. J. and WILLIAMS, R. E. O. (1969). *Gut* **10**, 334.

ARMINSKI, T. C. and McLEAN, D. W. (1964). *Diseases of the Colon and Rectum* **7**, 249.

BOCKUS, H. L., TACHDJIAN, V., FERGUSON, L. K., MOUHRAN, Y. and CHAMBERLAIN, C. (1961). *Gastroenterology* **41**, 225.

BREMNER, C. G. and ACKERMAN, L. V. (1970). *Cancer* **26**, 991.

BUCKLEY, R. M. (1967). *East African Medical Journal* **44**, 465.

BURKITT, D. P. (1971). *Cancer* **28**, 3.

CAMAIN, R. and LAMBERT, D. (1964). *In* "The Lymphoreticular Tumours in Africa". A symposium organised by UICC, pp. 42–53. Karger, Basel.

CLEVELAND, J. C., LITVAK, S. F. and COLE, J. W. (1967). *Cancer Research* **27**, 708.

DAVIES, J. N. P., KNOWELDEN, J. and WILSON, B. A. (1965). *Journal of the National Cancer Institute* **35**, 789.

DENUES, A. R. T. and MUNZ, W. (1967). *International Journal of Cancer* **2**, 1.

DOLBEY, R. V. and MOORO, A. W. (1924). *Lancet* **1**, 587.

DOLL, R. (1969). *British Journal of Cancer* **23**, 1.

DOLL, R., PAYNE, P. and WATERHOUSE, J. (eds) (1966). "Cancer Incidence in Five Continents", Vol. I. U.I.C.C. Springer-Verlag, Berlin, Heidelberg and New York.

DOLL, R., MUIR, C. and WATERHOUSE, J. (eds) (1970). "Cancer Incidence in Five Continents", Vol. II. U.I.C.C. Springer-Verlag, Berlin, Heidelberg and New York.

DRASAR, B. S. and HILL, M. J. (1972). *American Journal of Clinical Nutrition* **25**, 1399.

EDINGTON, G. M. (1956). *British Journal of Cancer* **10**, 595.

EDINGTON, G. M. and GILLES, H. M. (1969). "Pathology in the Tropics." Edward Arnold, London.

ESHLEMAN, J. L. (1966). *East African Medical Journal* **43**, 273.

HAENSZEL, W. and DAWSON, E. A. (1965). *Cancer* **18**, 265.

HALLS, J. (1965). *Proceedings of the Royal Society of Medicine* **58**, 859.

HELWIG, E. B. (1947). *Surgery, Gynecology and Obstetrics* **84**, 36.

HIGGINSON, J. (1967). *In* "Tumors of the Alimentary Tract in Africans", p. 191. National Cancer Institute Monograph 25, Bethesda.

HILL, M. J. and ARIES, V. C. (1971). *Journal of Pathology* **104**, 129.

HILL, M. J., CROWTHER, J. S., DRASAR, B. S., HAWKSWORTH, G., ARIES, V. and WILLIAMS, R. E. O. (1971). *Lancet* **1**, 95.

LACASSAGNE, A., BUU-HOÏ, N. P. and ZAJDELA, F. (1961). *Nature* **190**, 1007.

LACASSAGNE, A., BUU-HOÏ, N. P. and ZAJDELA, F. (1966). *Nature* **209**, 1026.

LAGUEUR, G. L. (1964). *Federation Proceedings* **23**, 1386.

LINSELL, C. A. (1967). *British Journal of Cancer* **21**, 465.

LOW-BEER, T. S. (1974). *British Medical Journal* **2**, 119.

LOWENFELS, A. B. (1973). *Lancet* **1**, 24.

LYNCH, J. B., HASSAN, A. M. and OMAR, A. (1963). *Sudan Medical Journal* **2**, 29.

MARTINEZ, I. (1968). "Cancer in Puerto Rico." Report from the Central Cancer Registry, Department of Health, Puerto Rico.

MOERTEL, C. G., DOCKERTY, M. B. and BAGGENSTOSS, A. H. (1961). *Cancer* **14**, 238.

MORSON, B. C. and BUSSEY, H. J. R. (1970). "Current Problems in Surgery." Year Book Medical Publishers, Chicago.

MULLIGAN, T. O. (1969). *British Journal of Cancer* **24**, 1.

NASR, A. L. A. (1967). *In* "Tumors of the Alimentary Tract in Africans", p. 1. National Cancer Institute Monograph 25, Bethesda.

NAVARRETE, A. and SPJUT, H. J. (1967). *Cancer* **20**, 1466.

NIGRO, N. D. BHADRACHARI, N. and CHOMCHAI, C. (1973). *Diseases of the Colon and Rectum* **16**, 438.

OETTLE, A. G. (1967). *In* "Tumors of the Alimentary Tract in Africans", p. 97. National Cancer Institute Monograph 25, Bethesda.

POMARE, E. W. and HEATON, K. W. (1973). *British Medical Journal* **4**, 262.

PRATES, M. D. and TORRES, F. O. (1965). *Journal of the National Cancer Institute* **35**, 729.

QUINLAND, W. S. and CUFF, J. R. (1940). *Archives of Pathology* **30**, 393.

REGISTRAR-GENERAL (1962). Statistical Review of England and Wales. Tables Medical. Her Majesty's Stationery Office, London.

RIDER, J. A., KIRSNER, J. B., MOELLER, H. C. and PALMER, W. L. (1954). *American Journal of Medicine* **16**, 555.

RIDER, J. A., KIRSNER, J. B., MOELLER, H. C. and PALMER, W. L. (1959). *Journal of the American Medical Association* **170**, 633.

RINGERTZ, N. (1967). *In* "Tumors of the Alimentary Tract in Africans", p. 219. National Cancer Institute Monograph 25, Bethesda.

ROBERTSON, J. (1972). *Nature* **238**, 290.

ROBERTSON, M. A. (1969). *South African Medical Journal* **43**, 915.

ROSE, G., BLACKBURN, H., KEYS, A., TAYLOR, H. L., KANNEL, W. B., PAUL, O., REID, D. D. and STAMLER, J. (1974). *Lancet* **1**, 181.

SCHONLAND, M. and BRADSHAW, E. (1968). *International Journal of Cancer* **3**, 304.

SILVERBERG, E. and HOLLEB, A. I. (1972). *Ca—A Cancer Journal for Clinicians* **22**, 2.

SKINNER, M. E. G. (1967). *In* "Tumors of the Alimentary Tract in Africans", pp. 57–71. National Cancer Institute Monograph 25, Bethesda.

SOUTHGATE, D. A. T. (1969). *Journal of the Science of Food and Agriculture* **20**, 331.

SPIRO, H. M. (1970). "Clinical Gastroenterology." Macmillan, London.

SPJUT, H. J. and SPRATT, J. S., Jr. (1965). *Annals of Surgery* **161**, 309.

STEINER, P. E. (1954). "Cancer: Race and Geography." The Williams and Wilkins Company, Baltimore.

STEMMERMANN, G. N. (1970). *Archives of Environmental Health* **20**, 266.

SUTHERLAND, J. C. (1968). *Cancer* **22**, 372.

TEMPLETON, A. C. (1973) (editor). "Tumors in a Tropical Country." Heinemann Medical Books, London.

THIJS, A. (1957). *Annales de la Société belge de médecine tropicale* **37**, 483.

TROWELL, H. C. (1960). "Non-infective Disease in Africa", p. 219. Edward Arnold, London.

WYNDER, E. L. and SHIGEMATSU, T. (1967). *Cancer* **20**, 1520.

WYNDER, E. L., KAJITANI, T., ISHIKAWA, S., DODO, H. and TAKANO, A. (1969). *Cancer* **23**, 1210.

Chapter 11

Ulcerative colitis and Crohn's disease

HUGH TROWELL

I. Ulcerative colitis 135
  A. Geographical distribution 135
  B. Experimental studies 138
  C. Association with bowel cancer. 138
II. Crohn's disease 138
References 139

I. Ulcerative colitis

In Britain no clear description of ulcerative colitis was made before 1859. There were few reports of this condition in the last century or indeed until the 1920s (*Proceedings of the Royal Society of Medicine*, 1909). In 1932 Crohn's disease was separated as a clinical entity.

A. Geographical distribution

Like many other non-infective diseases of the bowel, ulcerative colitis has its highest prevalence in the advanced countries of north-west Europe, North America, New Zealand and Australia. Prevalence rates appear to vary considerably even in advanced countries. It is less prevalent in southern and eastern Europe, and in Japan (Goligher *et al.*, 1968). In England prevalence has been assessed at roughly 80/100,000 population and incidence at approximately 6·5/100,000 per year. These figures were suggested by a careful survey of the Oxford area by Evans and Acheson (1965) and were the highest prevalence rates obtained in a planned prospective survey in any country.

It is not proposed to discuss the prevalence of ulcerative colitis in North America, except to note that incidence among U.S. whites is comparable

135

to that in Britain. At one time the disease was very uncommon in U.S. negroes (Bacon, 1958), but it is now encountered more frequently (Goligher *et al.*, 1968).

In complete contrast the disease is rare among the indigenous inhabitants of all developing countries from which data has been obtained. Table 11.1, compiled from many areas, shows some interesting details. In Africa the disease among the Africans of tropical Africa and the Bantu of South Africa has only been described in the largest cities, no cases having been reported from rural areas. On the other hand, ulcerative colitis occurs among South African whites, but its prevalence is uncertain. O. A. A. Brock (p.c., 1973) considered it to be fairly common, and D. J. du Plessis and L. M. Wessels (p.c., 1973) believed it was still less common among South African whites than in the United States and Britain. The rarity of ulcerative colitis in rural areas of Turkey, as opposed to its frequency in urban areas in that country, was stressed by Aktan *et al.* (1970) and the same situation has been found in Kuwait (Salem and Shubair, 1967). When the disease occurred in Africans (Billinghurst and Welchman, 1966) and in Indians (Tandon *et al.*, 1965) it often appeared in a mild form, for it appeared to be confined to the rectum and sigmoid colon. In Asia ulcerative colitis is fairly common in Japan (Goligher *et al.*, 1968) but uncommon in India, where reports are restricted to the cities (Tandon *et al.*, 1965; Chuttani *et al.*, 1967). Ulcerative colitis is also rare in New Zealand Maoris (Wigley and MacLaurin, 1962), likewise among Indonesians (Zuidema, 1959). In South America J. Berrios (p.c., 1974) stated that ulcerative colitis was very rare in Lima, Peru; Professor H. Miziara (p.c., 1974) considered that it was rare in Brasilia and A. de Carvalho (p.c., 1974) that it was rare in Recife, Brazil.

In Israel there is considerable difference between the prevalence of ulcerative colitis in the two main ethnic groups. None of the Jews who had lived in the Middle East before emigrating to Israel had ulcerative colitis prior to arrival there; some 18 developed the illness during the 5 years of observation 1952–56. Fourteen of these Jews who had lived in Europe or North America before emigrating to Israel had developed ulcerative colitis prior to arrival. Of the total population of Israel, occidental Jews comprised 60% and accounted for 76% of the total ulcerative colitis hospital admissions, whereas oriental Jews, who comprised 40% of the total population, accounted for only 24% of the ulcerative colitis hospital admissions (Birnbaum *et al.*, 1960). In a study in Baltimore, U.S.A., it was found that Jews had an unduly high prevalence of ulcerative colitis, compared to non-Jews (Monk *et al.*, 1967), as they had in the U.S.A. Army in 1944 (Acheson and Nefzger, 1963).

Contact with city life and with refined carbohydrate foods of a western type coincide with an increase of this disease, and in relating the disease to dietary changes in urban situations Awori *et al.* (1972) specifically mentioned white bread in the African diet, Salem and Shubair (1967) refined carbohydrates in the Arab diet, and Sobel and Schamroth (1970) the influence of a western-type diet on South African Bantu. The occidental Jews who

TABLE 11.1. Prevalence of ulcerative colitis in developing communities

Group	Reference	Date	Comments
AFRICA			
Africans south of Sahara	Trowell	1960	No reported cases
Uganda Africans	Billinghurst and Welchman	1966	First 4 cases at Kampala
Rhodesian Africans	Sealey and Gelfand	1968	First definite case
South African Bantu	Pillay	1964	First 4 cases at Durban
South African Bantu	Sobel and Schamroth	1970	First 2 cases at Johannesburg
Kenya Africans	Awori *et al.*	1972	First 4 cases at Nairobi
Tanzania Africans	Spencer and Nhonoli	1972	First 3 cases at Dar-es-Salaam
MIDDLE EAST			
Bedouin Arabs	Salem and Shubair	1967	First cases, all urban
Israeli groups	Birnbaum *et al.*	1960	Common in occidental Uncommon in oriental
Shiraz, Iran	Goligher *et al.*	1968	Rare disease
Egyptians	Abd-el-Ghaffar and Wahra	1959	Rare disease
Turkey	Aktan *et al.*	1970	Common in urban areas
OTHER AREAS			
Delhi Indians	Tandon *et al.*	1965	28 cases/year, often mild
Delhi Indians	Chuttani *et al.*	1967	Fairly common, mild
Japanese	Goligher *et al.*	1968	Fairly common, increasing
Indonesians	Zuidema	1959	Rare disease
New Zealand Maoris	Wigley and MacLaurin	1962	First 2 cases
North American Indians	Bebchuk *et al.*	1961	First case

had no ulcerative colitis prior to arrival in Israel came from countries where the consumption of bread had been high and it had been baked from fibre-rich coarse flour (Birnbaum *et al.*, 1960).

Many consider that auto-immune factors operate in the pathogenesis of ulcerative colitis; the apparent rarity of many auto-immune diseases in certain communities who consume high-fibre starchy carbohydrate foods is discussed in Chapter 20.

B. Experimental studies

It has not proved possible to identify aetiological factors in man, and more attention should therefore be paid to the carbohydrate intolerance present in ulcerative colitis. Fraser *et al.* (1966) ascertained that liquid stools, containing much lactic acid, were passed if the diet contained lactose (present in milk), sucrose, or flour (presumably white, for its cellulose content was negligible). Elimination of these items of diet produced great improvement in all respects; relapse occurred if these foods were re-introduced. In view of the fact that dietary fibre influences digestion in the small intestine and bacterial flora in the large bowel, its role should be investigated. The disease usually follows an erratic course which makes it difficult to evaluate a clinical trial; prospective controlled trials appear desirable.

C. Association with bowel cancer

The evidence suggesting that dietary factors may play a part in the aetiology of ulcerative colitis is partly derived from the very close relationship between this condition and bowel cancer, both in their geographical distribution and in their association in individual patients.

It is usually assumed that the malignant bowel tumours, which have a much higher incidence in patients with ulcerative colitis, represent neoplastic transformation in the inflammatory process. The possibility that the two conditions are associated because they are a result of a common cause seems a plausible alternative. Other chronic ulcers of the bowel, such as schistosomiasis or amoebiasis, exhibit no tendency to malignant transformation, and in fact no ulcerative process of the small or large intestine or elsewhere is known to undergo commonly malignant transformation.

If there is a causative factor common both to bowel tumours and ulcerative colitis there must be additional aetiological factors peculiar to each condition. The virtual or total absence of ulcerative colitis in all communities with a low incidence of bowel tumours demands explanation.

II. Crohn's disease

It is almost certain that a few cases of Crohn's disease were recorded in Britain towards the end of the last century and early in the present century, even before the disease was clearly described in 1932 in the

United States (Kyle, 1972a). This disease still appears to be usually more rare than ulcerative colitis among Africans throughout Africa south of the Sahara. In the Cape Province of South Africa, 14 cases of Crohn's disease were diagnosed among whites, eight cases among Asians or coloured persons, but not a single patient among the Bantu (Brom *et al.*, 1968). In over half a million admissions to the Baragwanath Hospital, Johannesburg, between 1958 and 1968, only four cases of Crohn's disease were diagnosed, and not a single case of ulcerative colitis (Giraud *et al.*, 1969). Kibaya (1946) described a possible case in Uganda. Many doctors can testify to having seen not a single case in 15–30 years' medical experience in East Africa (Trowell, 1960).

In the United States Crohn's disease was seldom diagnosed in the negro population before the 1950s; thus the Mayo Clinic reported only one case among a series of 600 patients (Van Patter *et al.*, 1954), but the incidence has probably risen in recent years (Ratzloff and Jacobs, 1970). Several reports from the United States would suggest that Jews have a higher incidence of the disease. Among the various Jewish ethnic groups who emigrate to Israel, Crohn's disease is encountered among those coming from North America and Europe, but it is practically unknown among those coming from the Middle East or North Africa (Kyle, 1972b). It is therefore of considerable interest that no case has been diagnosed at Shiraz among Iranians (Kyle, 1972b).

In India, Crohn's disease is encountered in the larger towns, such as Calcutta, but is possibly milder and more amenable to surgical treatment (Gupta *et al.*, 1962). On the other hand the disease has not been diagnosed in Burma or Nepal (Kyle, 1972b).

In Brazil Professor H. Miziara (p.c., 1974) reported only three cases of Crohn's disease in 10 years in a large hospital in Brasilia, and A. de Carvalho (p.c., 1974) considered it was very rare at Recife.

Clearly much more epidemiological data is required, but all available evidence suggests that environmental factors affect the incidence of Crohn's disease, which is very rare in less developed nations, even among those taking a fair amount of sugar, such as the Bantu in Cape Province and in Johannesburg. Crohn's disease appears to follow a pattern already discussed many times in this study and the role of refined starchy carbohydrates should be carefully investigated. Evaluation may be difficult, but it might prove possible to assess the progress of patients taking whole cereal products compared to those taking refined starchy carbohydrates.

References

ABD-EL-GHAFFAR, Y. and WAHRA, M. E. (1959). *Journal of the Egyptian Medical Association* **42**, 509.

ACHESON, F. D. and NEFZGER, M. D. (1963). *Gastroenterology* **44**, 7.

AKTAN, H., PAYKOE, Z. and ENTAN, A. (1970). *Diseases of Colon and Rectum* **13**, 62.

AWORI, N. W., REES, P. H. and ROY, A. D. (1972). *East African Medical Journal* **49**, 604.

BACON, H. E. (1958). "Ulcerative Colitis", p. 8. Lippincott, Philadelphia.

BEBCHUK, W., ROGERS, A. C. and DOWNEY, J. L. (1961). *Gastroenterology* **40**, 138.

BILLINGHURST, J. R. and WELCHMAN, J. M. (1966). *British Medical Journal* **1**, 211.

BIRNBAUM, D., GROEN, J. J. and KALLNER, G. (1960). *Archives of Internal Medicine* **105**, 843.

BROM, B., BANK, S., MARKS, I. N., BARBEZAT, G. O. and RAYNHAM, B. (1968). *South African Medical Journal* **42**, 1099.

CHUTTANI, H. K., NIGAM, S. P., SAMA, S. K., DHANDA, P. C. and GUPTA, P. S. (1967). *British Medical Journal* **4**, 204.

EVANS, J. G. and ACHESON, E. D. (1965). *Gut* **6**, 311.

FRASER, A. C., HOOD, C., MONTGOMERY, R. D., DAVIES, A. G., SCHNEIDER, R., CARTER, P. A. and GOODHART, J. (1966). *Lancet* **1**, 503.

GIRAUD, R. M. A., LUKE, I. and SCHMAMAN, A. (1969). *South African Medical Journal* **43**, 610.

GOLIGHER, J. C., DE DOMBAL, F. T., WATTS, J. McK. and WATKINSON, G. (1968). "Ulcerative Colitis", pp. 1–4, 47–61, 265. Baillière, Tindall and Cassell, London.

GUPTA, R. S., CHATTERJEE, A. K., ROY, R. and GHOSH, B. N. (1962). *Indian Journal of Surgery* **24**, 797.

KIBAYA, A. K. (1946). *East African Medical Journal* **23**, 317.

KYLE, J. (1972). "Crohn's Disease." Heinemann, London. (a) p. 4; (b) pp. 10–11.

MONK, M., MENDELOFF, A. I., SIEGEL, C. I. and LILIENFELD, A. (1967). *Gastroenterology* **53**, 198.

PILLAY, V. K. G. (1964). *British Medical Journal* **2**, 689.

Proceedings of the Royal Society of Medicine (1909) **2**, ii, Medical Section, 100.

RATZLOFF, N. and JACOBS, W. H. (1970). *American Journal of Gastroenterology* **53**, 252.

SALEM, S. N. and SHUBAIR, K. S. (1967). *Lancet* **1**, 473.

SEALEY, B. J. and GELFAND, M. (1968). *Central African Medical Journal* **14**, 173.

SOBEL, J. D. and SCHAMROTH, L. (1970). *Gut* **11**, 760.

SPENCER, S. S. and NHONOLI, A. M. (1972). *East African Medical Journal* **49**, 163.

TANDON, B. M., MATHUR, A. K., MOHAPATRA, L. N., TANDON, H. D. and WIG, K. L. (1965). *Gut* **6**, 448.

TROWELL, H. (1960). "Non-infective Disease in Africa", pp. 216–219. Edward Arnold, London.

VAN PATTER, W. N., BARGEN, J. A., DOCKERTY, M. B., FELDMAN, W. H., MAYO, C. W. and WAUGH, J. M. (1954). *Gastroenterology* **26**, 347.

WIGLEY, R. D. and MACLAURIN, B. P. (1962). *British Medical Journal* **2**, 228.

ZUIDEMA, P. J. (1959). *Tropical and Geographical Medicine* **11**, 246.

Part V

Other diseases associated with constipation and straining at stool

Chapter 12

Varicose veins, deep vein thrombosis and haemorrhoids

DENIS BURKITT

I. Prevalence in the western world 143
II. Rarity in developing countries 144
    A. Varicose veins 145
    B. Venous thrombosis 146
    C. Pulmonary embolism 148
    D. Haemorrhoids 149
III. Association between these venous disorders 149
IV. A new look at conventional speculation on possible aetiology . . 149
    A. Varicose veins 149
    B. Deep vein thrombosis and pulmonary embolism . . . 151
    C. Haemorrhoids 152
V. Possible dietetic factors in venous disorders 152
    A. Varicose veins 153
    B. Deep vein thrombosis 155
    C. Haemorrhoids 157
VI. Conclusion 157
References 158

I. Prevalence in the western world

At the present time varicose veins and haemorrhoids are among the commonest ailments in the western world. Varicose veins have been estimated to affect 10–17% of adults in England (De Takats and Quint, 1930; Dodd and Cockett, 1956; Martin *et al.*, 1956; Allen *et al.*, 1962) and in North America (Davis-Christopher, 1972). In a recent careful study of 610 subjects in Switzerland, Rougemont found 29% to have varicose veins (all nationalities). The prevalence was 32% in the 456 central European women and 18% in the 154 of Mediterranean origin. In the two groups combined the prevalence in those over 55 years of age was 64%

(Guberan *et al.*, 1973). The prevalence of haemorrhoids is more difficult to assess, but it has been estimated that 50% of people over 50 years of age in North America suffer from them in some degree. According to the Ministry of Pensions and National Insurance, Cmnd. 1764 (1961), nearly three million working days were lost in Britain during the year June 1959 to June 1960 due to these two conditions. Alexander (1972a) studied the prevalence of varicose veins in the western world, and concluded "it seems likely that something of the order of half the population in this western urbanised society will develop varicose veins if they live long enough".

The prevalence of deep vein thrombosis (DVT) in hospital patients varies according to the criteria by which diagnosis is made. Flanc *et al.* (1969) found that more than a third of all hospital patients over the age of 40 years developed some venous thrombosis. Kakkar *et al.* (1970) estimated that it occurred in 20–30% of all surgical patients and in 40–45% of older patients undergoing major surgery. Lambie *et al.* (1970), using ^{125}I-labelled fibrinogen, were able to demonstrate that nearly half of all "high risk" surgical patients developed some venous thrombosis which can be equally common in severe medical illnesses (Nicolaides *et al.*, 1971).

Not only is DVT an important cause of post-operative disability but it is the root cause of pulmonary embolism—one of the most dreaded complications of surgery—which kills about 2500 people in Britain every year (Registrar-General, 1969). Figures from the Registrar-General's Statistical Review (1969) show an annual rise in deaths from the disease. In 1969 the figure was 2447. It has in fact been estimated that some degree of pulmonary embolism occurs in half the patients who develop ileo-femoral thrombosis (Mavor, 1969). Not only does DVT prolong convalescence but its late sequelae are some of the most intractable problems in medicine (*Lancet* leader, 1971). Pulmonary emboli, more than 95% of which are believed to originate in the lower limbs, have been estimated to be responsible for 5–9% of hospital deaths (Davis-Christopher, 1972). Coon and Coller (1959) found pulmonary emboli in 14% of autopsies. Roberts (1971) has estimated that if deaths from venous thrombosis and pulmonary embolism continue to rise at their present rate there would, by 1973, have been a 10-fold increase in the previous 30 years.

II. Rarity in developing countries

The geographical distribution of varicose veins, DVT and haemorrhoids appears to be similar. All three conditions have their lowest incidence in communities who have deviated least from their traditional way of life. It appears that the prevalence of haemorrhoids always rises before that of varicose veins and DVT, which means they can be relatively common where varicose veins and DVT are still rare, and the reverse has not been observed.

A. Varicose veins

1. Africa

Varicose veins are very rare in rural Africa but are becoming commoner in communities influenced by western customs. During 1958 in an area of Uganda where at that time western culture had little impact, I specifically looked for varicose veins in over 4000 adults during an inspection of an entire community for evidence of trypanosomiasis. Only five cases were found, an incidence of 0·12%, which is about one-hundredth of the incidence in Britain or the U.S.A. In the Charles Johnson Memorial Hospital in Zululand (Natal), Barker (1964) saw only five patients with varicose veins among 14,000 in-patients. In a more developed area in Malawi, R. S. Harvey (p.c., 1971) found an incidence of approximately 0·2% in males aged 18–40 years applying for work in South African mines. J. Gildenhuys (p.c., 1973) reports that labour recruits in South West Africa are specifically examined for any evidence of varicose veins. Between the years 1968 and 1972 varicose veins were detected in 656 of 161,754 men examined (0·405%). Presumably these were relatively young men. Gildenhuys expressed the opinion that they were less common in women.

Replies to a questionnaire presented personally or through the post to doctors in 114 mission hospitals in 20 countries in Africa south of the Sahara indicated that in 89 hospitals (78%) less than five patients with varicose veins were seen annually. Only in three hospitals, all in South Africa or Rhodesia, were more than 20 cases of varicose veins seen annually. On average these hospitals admit 2000–3000 patients annually and see 20,000–30,000 out-patients (Burkitt, 1972). During 20 years' surgical practice in East Africa I never saw or heard of a case of varicose ulcer in an African. In contrast to this experience Rougemont (1973) found a prevalence of 10·9% of varicose veins in Mali villagers, but these included dilated subcutaneous veins, and no evidence of chronic venous insufficiency or any other complication was found. This prevalence, although high for Africa, was only a third of that found in Europeans, as quoted on p. 143. Daynes and Beighton (1973), in a carefully conducted survey in South African village women, found that 7·7% had varicose veins.

These recent figures suggest that more careful studies may show the prevalence of varicose veins in Africa to be greater than impressions have indicated but significantly less than in western countries.

2. India and Pakistan

In rural India and Pakistan the incidence appears to be only slightly higher. Sixteen of 33 mission hospitals estimated that they saw less than five patients with varicose veins annually, and only five saw over 20 cases. In urban India the figure is significantly higher (M. J. Joshi, p.c. 1972).

3. Indonesia

Fick (1965) in an 8 year period in Indonesia, during which he was medically responsible for about 10,000 people, saw no severe and only occasionally mild varicose veins.

4. New Guinea

Alexander (1972a) quotes workers in six different areas in New Guinea, all of whom stressed the extreme rarity of varicose veins in the inhabitants of that country.

5. Japan

More than half a century ago Miyauchi (1913) found that varicose veins were six times commoner in young German soldiers compared with Japanese soldiers of the same age.

There can be no doubt that varicose veins are very much more prevalent in the western world than they are in developing countries. Accurate assessment of these differences must await careful surveys in which the same diagnostic criteria are used. The term "varicose veins" is variously interpreted.

B. Venous thrombosis

1. Africa

Thomas et al. (1960) contrasted the 2% necropsy incidence of thromboembolic phenomena they found in Ugandan Africans with 24% and 22% in American whites and negroes respectively (Fig. 12.1). Kemble (1971) quoted an incidence of over 40% in Britain. These figures emphasize environmental rather than genetic causative factors. The incidence found at autopsy, as in life, depends very much on the methods used to discover the condition. Kallichurum (1969) in very detailed autopsy studies in which the veins of the leg were carefully dissected found a much higher incidence in Bantu than reported by other workers.

More than half of the 114 African mission hospitals referred to above did not diagnose one case of DVT annually. Following a visit to the Charles Johnson Memorial Hospital in Zululand, Dodd (1964) reported only three patients with femoral thrombosis over a period in which 11,000 patients, including 3000 for confinement, had been admitted. This would suggest that clinically overt DVT occurred in only one case in 5000–10,000 admissions in up-country hospitals in Africa. Monthly returns from 99 hospitals in 14 countries in Africa indicate that on average less than one case of deep vein thrombosis is clinically detected per hospital per year. There is some evidence that the prevalence of DVT, like that of varicose veins, is increasing, particularly in urban communities in Africa.

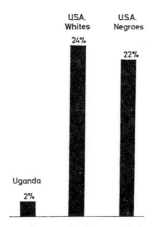

FIG. 12.1. Contrast between necropsy incidence of thrombo-embolic phenomena in lungs and veins found in Ugandan Africans with that found in American whites and negroes (compiled from Thomas *et al.*, 1960).

Luyombya-Sengero (1968) showed that thrombo-embolic episodes found at autopsy in Uganda rose from 2·4% in the period 1951–56 to 6% in the years 1965–67.

Recently the prevalence of DVT in Khartoum was measured by radio-isotope scanning techniques (Hassan *et al.*, 1973) and it was estimated to be less than half that of Britain. Patterns of other diseases associated with westernization show a much greater prevalence in the Sudan than in sub-Saharal Africa and it seems likely that the same applies to DVT.

2. India and Pakistan

Doctors in 13 of the 33 hospitals in India and Pakistan estimated that they saw less than one patient suffering from clinically recognizable DVT annually, and only five hospitals saw more than five cases. Monthly returns from ten hospitals in a prospective study indicate that the yearly average was just over two cases per hospital. Although figures are not available, M. J. Joshi (p.c., 1972) and P. K. Sen (p.c., 1971), who are heads of surgical departments at Sasoon Hospital, Poona, and the King Edward Memorial

Hospital, Bombay, respectively, have emphasized the rarity of DVT even in the urban communities in India which these hospitals serve.

3. Hong Kong and Japan

D. F. Hickock (p.c., 1972) found DVT to be very rare in maternity patients in Hong Kong.

Pulmonary embolism and infarction is uncommon in Japan. Stemmermann (1970) quotes a necropsy rate of 1·5% in Fukuoka in contrast to 23% for Los Angeles whites.

4. Thailand

From an examination of clinical charts at the Chulalongkorn Hospital for the years 1970–71, the prevalence of post-partum thromboembolic complication was 1·7 per 10,000 deliveries. The results of a similar study at the Mayo Clinic indicated a prevalence of 134·7 per 10,000 deliveries (Chumnijarakij, 1974).

5. Contrasting rates in indigenous and immigrant Britons

Among 46,500 patients known to have been born in Britain and discharged from Birmingham hospitals in 1969 there were 138 recorded cases of venous thrombosis and embolism. No case of either disease was recorded among 1976 immigrant patients known to have been born in India and Pakistan. Although the place of birth was recorded in only two-thirds of all admissions, this suggests a lower thrombosis rate in the immigrant population (G. Slaney, p.c. 1971).

C. Pulmonary embolism

Davies (1948), when reviewing autopsy records of 159 cases of sudden death in Africans in Uganda, found only one case of fatal pulmonary embolism. S. G. Browne (p.c., 1971) and J. Wilkinson (p.c., 1971), who both have more than 20 years' experience in mission hospitals in Africa, could each recall only one case of fatal pulmonary embolism. I remember no case in the surgical wards during my 20 years in Uganda. In Johannesburg only three cases were seen following over 10,000 operations on Africans (Barlow et al., 1953). At the King Edward Memorial Hospital, Bombay, where over 61,000 patients from lower income groups are admitted annually, fatal pulmonary embolism is almost unknown (P. K. Sen, p.c. 1971).

D. Haemorrhoids

In Africa haemorrhoids appear to be extremely rare in the primitive communities, and more prevalent in those who have had considerable contact with western civilization, although they are everywhere rare in comparison with the western world. Dodd (1964) reported one case at the Charles Johnson Memorial Hospital in Zululand over a 3 year period during which 11,000 patients were admitted. Trowell (1960) during 30 years saw only two Africans with anaemia due to bleeding haemorrhoids and one of these was a prince on semi-European diet.

In parts of southern Nigeria where European influences have been present for much longer than in East or Central Africa haemorrhoids appear to be quite common although varicose veins and DVT are still rare. An 11-fold increase in haemorrhoidectomies at Baragwanath Hospital, Johannesburg, during the period 1960–69 (C. G. Bremner, p.c. 1971) suggested that the condition was becoming more common in urban Africans.

Although the accuracy of some of the personal experiences quoted might be questioned there can be no doubt that varicose veins, DVT and pulmonary embolism are rare in developing countries, and that haemorrhoids are much less common than in the western world.

III. Association between these venous disorders

As with the non-infective diseases of the bowel there is a close similarity between the geographical distribution of these venous disorders. Just as appendicitis becomes a clinical problem at an earlier stage of economic development than do the other non-infective bowel diseases, so haemorrhoids appear to become relatively common before the other venous disorders. These observations would seem to suggest some common causative factor.

IV. A new look at conventional speculation on possible aetiology

A. Varicose veins

The causes most often suggested include:

1. Maladjustment to evolutionary changes

It has frequently been suggested that varicose veins reflect a failure of veins to adapt to man's erect posture. As Cleave (1960) and Cleave et al.

(1969) have pointed out, this view is totally untenable in the light of current epidemiological evidence. It is in communities whose women stand most erect, carrying burdens on their heads, that varicose veins are least common.

2. Hereditary factors

Many standard works (Martin et al., 1956; Allen et al., 1962) suggest that some inherited defect in the walls or valves of the leg veins is largely responsible for the development of varicosities. The present comparable incidence in U.S. whites and negroes (Stamler, 1958; Menendez, quoted by Cleave, 1960), the greater incidence in New Zealand Maoris than in less westernized Polynesian Islanders (I. Prior, p.c. 1970), and in urban than village Africans, refutes any suggestion that heredity is a primary causative factor, although it may be contributory.

3. Prolonged standing

This may well be an aggravating factor, but there is no evidence that it is a primary cause. It has been shown that there is constant minor muscle activity involved in normal standing (Smith, 1953). Under these repeated movements the venous pressures are much less than those expected from hydrostatic pressures (Henry and Gauer, 1950).

4. Pregnancy

Unlike varicose veins, pregnancy has no pattern of distribution, but women in countries with a low incidence of varicose veins have, on average, many more pregnancies than women in more economically developed countries where varicose veins are much more common. Moreover, as Cleave (p.c., 1971) has pointed out, the human race has adapted well to the physiological process of normal pregnancy. Guberan et al. (1973) have recently shown that when the age factor is taken into consideration there is no significant association between varicose veins and childbirth.

5. Constrictive clothing

Guberan et al. (1973) found when comparing women who wore corsetry with those who did not, there was a higher prevalence of varicose veins in the first group. But once again the difference was only due to a higher average age of this group.

6. *Femoral thrombosis*

This cannot be a fundamental cause of varicose veins, because in any community the incidence of varicose veins always appears to rise before that of DVT.

All of these postulated causes may well contribute to or aggravate varicose veins, but they cannot be considered as fundamental causes. The well-recognized tendency for varicosities to run in families might be due to a genetic susceptibility to certain environmental factors, or might merely depend on environmental factors to which some families are unduly exposed, or might be due to chance association.

B. *Deep vein thrombosis and pulmonary embolism*

Virchow (1856) suggested that the fundamental causes of venous thrombosis must be the changes in the vessel walls, an increased tendency for the blood to clot, or venous stasis. To these should be added changes in fibrinolysis, a matter discussed in Chapter 15.

An increased tendency for the blood to clot (Doran, 1971) or on the other hand less active fibrinolysis, may be contributory factors but would not alone explain the almost total exemption of the upper limbs even in unconscious or quadriplegic patients. The normal slowing of venous return during operation (Doran *et al.*, 1964; Clark and Cotton, 1968) or even during post-operative bed recumbency (Wright *et al.*, 1951) cannot, by itself, account for the different incidences in hospitals in western countries and in teaching hospitals in Africa and India, in all of which operating theatre circumstances are similar, but prophylactic measures are taken only in western countries.

Many of the prophylactic measures at present advocated are based on the assumption that certain circumstances attending surgery are responsible. These measures include early post-operative ambulation and active physiotherapy, intermittent pressures applied to the lower limbs to aid circulation (Calnan *et al.*, 1970; Sabri *et al.*, 1971), mechanical maintenance of foot movements (Roberts, 1971; Roberts *et al.*, 1971) and electrical stimulation of the calf muscles (Browse and Negus, 1970; Doran *et al.*, 1970).

Slowing of venous blood flow during enforced immobilization as demonstrated by Gibbs (1959–1960) and Sevitt and Gallagher (1959) undoubtedly contributes to venous thrombosis. Nicolaides *et al.* (1972) emphasize that most thrombi originate in the deep veins of the calf muscles. The fundamental factor must explain localization in the legs, both of which have been shown to be affected with equal frequency when studied by phlebography or with radioactive fibrinogen (Browse and Negus, 1970; Kakkar *et al.*, 1970; Sripad *et al.*, 1971; Kemble, 1971). On the other hand clinically recognizable cases, particularly ileofemoral thrombosis, have been reported to be two or three times commoner in the left than in the right leg (Atkins, 1938; Barker *et al.*, 1941; Negus, 1970). The prophylactic measures referred to above are doubtless of value in reducing the incidence of deep vein thrombosis in the presence of a primary factor.

The cause of pulmonary embolism is fundamentally the cause of the thrombus which, when dislodged, produces the embolism. There may be other contributing factors.

C. Haemorrhoids

These have been attributed to man's erect posture, heredity and anatomical features such as the arrangement of the collecting veins in the lax rectal sub-mucosa, and their liability to compression as they traverse the muscular wall of the rectum. It has generally been assumed that a valve-less portal venous system was satisfactory for quadrupeds but inadequate for man. Suggested subsidiary causes include strenuous work, prolonged standing, pregnancy and horse-riding.

None of these suggested primary or subsidiary causes, with the exception of straining at stool, explains the geographical distribution of this disorder as outlined above.

V. Possible dietetic factors in venous disorders

Straining at stool is inevitably associated with, and caused by, constipation; it is much less common in communities on a high-fibre diet than in those, for example in North America and Great Britain, where a low-fibre diet is now recognized as the most important single cause of constipation (Avery Jones, 1972).

The contraction of abdominal muscles, including fixation of the diaphragm which accompanies efforts to evacuate firm faeces, causes raised intra-abdominal pressures that are transmitted to the vena cava and its tributaries and to the veins of the lower limb when the protective valves have become incompetent.

Intra-abdominal pressures can certainly be raised to over 200 mmHg when straining (Dodd, 1964; D. Edwards, p.c. 1971; A. Connell, p.c. 1972) and Sharpey-Schafer (quoted by Shemilt, 1972) has stated that coughing can raise the pressure in the abdominal vena cava to over 400 mmHg. Presumably strong straining may raise it even higher.

The fact that these pressures are readily transmitted to the veins of the lower limb in the absence of competent valves (Fig. 12.2) is the basis of the clinical test for incompetency, an impulse transmitted down the saphenous vein on coughing.

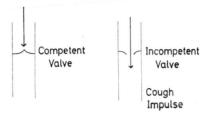

FIG. 12.2. Showing that raised intra-abdominal pressures are sustained by competent valves in the veins of the leg, but are transmitted through the veins when the valves become incompetent.

A. Varicose veins

Any adequate hypothesis concerning the aetiology of varicose veins, DVT and haemorrhoids must take account of the following established facts:

1. the low prevalence of varicose veins, DVT and haemorrhoids in developing countries, especially Africa;

2. the high prevalence of all these conditions in white and coloured Americans;

3. the rise in prevalence of haemorrhoids before that of varicose veins and DVT;

4. the higher prevalence of DVT in the legs than in the arms.

As mentioned above raised intra-abdominal pressures, consequent on straining at stool, are readily transmitted down the leg veins as soon as the valves become incompetent. It must therefore be assumed that as long as the valves remain competent they and the venous walls above them are subjected to any increase in intra-abdominal pressure (Fig. 12.2). It seems reasonable to suspect that vein valves which are repeatedly subjected to these abnormal pressures may become incompetent, a reflux of blood being forced back into the leg veins (Burkitt, 1972). This might initiate a process leading to venous dilatation and varicosities. Edwards and Edwards (1940) have shown that changes are not histologically detectable in the cusps of the valves after they have become incompetent, but that the fundamental change is the dilatation of the lumen of the vein with stretching of the portion of the vein wall between the attachment of the cusps. This leads to evagination of the wall and separation of the cusps with resultant incompetence of the valves (Fig. 12.3). These authors "feel that the varicose change can be regarded as resulting from a disproportion between the venous pressure and the resistance force of the venous wall". With the latter they include the pressure of surrounding structures. This would be consistent with the explanation of transmitted pressures outlined above. In the early stages the incompetence need not necessarily allow sufficient venous return to result in a clinically detected cough impulse. This would explain why visible varicosities are not always accompanied by a clinically detectable reverse flow of venous blood on coughing.

An important contributory factor may well be the position adopted during defaecation (Osman, p.c. 1971). In developing countries the traditional squatting position is usually retained; this means that the veins of the lower limb are protected from abdominal pressures by compression.

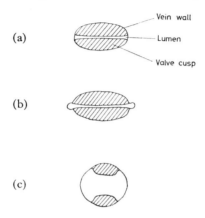

(a)

Vein wall

Lumen

Valve cusp

(b)

(c)

FIG. 12.3. Cross-section of veins: (a) normal; (b) early incompetence, with slight separation of attachments of valve cusps with vein dilatation; (c) gross incompetence with wide separation of attachments of valve cusps and further dilatation. (Modified from Edwards and Edwards, 1940.)

In patients in whom a cough impulse can be elicited when standing, or even sitting, the impulse is far less, and may not be detected by clinical means, when squatting. The modern raised toilet does not offer this protection to leg veins; and it has moreover been suggested that in the squatting position less muscular effort is required to evacuate the bowel than when sitting. A further contributory factor has been suggested by Alexander (1972b), who has shown a correlation between the geographical distribution of chair-sitting and that of varicose veins. He believes that the additional hydrostatic pressure in the veins of the leg imposed by sitting in chairs rather than, as traditionally, on the ground helps to explain the preponderance of this condition in economically more developed countries.

Cleave (1956, 1960) was the first to associate varicose veins with the faecal arrest resultant on a low-fibre diet, but he postulated a different mechanism from the one suggested here. He believed that an unnaturally loaded iliac colon on the left, and caecum on the right, exert small but unnatural pressures on the external iliac veins.

Latto *et al.* (1973) have recently demonstrated an association between varicose veins and diverticular disease in individual patients which suggests causative factors common to each (Fig. 12.4). The relationship between faecal arrest and diverticular disease is well established (Chapter 9). It therefore seems reasonable to suspect that a similar mechanism may operate in the pathogenesis of varicose veins.

The argument relating varicose veins to factors raising intraluminal pressures may be summarized as follows:

By their very nature the varicosity and dilatation of veins implies reversed blood flow, which denotes valve incompetence. Histological studies have shown no structural changes in the valve cusps but have shown stretching

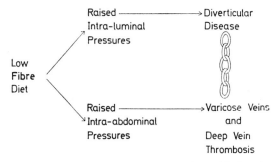

Fig. 12.4. Postulated explanation of the observed association between varicose veins and diverticular disease.

of the vein walls in the region of the valves, particularly between the attachments of the valve cusps. This separation of the valve cusps causes incompetence. It seems likely that above the valves, veins are also dilated, as a result of increased intraluminal pressure relative to external support (Edwards and Edwards, 1940). The cause of varicose veins must therefore be sought in the cause of raised intraluminal pressure, as in the case of diverticular disease of the colon. Gravity may play a role but cannot be the fundamental factor. Raised intra-abdominal pressures from straining or other causes could be responsible for the raised intravenous pressures. I am not aware of any study relating varicose veins to chronic pulmonary disease or of any efforts to determine the relative effects of momentary pressure rises in coughing with the more prolonged pressures of straining.

B. Deep vein thrombosis

The aetiological factors first suggested by Virchow (1856) are still valid, but the possible changes in the veins or blood which he postulated as causative factors themselves need explanation. Damaged vessel walls can lead to thrombosis, but does such damage usually precede DVT and, if so, why?

If an increased tendency for the blood to clot is a primary factor (Doran, 1971), why is thrombosis in the veins of a limb almost limited to those in the leg? Even when the upper limbs are immobilized for long periods through unconsciousness or quadriplegia they are seldom the site of venous thrombosis. This virtual exemption of the upper limbs makes it seem unlikely that abnormal fibrinolytic activity in different racial groups (Shaper et al., 1966; Shaper, 1970) or in individuals (Chakrabarti et al., 1968) is the primary factor, although it may be contributory (Chapter 15). Even if changes in thrombotic or fibrinolytic activity predispose to variations in the prevalence of DVT, gravity alone seems unlikely to account for the almost exclusive selection of the lower limbs, particularly in view of the geographical distribution of the diseases outlined above.

Virchow's third factor, venous stasis, seems the most likely explanation and this would also be consistent with the relative rarity of DVT outside more economically developed communities.

Any factor that could account for an undue tendency to venous stasis in the lower limb would offer a plausible explanation of venous thrombosis. It must account for both legs being equally affected (Browse and Negus, 1970; Kakkar et al., 1970; Kemble, 1971; Sripad et al., 1971) and the greater tendency for thrombosis to spread and become clinically detectable in the left leg.

If it is accepted that intra-abdominal pressures caused by straining could lead to valvular incompetence with resultant changes in the superficial veins, it would seem reasonable to postulate that similar changes may result in the deep venous plexuses. Dilatation or elongation of these veins may well predispose to a degree of venous stasis during enforced recumbency which might result in thrombosis under these conditions whereas normal veins would be less affected. This hypothesis could be tested if a sufficient number of venograms, particularly in elderly patients, from communities with a high and low prevalence of DVT, were available for comparison.

Cleave (1956, 1960) has propounded an alternative hypothesis. In his view it is the direct pressure of a loaded colon or prolapsed caecum on the underlying veins that is responsible for slight but unnatural pressure retarding the venous flow. In this connection he attributed the great rise in incidence of DVT since the Second World War to the abandonment of pre-operative enemas and laxatives. Cleave is obviously right in refusing to accept as a primary cause pressure on the left common iliac vein where it is crossed by the right common iliac artery, since this is a normal anatomical relationship; however, any narrowing of the vein at this point might contribute to extension of thrombosis on the left side.

The cause of these venous conditions may be associated with the geographical distribution of pelvic phleboliths which, it has been agreed, are calcified thrombi probably caused by rupture of the endothelium in the small pelvic veins due to raised intra-venous pressures (Shemilt, 1972). There is some evidence that phleboliths are less common in communities with a low incidence of varicose veins and DVT than they are in the western world. Scott Brown (1943) saw only two phleboliths in Africans during many years experience as a radiologist in Uganda. J. I. Levy (p.c., 1972) has seen far fewer in South African Bantu than in whites. These observations would be consistent with the hypothesis that both the pelvic and leg venous anomalies are related to unnaturally raised intra-abdominal pressure.

C. Haemorrhoids

Theories concerning the aetiology of haemorrhoids which are based on anatomical relationships of the haemorrhoidal veins or supposed structural defects such as the absence of valves in the portal venous system are unacceptable as primary causative factors since they are not peculiar to, or more pronounced in, western communities. It is well known that abdominal straining causes dilatation of haemorrhoidal veins, and that haemorrhoidal prolapse is often precipitated by such straining. Cleave et al. (1969) have postulated that haemorrhoids result from faecal arrest, blaming straining at stool and the direct pressure of unnaturally firm faecal masses on the veins in the rectal wall. Whatever the precise mechanism, it seems likely that constipation plays a prominent causative role. Epidemiological observations that the frequency of haemorrhoids in any community increases before that of varicose veins could be explained by the fact that haemorrhoidal veins are unprotected from raised intra-abdominal pressures, whereas the veins of the lower limb are protected by valves and, in those who squat at stool, by pressure from without.

VI. Conclusion

An attempt has been made to determine the fundamental cause of these venous disorders. All the factors traditionally listed as causes of these conditions almost certainly contribute to their development when acting in association with the primary factor suggested, or aggravate the disease once it has been established.

Alexander (1972a), after showing the inadequacy of conventional concepts of the aetiology of varicose veins, wrote, "We need to look for some factor in western civilization which either results in a weak wall or raises saphenous wall stress, and renders us suceptible to accelerating factors which have no effect on primitive communities". He concluded another communication with these words "It appears, too, that all the factors known to be associated with increased incidence—female sex, parity, tight clothing and long-continued standing—must be dismissed as primary causes. They can be no more than accelerators, acting on veins already rendered susceptible by some effect of the western style of living."

A deficiency in dietary fibre may be a causative factor common to all these venous disorders.

References

ALEXANDER, C. J. (1972a). *Medical Journal of Australia* **1**, 215.

ALEXANDER, C. J. (1972b). *Lancet* **1**, 822.

ALLEN, E. V., BARKER, N. W. and HINES, E. A. (1962). "Peripheral Vascular Diseases", p. 636. W. B. Saunders, Philadelphia.

ATKINS, H. J. B. (1938). *Guy's Hospital Reports* **88**, 92.

AVERY JONES, F. (1972). *In* "Management of Constipation" (F. Avery Jones and E. W. Godding, eds), Chapter 4. Blackwell Scientific Publications, Oxford.

BARKER, A. (1964). *Lancet* **2**, 970.

BARKER, N. W., NYGAARD, K. K., WALTERS, W. and PRIESTLEY, J. T. (1941). *Proceedings of the staff meetings of the Mayo Clinic* **16**, 1.

BARLOW, M. B., GINSBERG, H. and GOTTLICH, J. (1953). *South African Medical Journal* **27**, 242.

BROWSE, N. L. and NEGUS, D. (1970). *British Medical Journal* **3**, 615.

BURKITT, D. P. (1972). *British Medical Journal* **2**, 556.

CALNAN, J. S., PFLUG, J. J. and MILLS, C. J. (1970). *Lancet* **2**, 502.

CHAKRABARTI, R., HOCKING, E. D., FEARNLEY, G. R., MANN, R. D., ATTWELL, T. N. and JACKSON, D. (1968). *Lancet* **1**, 987.

CHUMNIJARAKIJ, T. (1974). *British Medical Journal* **1**, 245.

CLARK, C. and COTTON, L. T. (1968). *British Journal of Surgery* **55**, 211.

CLEAVE, T. L. (1956). *Journal of the Royal Naval Medical Service* **42**, 55.

CLEAVE, T. L. (1960). "On the Causation of Varicose Veins." John Wright, Bristol.

CLEAVE, T. L., CAMPBELL, G. D. and PAINTER, N. S. (1969). "Diabetes, Coronary Thrombosis and the Saccharine Disease", 2nd edition. John Wright, Bristol.

COON, W. W. and COLLER, F. A. (1959). *Surgery, Gynecology and Obstetrics* **109**, 487.

DAVIES, J. N. P. (1948). *East African Medical Journal* **25**, 322.

"Davis-Christopher Textbook of Surgery" (1972) (D. C. Sabiston, ed.) 10th edition, pp. 1600, 1623. W. B. Saunders, Philadelphia.

DAYNES, G. and BEIGHTON, P. (1973). *British Medical Journal* **3**, 354.

DE TAKATS, G. and QUINT, H. (1930). *Surgery, Gynecology and Obstetrics* **50**, 545.

DODD, H. (1964). *Lancet* **2**, 809.

DODD, H. and COCKETT, F. B. (1956). "The Pathology and Surgery of the Veins of the Lower Limb", p. 3. Livingstone, Edinburgh.

DORAN, F. S. A. (1971). *British Journal of Hospital Medicine* 6, 773.
DORAN, F. S. A., DRURY, M. and SIVYER, A. (1964). *British Journal of Surgery* 51, 486.
DORAN, F. S. A., WHITE, M. and DRURY, M. (1970). *British Journal of Surgery* 57, 20.
EDWARDS, J. E. and EDWARDS, E. A. (1940). *American Heart Journal* 19, 338.
FICK, W. (1965). "Zur Entstehung und Prophylaxe der Krampfadem. Ein Beitrag zur vergleichenden Medizin", Hippokrates, 36, 229.
FLANC, C., KAKKAR, V. V. and CLARKE, M. B. (1969). *Lancet* 1, 447.
GENERAL REGISTER OFFICE (1969). Statistical Review of England and Wales: Part 1, Tables Medical. Her Majesty's Stationery Office, London.
GIBBS, N. M. (1959–1960). *British Journal of Surgery* 47, 282.
GUBERAN, E., WIDMER, L. K., GLAUS, L., MULLER, R., ROUGEMONT, A., DA SILVA, A. and GENDRE, F. (1973). *Journal for Vascular Disease* 2, 115.
HASSAN, M. A., RAHMAN, E. A. and RAHMAN, I. A. (1973). *British Medical Journal* 1, 515.
HENRY, J. P. and GAUER, O. H. (1950). *Journal of Clinical Investigation* 29, 855.
KAKKAR, V. V., HOWE, C. T., NICOLAIDES, A. N., RENNEY, J. T. G. and CLARKE, M. B. (1970). *American Journal of Surgery* 120, 527.
KALLICHURUM, S. (1969). *South African Medical Journal* 43, 358.
KEMBLE, J. V. H. (1971). *British Journal of Hospital Medicine* 6, 721.
LAMBIE, J. M., MAHAFFY, R. G., BARBER, D. C., KARMODY, A. M., SCOTT, M. M. and MATHESON, N. A. (1970). *British Medical Journal* 2, 142.
Lancet leader (1971). *Lancet* 2, 693.
LATTO, C., WILKINSON, R. W. and GILMORE, O. J. A. (1973). *Lancet* 1, 1089.
LUYOMBYA-SENGERO, J. M. (1968). *Makerere Medical Journal* 12, 20.
MARTIN, P., LYNN, P. B., DIBLE, J. H. and AIRD, I. (1956). "Peripheral Vascular Disorders", p. 664. Livingstone, Edinburgh.
MAVOR, G. E. (1969). *British Medical Journal* 4, 680.
MINISTRY OF PENSIONS AND NATIONAL INSURANCE, Cmnd. 1764 (1961). Her Majesty's Stationery Office, London.
MIYAUCHI, K. (1913). *Archiv für klinische Chirurgie*, Berlin 100, 1079.
NEGUS, D. (1970). *Annals of the Royal College of Surgeons of England* 47, 92.
NICOLAIDES, A. N., KAKKAR, V. V., RENNEY, J. T. G., KIDNER, P. H., HUTCHISON, D. C. S. and CLARKE, M. B. (1971). *British Medical Journal* 1, 432.
NICOLAIDES, A. N., KAKKAR, V. V., FIELD, E. S. and FISH, P. (1972). *British Journal of Surgery* 59, 713.
ROBERTS, C. (1971). *New Scientist and Science Journal* 51, 620.
ROBERTS, V. C., SABRI, S., PIETRONI, M. C., GUREWICH, V. and COTTON, L. T. (1971). *British Medical Journal* 3, 78.
ROUGEMONT, A. (1973). *British Medical Journal* 2, 547.
SABRI, S., ROBERTS, V. C. and COTTON, L. T. (1971). *British Medical Journal* 3, 82.
SCOTT BROWN, J. (1943). *East African Medical Journal* 20, 122.
SEVITT, S. and GALLAGHER, N. G. (1959). *Lancet* 2, 981.
SHAPER, A. G. (1970). "Atherosclerosis: Proceedings of the 2nd International Symposium" (R. J. Jones, ed.), pp. 314–320. Springer-Verlag, Heidelberg.

SHAPER, A. G., JONES, K. W., KYOBE, J. and JONES, M. (1966). *Journal of Atherosclerosis Research* **6**, 313.

SHEMILT, P. (1972). *British Journal of Surgery* **59**, 695.

SMITH, J. W. (1953). *Acta orthopaedica scandinavica* **23**, 159.

SRIPAD, S., ANTCLIFF, A. C. and MARTIN, P. (1971). *British Journal of Surgery* **58**, 563.

STAMLER, J. (1958). *Journal of the National Medical Association* **50**, 161.

STEMMERMANN, G. N. (1970). *Archives of Environmental Health* **20**, 266.

THOMAS, W. A., DAVIES, J. N. P., O'NEAL, R. M. and DIMAKULANGAN, A. A. (1960). *American Journal of Cardiology* **5**, 41.

TROWELL, H. C. (1960). "Non-infective Disease in Africa", p. 218. Edward Arnold, London.

VIRCHOW, R. (1856). *In* "Gesammelte abhandlungen zur wissenschaftlichen Medicin", p. 219. Meidinger, Frankfurt.

WRIGHT, H. P., OSBORN, S. B. and EDMONDS, D. G. (1951). *Lancet* **1**, 22.

Chapter 13

Hiatus hernia

DENIS BURKITT

I. Historical emergence. 162
II. Current prevalence 162
   A. Western world 162
   B. Developing countries 163
III. Current concepts of the aetiology of hiatus hernia, and reappraisal in
   the light of aetiological evidence 165
   A. Conventional concepts of the possible causes of hiatus hernia . 165
   B. Examination of postulated causes in the light of epidemiological
   evidence 166
IV. The possible significance of relationships with other diseases . . 167
V. Postulated dietary factors 168
References 168

When first recognized, what is now known as hiatus hernia was considered to be a development defect and was called "congenital short oesophagus".

There are two main types of hiatus hernia. The less common para-oesophageal hernia may be symptomless or may show such symptoms as pain, regurgitation and borborygmi, due to intermittent obstruction, or breathlessness from enlargement of the intrathoracic portion of the stomach.

"Sliding" hernia, which is usually much more common, only causes symptoms when oesophagitis results from reflux of gastric juices into the oesophagus through the now incompetent cardia. The most prominent symptoms are retrosternal pain and haemorrhage, and also ulceration which may lead to gross fibrosis and stricture formation frequently enhanced by accompanying inflammatory oedema.

Largely because of its rarity in early life, and also its increasing incidence with advancing age, it subsequently became evident that hiatus hernia must be an acquired defect.

I. Historical emergence

It is difficult to determine when hiatus hernia became a common clinical problem in the west, but there is no doubt that recognized cases were a rarity until 50 years ago. The increasing number of cases reported since the Second World War has usually been assumed to reflect merely increased awareness of the condition and improved diagnostic techniques, but the rarity of hiatus hernia in areas where good radiological facilities are available suggests that this was not the sole explanation.

II. Current prevalence

There is no doubt that hiatus hernia, though usually without symptoms, is one of the most common defects of the gastrointestinal tract in western nations at the present time. By contrast there is no indication of its being other than rare in the developing countries from which information is available. Studies carried out in many countries emphasize this difference.

A. Western world

Pridie (1966), reviewing the recorded experience of workers in many areas, has shown that hiatus herniae could be demonstrated in 2·1–11·8% of subjects during radiological examination of the gastro-oesophageal region, when intra-abdominal pressure was increased. He studied the prevalence of hiatus hernia in 500 consecutive barium meal examinations, none of which was performed on patients suspected of having this condition. The barium was swallowed whilst lying prone. "A film was taken of the oesophagus after it had emptied as much as it would and a hiatus hernia was diagnosed only if a ring or groove as described by MacLean (1959) could be identified above the diaphragm and the mucosal pattern of the supradiaphragmatic pouch was continuous with that of the infradiaphragmatic portion of the stomach." From these criteria the overall incidence of hiatus hernia was found to be 29·6%: 21% men and 39% women. The significance of this sex discrepancy will be discussed below. As with diverticular disease the frequency rose with age, in this case 9% in those under 40, to 69% in patients over 70 years of age.

Wolf and Guglielmo (1957) reported that when the barium is swallowed in the prone position with the abdomen compressed, the percentage of patients in whom herniae can be demonstrated is even higher than the above figures.

Hafter (1958) noted a frequency of 12·5% in 2402 barium meal examinations, and Stein and Finkelstein (1960) reported finding one of 50% in 100 consecutive barium examinations. In Miami, hiatus hernia was shown to be present in one in five patients undergoing radiological examination of the upper gastrointestinal tract (Zeppa and Polk, 1971).

Conversations with many American surgeons and radiologists have not revealed any gross disparity in the frequency of this condition in white and coloured Americans. A. Segel (p.c., 1972), head of the radiological department at Cuyahoga County Hospital, Cleveland, Ohio, wrote: "Our hospital's population is approximately equally divided between white and black patients, and I do not believe that there is any significant racial difference in the incidence of hiatus hernia".

B. Developing countries

1. Africa

(a) *Kenya, Nairobi.* Whittaker (1966) found only one case in a series of 1319 barium examinations in Kenyan Africans.

(b) *Uganda, Kampala.* Moore (1967) found 25 in 786 upper gastrointestinal tract investigations; almost all were of the "small stenosing type". During 7 years as the sole thoracic surgeon in Uganda, James did not see a single case of hiatus hernia or oesophageal stricture due to reflux oesophagitis in an African (Burkitt and James, 1973). No case of hiatus hernia was seen in Kampala 1953–58 by the radiologist A. G. M. Davies (Trowell, 1960).

(c) *Tanzania, Dar es Salaam.* Grech (1965) found only one in 733 barium examinations, and H. Diefental at Moshi (p.c., 1972) was able to demonstrate hiatus hernia in only two of 1200 radiological examinations of the upper gastrointestinal tract.

(d) *Nigeria, Lagos.* O. Bassey (p.c., 1974) found only four cases in over 1000 consecutive barium meal X-ray examinations on Africans.

(e) *Ivory Coast, Abidjan.* A. Renaud (p.c., 1974) detected less than one in every 500 upper gastrointestinal tract radiological examinations.

(f) *South Africa, Cape Town.* W. Silber (p.c., 1972) stated that hiatus hernia was "extremely uncommon in urban Africans".

Pretoria. It is almost unknown in the Bantu, but can be demonstrated in some 40% of white patients undergoing radiological investigation of the upper gastrointestinal tract (P. J. Kloppers, p.c. 1972).

(g) *Rhodesia, Bulawayo.* A. R. Watson (p.c., 1973) demonstrated hiatus hernia in only seven of 952 radiological examinations of the upper gastrointestinal tract of Africans, a frequency of 0·73%. Most of these were from the upper socio-economic groups, which suggests that the average figure for Africans was much lower. He found the condition in 27 of 697 barium examinations in Europeans, a frequency of 3·87%, which is low compared with western countries, but the discovery of herniae depends on the techniques used. The two series carried out by the same investigator do indicate that herniation is much more prevalent in Rhodesian whites than even in the most westernized Africans.

2. India

(a) *Ludhiana, north-east India.* E. R. F. Rebello (p.c., 1972) demonstrated hiatus hernia in not more than 1% of his barium meal studies.

(b) *Delhi.* O. P. Bhardwaj (p.c., 1973), who has studied hiatus herniation intensively in an exceptionally large university radiological department, where over 3000 upper gastrointestinal tract examinations are performed annually, has demonstrated the condition in 2·8% of his patients when using techniques to raise intra-abdominal pressures.

(c) *Calcutta.* N. M. Bannerjee (p.c., 1973) has seen only eight cases in 7 years in a department doing between 300 and 400 upper gastrointestinal tract examinations annually. In the same city, B. Chatterjee (p.c., 1973), although specifically looking for the condition, has been unable to demonstrate it in nearly 800 barium meal examinations.

(d) *Vellore, South India.* Johnson and Johnson (1969) specifically endeavouring to demonstrate hiatus hernia, found it in over 30% of their patients.

3. Iraq—Baghdad

Mohammed Abu-Tabikh (p.c., 1973) in the University Radiology Department, demonstrated hiatus hernia in less than 1·0% of patients X-rayed in a Trendelenberg position to raise intra-abdominal pressures.

4. South Korea—Seoul

Kim (1964), specifically searching for evidence of hiatus hernia in 1000 consecutive radiological examinations of the gastro-oesophageal junction, found only 14 cases of minimal hiatus hernia, mostly in persons over the age of 50 years.

The discovery of cases of hiatus hernia in any barium series is dependent on the effort made to detect them. There is obviously a need for prospective studies in areas of high and low incidence, using standard techniques and diagnostic criteria.

III. Current concepts of the aetiology of hiatus hernia, and reappraisal in the light of aetiological evidence

Fundamentally all postulated causes must fall into three different categories or a combination of them. The rise of the upper part of the stomach into the thorax could be due to increased pressure from below, or an upward pull from the thorax, or a derangement of the hiatus in the diaphragm allowing the stomach to move more freely through it. Sir David Smithers (1961) has summarized this as follows: "The normal sub-diaphragmatic position of the vestibule is maintained by a fine balance between opposing forces at the level of the diaphragm. The anatomical arrangements are normally sufficient to prevent the variable lower pressures in the thorax and higher pressures in the abdomen from displacing the vestibule upwards through the hiatus."

A. Conventional concepts of the possible causes of hiatus hernia

1. A "pulling-up" mechanism

Von Bergmann and Goldner (1932) suggested that hiatus herniations might be due to the pull of oesophageal contractions in response to a vago-vagal reflux. Johnstone (1941, 1943) and Harrington (1940) suggested that gastric reflux leading to oesophagitis was the primary condition and that the subsequent oesophageal fibrosis pulled the stomach upwards into the thorax. Cleave et al. (1969) have postulated that gastric stasis resultant on faulty eating habits leads to oesophageal reflux with subsequent oesophageal contraction pulling up the stomach.

2. A "pushing-up" mechanism

This implies abnormally raised intra-abdominal pressures (Fig. 13.1) for which the most frequently suggested causes are: tumours, pregnancy, obesity and constrictive clothing.

3. A combination of these two mechanisms

Smithers (1945) considered that the development of a lax hiatus was the primary defect and that this was followed by herniation which in turn resulted in reflux with irritation of the oesophagus and subsequent contraction pulling up the stomach.

4. Defects in the diaphragmatic control mechanism

As the prevalence of hiatus hernia increases with advancing age, it has been suggested that atrophy of the muscles providing the diaphragmatic sphincter might be primarily responsible. It has also been suggested that fat deposits may stretch the sphincter.

INTRA – ABDOMINAL PRESSURES

and

HIATUS HERNIA

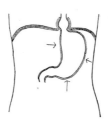

Fɪɢ. 13.1. Diagrammatic representation of postulated relationship between raised intra-abdominal pressures and hiatus hernia.

B. Examination of postulated causes in the light of epidemiological evidence

1. The "pull-up" theory

It is difficult to postulate reflux as the cause of oesophageal contraction since it is only present in a minority of cases.

2. The "push-up" theory

Increased intra-abdominal pressure is almost certainly a major causative factor, but for the reasons listed below is seldom likely to result from the causes traditionally suggested.

(a) *Tumours.* Much larger ovarian cysts and other abdominal tumours are encountered in developing countries where surgical facilities are more limited than in the western world, yet it is in these very communities that hiatus hernia is most unusual.

(b) *Pregnancy.* This is a normal physiological condition, and as pointed out by Cleave (1960) when discussing the aetiology of varicose veins, failure to adapt to it would be strange. Moreover, the number of pregnancies is higher in communities with the lowest prevalence of hiatus hernia.

(c) *Obesity.* Increased weight certainly tends to be associated with hiatus hernia, but it seems doubtful whether obesity does, in fact, significantly raise intra-abdominal pressure. Reasons why it appears more likely that both hiatus hernia and obesity result at least in part from common or related causes, will be given below and in Chapter 16.

(d) *Constrictive clothing* has never been demonstrated as having any relationship to hiatus hernia; in any case this type of hernia might have been expected to decrease rather than increase with less formal and less restrictive clothing in western countries during the present century.

3. *Defective sphincteric mechanism*

There is no evidence to incriminate the muscular degeneration which results from increasing age. If this were a major causative factor, hiatus hernia might be expected to have a similar incidence in elderly people in different countries, whereas in developing countries it is rare irrespective of age.

To blame fat deposits at the hiatus demands a cause for the fat. It is considered more likely that this deposition of fat and hiatus hernia share a common cause rather than that there is here a cause and effect relationship.

It is postulated that hiatus hernia is caused by raised intra-abdominal pressures which result not from the factors listed above but from straining at stool (Burkitt and James, 1973).

IV. The possible significance of relationships with other diseases

Epidemiological relationships between one disease and another can often provide valuable clues as to their possible cause (Burkitt, 1969, 1970a, b). The close association between diverticular disease and cancer of the colon and rectum has thus suggested possible factors that may be causative in the latter disease (Burkitt, 1971). Similarly, the recognition of a close relationship between diverticular disease and varicose veins and deep vein thrombosis (Burkitt, 1972, 1973; Latto *et al.*, 1973) and between diverticular disease and ischaemic heart disease (Trowell *et al.*, 1974) has thrown light on their possible causes.

Hiatus hernia has a similar geographical distribution to all these diseases which are believed to be related to western-type diets. Furthermore, diverticular disease and hiatus hernia have been the last two diseases to appear in all situations examined. Hiatus hernia has also been associated with diverticular disease and gallstones in individual patients in Saint's triad (Muller, 1948) and is known to be associated with obesity. Like diverticular disease it has a marked female preponderance and in the west becomes increasingly prevalent with advancing age. These associations inevitably suggest some common causative factor.

V. Postulated dietary factors

Any adequate hypothesis concerning the aetiology of hiatus hernia must explain the very great disparity in prevalence between more affluent communities and developing countries, and the close associations between hiatus hernia and certain other diseases characteristic of modern western civilization, especially of diverticular disease (Burkitt, 1972, 1973). This latter condition is now believed to be caused by unnaturally raised intra-luminal pressures in the colon resulting from a fibre-depleted diet (Painter, 1964, 1967). Not only does the faecal arrest which is associated with a fibre-depleted diet (Burkitt *et al.*, 1972) lead to raised intraluminal pressures, but it is also responsible for abnormally raised intra-abdominal pressures during straining at stool. These often exceed 100 mmHg (N. S. Painter, p.c. 1973), and can exceed 200 mmHg (D. Edwards, p.c. 1971). It seems likely that these pressures could well be a major contributory factor in the development of any abdominal hernia and have a much greater significance than pressures postulated to result from other causes (Fig. 13.1).

Muller (1948), discussing Saint's triad of hiatus hernia, diverticular disease and gallstones, suggested that intra-abdominal pressures raised when straining at stool might be a causative factor in hiatus hernia.

The hypothesis that hiatus hernia is in part caused by raised intra-abdominal pressures resulting from a fibre-depleted diet would explain its geographical distribution. It could also explain the geographical relationship between this condition and some other diseases such as the non-infective diseases of the bowel and certain venous disorders (Burkitt, 1973).

Since a fibre-depleted diet almost invariably implies a high consumption of starches and sugars, it tends to impose obesity (Chapter 16), and is believed to be an important cause of cholesterol gallstones (Heaton, 1973). This could account for the association between these diseases and hiatus hernia, not only geographically but also in individual patients. Moreover, it would explain the deposition of fat at the oesophageal hiatus.

We are aware of no alternative hypothesis that explains both the epidemiological and clinical observations. This postulated aetiology, as well as satisfying all the requirements posed by known facts about the disease, points to simple preventive measures, which would merely entail the restoration of an adequate amount of dietary fibre to western diets.

References

BERGMANN, G. VON and GOLDNER, M. (1932). "Funktionelle Pathologie, eine klinische Sammlung von Ergebnissen und Anschauungen einer Arbeitsrichtung", p. 70. Julius Springer, Berlin.

BURKITT, D. P. (1969). *Lancet* **2**, 1229.
BURKITT, D. P. (1970a). *Lancet* **2**, 1237.
BURKITT, D. P. (1970b). *International Pathology* **11**, 3.
BURKITT, D. P. (1971). *Cancer* **28**, 3.
BURKITT, D. P. (1972). *In* "The Medical Annual" (R. B. Scott and R. M. Walker, eds), p. 5. John Wright, Bristol.
BURKITT, D. P. (1973). *Clinical Radiology* **24**, 271.
BURKITT, D. P. and JAMES, P. A. (1973). *Lancet* **2**, 128.
BURKITT, D. P., WALKER, A. R. P. and PAINTER, N. S. (1972). *Lancet* **2**, 1408.
CLEAVE, T. L. (1960). "On the Causation of Varicose Veins." John Wright, Bristol.
CLEAVE, T. L., CAMPBELL, G. D. and PAINTER, N. S. (1969). "Diabetes, Coronary Thrombosis and the Saccharine Disease." John Wright, Bristol.
GRECH, P. (1965). *East African Medical Journal* **42**, 106.
HAFTER, E. (1958). *American Journal of Digestive Diseases* **3**, 901.
HARRINGTON, S. W. (1940). *American Journal of Surgery* **50**, 377.
HEATON, K. W. (1973). *Nutrition, London* **27**, 170.
JOHNSON, A. C. and JOHNSON, S. (1969). *Australian Radiology* **13**, 287.
JOHNSTONE, A. S. (1941). *Lancet* **2**, 18.
JOHNSTONE, A. S. (1943). *British Journal of Radiology* **16**, 357.
KIM, E. H. (1964). *New England Journal of Medicine* **271**, 764.
LATTO, C., WILKINSON, R. W. and GILMORE, O. J. A. (1973). *Lancet* **1**, 1089.
MACLEAN, C. D. T. (1959). *British Journal of Clinical Practice* **13**, 849.
MOORE, E. W. (1967). *East African Medical Journal* **44**, 513.
MULLER, C. J. B. (1948). *South African Medical Journal* **22**, 376.
PAINTER, N. S. (1964). *Annals of the Royal College of Surgeons of England* **34**, 98.
PAINTER, N. S. (1967). *American Journal of Digestive Diseases* **12**, 222.
PRIDIE, R. B. (1966). *Gut* **7**, 188.
SMITHERS, D. W. (1945). *British Journal of Radiology* **18**, 199.
SMITHERS, D. W. (1961). *In* "Tumours of the Oseophagus" (N. C. Tanner and D. W. Smithers, eds), p. 67. Livingstone, Edinburgh.
STEIN, G. N. and FINKELSTEIN, A. (1960). *American Journal of Digestive Diseases* **5**, 77.
TROWELL, H. (1960). "Non-infective Disease in Africa", p. 198. Edward Arnold, London.
TROWELL, H., PAINTER, N. S. and BURKITT, D. P. (1974). *American Journal of Digestive Diseases* **19**, 864.
WHITTAKER, L. R. (1966). *East African Medical Journal* **43**, 336.
WOLF, B. S. and GUGLIELMO, J. (1957). *Medical Radiography and Photography* **33**, 90.
ZEPPA, R. and POLK, H. C. (1971). *Journal of the Florida Medical Association* **58**, 26.

Part VI

Other disorders related to refined carbohydrate foods

Chapter 14

Gallstones and cholecystitis

KENNETH HEATON

I. Introduction 173
II. Epidemiology of gallstones. 174
   A. Some general remarks 174
   B. Gallstones in the western world 175
   C. Gallstones in developing countries 176
   D. Changes in gallstone incidence with urbanization and western-
      ization 177
   E. Changes on emigration. 178
III. Diet and the aetiology of gallstones 179
   A. Theories for the aetiology of gallstones 179
   B. Diet and the epidemiology of gallstones 179
   C. Diet and the diseases associated with gallstones . . . 180
   D. Diet and experimental gallstones in animals 182
   E. Diet and the biochemical mechanisms leading to gallstone
      formation 183
IV. Summary 189
References 190

I. Introduction

Clinical disease of the gallbladder is secondary to gallstones in nearly all cases. Stones were present in 98% of cholecystectomy patients in England and America (Munster and Brown, 1967; Holland and Heaton, 1972), and in the remaining 2% it is possible that stones had been passed. In effect, the problem of gallbladder disease is the problem of gallstones.

The traditional classification of gallstones into cholesterol, mixed and pigment stones is now felt to be unhelpful, since chemical analysis shows that stones vary in composition continuously over a wide spectrum (*Lancet*, 1968). Pure pigment stones occur in the gallbladder in haemolytic states and cirrhosis of the liver. In the Orient these also occur in the common bile duct, probably as a result of biliary infection. With these exceptions, all

173

gallstones contain cholesterol in amounts varying continuously from a few per cent to 100%. In all western countries, cholesterol is the predominant component. In England, cholesterol comprises about 60% of the average stone, in the U.S.A. 74% and in Sweden 88%. Minor components are calcium carbonate, calcium palmitate and calcium phosphate (Sutor and Wooley, 1971). The problem of gallstones is to a large extent the problem of cholesterol precipitation from bile.

Current thinking considers gallstone formation to be a three-stage process. The basic metabolic defect is the production of bile supersaturated with cholesterol (lithogenic bile). This is followed by the precipitation of cholesterol microcrystals, which requires a seeding or nucleating agent, and finally the growth or agglomeration of the crystals to form calculi.

The aetiology of gallstones is traditionally regarded as a complex and obscure subject lacking a coherent hypothesis. This is probably because: (1) aetiology (cause) has often been confused with pathogenesis (mechanism); an aetiological hypothesis is obviously more plausible if it fits into a detailed scheme of pathogenesis, but it can stand alone when it fits the epidemiology and clinical associations of the disease; recent research has clarified the mechanism of gallstone formation but has largely ignored its cause; (2) not enough attention has been paid to the epidemiology of gallstones, although this provides powerful clues to their aetiology; (3) while many workers have suspected that diet is the major factor, their thinking about diet has been imprecise or preoccupied with fat. The new concepts of carbohydrate-refining and fibre depletion provide an entirely new perspective on the relationship between diet and gallstone formation.

II. Epidemiology of gallstones

A. Some general remarks

In no country is the exact prevalence of cholelithiasis known. This is because the disease is non-fatal and because about 70% of patients are asymptomatic and so undiagnosed. Autopsy surveys provide the best indication of prevalence, but autopsied subjects are a selected and atypical sub-group of the population. In comparing autopsy surveys, allowance has to be made for the steady increase of gallstone incidence with advancing age and for the usually 2-fold greater frequency in women, factors which are well-known determinants of gallstone incidence in at least western countries. Clinical records, especially operation registers, supply some indication of gallstone frequency in a community, but these are influenced by extraneous factors such as diagnostic skill, radiological facilities and attitudes to surgical treatment.

In spite of these limitations, some generalizations can be made about the frequency of gallstones in different places and at different times (Heaton, 1973a).

B. Gallstones in the western world

Gallstones are common or very common in all western countries for which statistics are available. A much-quoted figure is the one-third of a million gallbladders removed each year in the U.S.A. (Glenn, 1970). In female Americans, cholecystectomy is a commoner operation than appendicectomy (Pearson et al., 1968). In a 10 year survey at Framingham, Massachusetts, 8% of the population in the age-group 30–62 had symptoms of gallbladder disease, or after death were found to have it at autopsy (Friedman et al., 1966). In a large autopsy series at Philadelphia, covering the period 1920 to 1949, gallstones were found in 16·8% of women and 7·8% of men aged over 20 (Lieber, 1952). American Indians have the highest known prevalence of cholelithiasis of any population, and Indian women develop the disease at an extraordinarily early age. A cholecystographic survey of Pima Indians in Arizona revealed gallstones in no less than 73% of women aged 25–34 (Sampliner et al., 1970). American negroes probably get gallstones as often as the white population. In Philadelphia, negroes provide 36% of all hospital admissions and 42% of admissions for treatment of cholesterol gallstones (Trotman and Soloway, 1973).

In England, cholecystectomy is probably the commonest elective abdominal operation (Dawson, 1973). Autopsy surveys suggest that 21–41% of women and 12–20% of men are destined to develop gallstones by their seventies (Gross, 1929; Horn, 1956; Bouchier, 1969). In Sweden, the odds on getting cholelithiasis are even higher. By the age of 70, gallstones had formed in 70% of women and 35% of men subjected to autopsy in the city of Malmö (Sternby, 1968). In other European countries the situation is probably much the same, though less well documented. In Australia, too, gallstones are very common, being present in 31% of autopsied subjects in Brisbane (Burnett, 1971) and accounting for 3% of female admissions to hospital in Melbourne (Wheeler et al., 1970). The situation is little better in New Zealand (Doouss and Castleden, 1973).

Have gallstones always been so common in western civilization? Almost certainly not. The present "epidemic proportions" have only been reached since the Second World War. In Bristol, the frequency of operations on the gallbladder rose 230% between 1950 and 1970, the main increase occurring in the 1950s (Holland and Heaton, 1972). In the same period even bigger increases were noted in two Swedish cities (Edlund and Olsson, 1956; van der Linden and Rentzhog, 1960). In America, the "increasing burden on surgical facilities" from gallstone disease has caused concern (Glenn, 1970) and has stimulated intensive research in recent years. Nevertheless, cholelithiasis was a common disease before the Second World War (Gross, 1929). Whether or not it was common before the present century is impossible to ascertain, since so few statistics were kept. In perhaps the earliest recorded autopsy series, Haller, in the mid eighteenth century, found gallstones in 14 out of 230 autopsies in Göttingen, Germany (Thudichum, 1863). At the same time the first English book about this disease was being written by Thomas Coe (1757), who ventured the opinion that gallstones "happen much oftener than is commonly supposed". Coe agreed, however, that gallstones had probably not been so common in the previous century, if only because that prolific seventeenth-century writer, the physician Thomas Sydenham, had failed to mention gallstones at all. Tentatively, therefore, one may hypothesize that cholelithiasis began to be reasonably common in England during the seventeenth and early eighteenth centuries. This is not necessarily true of other European countries; indeed, in Finland the overall autopsy incidence of gallstones was only 0·2% before 1879, but climbed to 14% by 1930–39 (Ehrström, 1942). Finland in the nineteenth century was of course a poorer and more rural country than England.

As gallstones have become commoner they have spread to affect a wider range of social classes. In America, cholelithiasis was regarded until the late nineteenth century as a disease of sedentary people, which presumably meant the middle and upper classes (Osler, 1892), but nowadays no class difference in gallstone incidence is recognized. As gallstones have become commoner they have spread to affect younger people. In Bristol, the under-30 age-group accounted for only 4% of gallbladder operations between 1933 and 1950, but by 1970 this figure had risen to over 9% (Holland and Heaton, 1972). In Östersund, Sweden, the under-30s' share of gallbladder surgery rose from 7% to 13% during the decade up to 1957 (van der Linden and Rentzhog, 1960). In Canada, where gallbladder operations have increased 2½-fold in 10 years, a recent survey showed that 26% of cholecystectomy patients are aged under 35 (Plant et al., 1973). In the affluent countries of the west, gallstones can no longer be regarded as a disease of the middle-aged and elderly. Indeed, in Sweden it is no longer a rarity for a child to require a gallbladder operation (Hagberg et al., 1962; Nilsson, 1966).

C. Gallstones in developing countries

There is relatively little published information on the frequency of gallstones in developing countries. This in itself suggests that the disease is uncommon, because absence of a disease naturally provokes less comment than its presence; also epidemiological statistics are far more tedious to collect if a disease is rare. However, more systematic evidence is required before absence or rarity can be used to support a hypothesis.

The developing communities with the best documentation of gallstone frequency are in sub-Saharal Africa. In Uganda, an autopsy survey showed gallstones to be present in only 1·35% of subjects aged 35–64 (Owor, 1964). Moreover, the calculi found were mostly pure pigment stones, which represent an entirely different disease from the cholesterol-rich stones of the west. In West Africa, too, gallstones are a rarity. When Edington (1957) reviewed 4395 autopsies performed in Ghana between 1923 and 1955, he did not find a single case of cholelithiasis. In the first 5 years of Ibadan University Hospital, only 27 patients were admitted to the surgical wards on account of this disease (Parnis, 1964). Such patients as do present with gallstones in these areas tend to be wealthy, obese and eating a westernized diet. Denis Burkitt (p.c., 1974) recalls that in 17 years' surgical practice in East Africa he operated on only two patients with gallstones, one of whom was a queen. At the time of writing, figures from replies to question-naires received by D. B. amply confirm personal impressions. Twelve hospitals in Uganda have supplied 109 monthly returns and have not reported a single case of gallstones. The same is true of Malawi after 102 hospital months. In Tanzania, 207 hospital months have yielded only two cases and in Kenya 67 hospital months have turned up just one case. In West Africa, 13 Nigerian hospitals have seen only two patients with gallstones in a total of 109 months.

Statistics from societies little influenced by western cultures outside Africa are inadequate, but a hospital in Papua has completed 12 monthly questionnaires without seeing a single case of gallstones.

In the Far East, pigment gallstones are not uncommon but cholesterol-rich stones are relatively rare, at least in rural areas (Yagi, 1960; Maki, 1961; Miyake and Johnston, 1968). Adequate statistics are lacking from India, but in the lowlands of Northern India at least, gallstones seem to be relatively common. However, the most striking finding of Malhotra (1968) was a marked class difference in incidence. In social classes I and II, cholelithiasis was diagnosed 13 times more often than in class III and 22 times more often than in class IV.

D. Changes in gallstone incidence with urbanization and western-ization

In developing countries and communities, urbanization and westernization are followed by an increase in gallstone incidence. This can be illustrated by the experience of such widely differing groups as the Japanese, the Eskimo, the African in Africa and, less securely, the negro in America.

Japanese workers in several centres have reported that since the Second World War there has been a substantial increase in cholesterol gallstones. This has been masked to some extent by a decrease in pigment stones (Yagi, 1960; Maki *et al.*, 1964; Kameda, 1967; Nakayama and Miyake, 1970). Nevertheless, at the University of Tokyo Department of Pathology, the autopsy incidence of gallstones rose from 2·5% in 1949 to 6·1% in 1964 (Kameda, 1967). In Japanese cities, cholesterol gallstones are now the commonest variety, but in the country pigment stones still predominate (Yagi, 1960; Maki, 1961; Kameda, 1967).

The Canadian Eskimo rarely suffered from cholelithiasis when he lived in his traditional nomadic way, but since he has taken to living in townships like Inuvik where western "culture" holds sway, gallstones have become so common that "operations for gallbladder disease have outnumbered all other operative procedures" (Schaefer, 1971).

Africans living in the cities of Africa seem to be much more prone to gallstones than their rural brothers. In Johannesburg, stones were found at autopsy in no less than 10% of Bantu females in their forties (Becker and Chatgidakis, 1952). This may be a relatively recent phenomenon. In Accra, gallstones were unknown up to 1955 (Edington, 1957), but in recent years they have accounted for 0·4% of surgical admissions (Archampong, 1969). In the southern United States in the early years of this century, negro males were regarded as virtually immune to gallstones (Cunningham and Hardenbergh, 1956), but in 1963 Hall found biliary calculi in 6·4% of autopsied male negroes in the Panama Canal Zone.

E. Changes on emigration

There have been no systematic investigations into the effect of emigration on gallstone incidence. However, Italians seem to acquire an increased incidence when they emigrate to Australia. In Melbourne, 4·8% of Italians entering hospital do so for the treatment of gallstones, whereas in Italy itself gallstones account for only 1·5% of hospital admissions (Hills, 1971). The Japanese who have emigrated to Hawaii are probably more prone to cholesterol gallstones than those in Japan (G. N. Stemmermann, p.c. 1973). American negroes seem as prone to gallstones as their white compatriots (Trotman and Soloway, 1973), although the disease is rare in their place of origin, West Africa.

In summary, the epidemiology of cholesterol-rich gallstones suggests that this is essentially a disease of modern western civilization. Western countries have experienced a rising incidence of the disease since the Second World War, and some western women now have a more than even chance of developing gallstones in their lifetime.

III. Diet and the aetiology of gallstones

A. Theories for the aetiology of gallstones

No credence is now given to old theories that gallstones are caused by biliary stasis due to a sedentary existence or to tight corseting. Infection of the gallbladder has been a popular theory in the last 100 years, but this has withered for lack of evidence, except in the case of typhoid. Today it is generally accepted that gallstone formation is a metabolic disease. Of exogenous influences on metabolism, only diet has received serious consideration.

B. Diet and the epidemiology of gallstones

In primitive societies where gallstones are rare or unknown, the diet is very variable. Most rural Africans live on cereals such as maize and millet, or roots such as cassava, but the Masai consume little except milk and blood, while the primitive Eskimo is virtually a pure carnivore. One common feature of these and all primitive diets is the absence of highly refined carbohydrate. Civilized diets have characteristic components other than refined carbohydrate, notably saturated animal fat and animal protein. However, animal foods are expensive and refined carbohydrate is cheap and in the affluent societies of today it is no longer the rich who have the highest risk of gallstones, but the poor. In America it is the deprived Indian who gets most gallstones, and in England it is probably the relatively poor Northerner (Heaton, 1973a). In past centuries, when refined carbohydrate was expensive, it was the higher social classes who were more prone to cholelithiasis. Similarly, in developing countries today it is townspeople and the professional classes who first learn to adopt western eating habits, and they who are first to develop cholelithiasis.

The big post-war increase in gallstone frequency in Europe was associated with a steady decline in the consumption of bread, potatoes and oatmeal (starchy and more or less fibrous carbohydrates) and steady increases in the use of fibre-free sucrose. At the same time, the incidence of obesity increased (Khosla and Lowe, 1968).

Some workers, especially in Japan, have postulated that it is deficiency of polyunsaturated fatty acids which causes cholesterol gallstones. However, this view has been rendered untenable by the recent finding of Sturdevant et al. (1973) that volunteers eating a diet rich in polyunsaturated fatty acids had an *increased* incidence of gallstones.

C. Diet and the diseases associated with gallstones

The diseases associated with cholesterol-rich gallstones (and not caused by the stones) are obesity, diabetes, probably coronary heart disease and ileal disease or resection (Heaton, 1973a). Ileal disease and resection need not be considered further since ileal dysfunction itself is believed to cause the gallstone-forming tendency (Heaton and Read, 1969; Dowling *et al.*, 1973).

The association of gallstones with obesity has long been recognized. For example, in a survey in Brisbane, gallstone patients weighed 5·5 kg

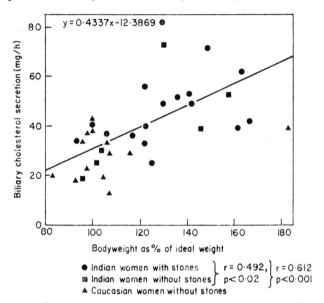

● Indian women with stones ⎫ r = 0·492, ⎫ r = 0·612
🖪 Indian women without stones ⎰ p< 0·02 ⎰ p<0·001
▲ Caucasian women without stones

FIG. 14.1. The relationship between excess body weight and bile cholesterol secretion. This graph was plotted from data published by Grundy *et al.* (1972a).

more than matched controls (Burnett, 1971). The relationship is at least partly explained by the recent finding that as body weight goes up, so does the secretion of cholesterol into bile (Fig. 14.1) (Grundy *et al.*, 1972a). Overnutrition is probably a crucial factor in gallstone formation. The mere fact of eating a high calorie diet promotes cholesterol secretion, and on dietary analysis gallstone patients have been shown to take in more calories than controls (Sarles *et al.*, 1968, 1970). The post-war tendency of the disease to spread more to men and to young people parallels a post-war increase of obesity in men and in the young (Montegriffo, 1971; Walker and Richardson, 1971). There are compelling reasons for blaming most overnutrition on eating foods with an artificially increased energy/satiety ratio, namely refined carbohydrates (Cleave *et al.*, 1969; Heaton, 1973b; see also Chapters 6 and 16).

Diabetics have an increased proneness to gallstones (Gross, 1929; Lieber, 1952; Newman and Northup, 1959), and gallstone patients are diabetic twice as often as expected (Watkinson, 1967). The world records for the prevalence of diabetes and of gallstones are both held by the same unfortunate community, the Pima Indians, who are also exceptionally obese (Kravetz, 1964). It is a well-known clinical fact that obesity and diabetes are closely associated. One may therefore regard obesity, diabetes and gallstones as three overlapping or interlinked diseases (Fig. 14.2). This suggests that they share a common aetiological factor. The evidence linking diabetes with refined carbohydrate is discussed elsewhere (Cleave *et al.*, 1969; see also Chapter 16).

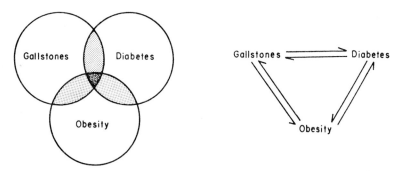

FIG. 14.2. Schematic representation of the clinical and biochemical overlap between obesity, diabetes and gallstones.

The association between gallstones and coronary heart disease (CHD) is controversial, but on balance the evidence does favour its existence (Heaton, 1973a). A major risk indicator for CHD is elevation of the plasma triglyceride level (Carlson and Böttiger, 1972). In gallstone patients, the plasma triglyceride level was found to be very significantly raised by Braunsteiner *et al.* (1966). The mean value was 163 mg/100 ml compared with 98 mg/100 ml in matched controls. Conversely, it has been found by T. Scherstén (p.c., 1973) that patients with high plasma triglycerides (type IV hyperlipoproteinaemia) have an increased risk of cholelithiasis. The link between these two conditions is apparent also in the finding that the contraceptive pill causes both an increased serum triglyceride level (Stokes and Wynn, 1971) and an increased risk of being operated on for gallstones (Report from the Boston Collaborative Drug Surveillance Programme, 1973). The relationship between gallstones and serum triglycerides could explain the link between gallstones and coronary disease (Chapter 15).

Sailer (1972) drew attention to the frequent coexistence in the same patient of obesity, diabetes and hypertriglyceridaemia and to the fact that all three conditions are ameliorated by weight reduction. He suggested that the triad of diseases should be regarded as a manifestation of overnutrition. I should like to propose that cholesterol-rich gallstones be included to make a tetrad of closely related diseases (Fig. 14.3) with a common aetiology in refined carbohydrate.

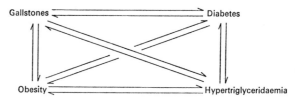

Gallstones · Diabetes

Obesity · Hypertriglyceridaemia

FIG. 14.3. An interlocking network of associated diseases. Each line represents a documented association.

D. Diet and experimental gallstones in animals

Cholesterol-rich gallstones can be induced in a variety of animals by feeding artificial diets. In the pioneer work of Dam and Christensen (1952) a diet containing 70% sucrose or glucose induced gallstones in most young hamsters. Later workers confirmed this finding and showed that this diet also induced diabetes (Hikasa *et al.*, 1969). The diet is most lithogenic if it is devoid of fat. It loses its effect if the sugar is replaced by an uncooked starchy carbohydrate.

Table 14.1 summarizes the composition of diets used to produce cholesterol-rich gallstones in six mammalian species by seven different groups of workers. It is obviously important to know if these diets have anything in common. All the diets are semi-synthetic and therefore highly abnormal for any animal. Otherwise, they appear at first sight to be very different from one another. However, they do all share one characteristic: the carbohydrate in the diet is always refined and fibre-depleted; consequently, no diet contains significant quantities of crude fibre. A low intake of fibre is grossly abnormal for herbivorous animals like the rabbit and prairie dog, but not abnormal at all for the domesticated dog. The common factor in these lithogenic diets is therefore not so much the absence of fibre as the presence of carbohydrate stripped of its natural complement of fibre, that is refined carbohydrate. (It may be added that the presence in two diets of some ground cellulose, probably derived from cotton, does not make them less abnormal, since the presence of intact dietary fibre cannot be equated with the addition of purified, powdered cellulose.) In the non-carnivorous species there is probably an absolute requirement for fibre or at least bulk. In the hamster the diet loses its lithogenic action if it is supplemented with artificial bulking agents such as agar and carboxy-

methylcellulose, or even if straw is laid on the floor of the animals' cages
(Hikasa *et al.*, 1969).

Other writers have suggested that the lithogenic factor in these diets is
deficiency of essential (polyunsaturated) fatty acids (Hikasa *et al.*, 1969).
However, in man addition of such fatty acids to the diet actually induces
gallstones (Sturdevant *et al.*, 1973).

TABLE 14.1. Diets used to produce cholesterol-rich gallstones in animals

mal	Carbohydrate in diet	Crude fibre in diet	Other features of diet	Reference
er	72% glucose or sucrose	Nil	Fat-free	Dam and Christensen (1952) Hikasa *et al.* (1969)
	51% glucose	Nil	31% fat, added cholesterol and cholic acid	Tepperman *et al.* (1964)
	34% sucrose, 14% corn-starch	Trace (0·03%)	41% calories as fat, added cholesterol, 2·6% ground cellulose	Brenneman *et al.* (1972)
	7% sucrose, 6½% glucose, 6% corn-starch	Trace (0·01%)	40% casein, 15% olive oil, 15% ground cellulose	Borgman and Haselden (1968)
el key	62% sucrose	Nil	45% calories as fat, added cholesterol	Osuga and Portman (1971)
	50% sucrose, 26% corn-starch	Trace (0·05%)	Low protein, added cholesterol	Englert *et al.* (1969)

Note: The figures for crude fibre are calculated on the basis that corn-starch
contains 0·2% fibre (Platt, 1962).

The writer knows of no unifying hypothesis to explain gallstone production in animals apart from the refined carbohydrate hypothesis.

Diet and the biochemical mechanisms leading to gallstone formation

In the last few years there has been intensive research into the biochemical
mechanisms leading to the precipitation of cholesterol in bile. It is now
generally agreed that the basic defect is oversaturation of the bile with
cholesterol, that is an excess of cholesterol relative to its solubilizers, bile
salt and lecithin (Admirand and Small, 1968). Bile with this lithogenic
property is present in the gallbladders of most patients with gallstones.*
It is also present in many non-gallstone patients if they live in a country

* The fact that a few gallstone patients have unsaturated gallbladder bile
(Smallwood *et al.*, 1972; Heller and Bouchier, 1973) can be explained on the basis
that the gallstone-forming diathesis is intermittent like the peptic ulcer diathesis,
so some samples are inevitably obtained in a normal period.

with a high incidence of cholelithiasis (Nakayama and van der Linden, 1970 1971; Redinger and Small, 1972; Dowling *et al.*, 1973), but not if they live in countries with a low incidence of cholelithiasis (Biss *et al.*, 1971 Nakayama and van der Linden, 1971). This shows first that the production of bile supersaturated with cholesterol is a prerequisite for gallstone formation and secondly that other conditions must be present for cholesterol to crystallize out and form into stones. Nothing is known of these other conditions (Holzbach *et al.*, 1972). However, a good deal is known about dietary manipulations which favour the fundamental abnormality, i.e formation of supersaturated bile.

Gallbladder bile becomes supersaturated either because it contains too much cholesterol or because it contains too little bile salt. A theoretical third possibility, deficiency of lecithin, will not be considered further because lecithin secretion is closely dependent upon bile salt secretion (Nilsson and Scherstén, 1969). Probably, both cholesterol excess and bile salt deficiency contribute to human gallstone formation, and both can be explained as effects of refined carbohydrate.

1. Bile salt deficiency and diet

The key factor determining the bile salt content of the relaxed gallbladder (in which, presumably, it is easiest for gallstones to form and grow), is the size of the circulating bile salt pool (Heaton, 1975). In patients with gallstones, the bile salt pool is only 50–60% of its normal size of 2–3 g (Vlahcevic *et al.*, 1970, 1972; Pomare and Heaton, 1973a). This shrinkage of the bile salt pool could be blamed in part on gallbladder dysfunction, but it probably does precede the formation of gallstones, since it has been demonstrated in stone-free subjects who have supersaturated bile (Bell *et al.*, 1973). The small bile salt pool is most probably due to inhibition of bile salt synthesis by the liver (Grundy *et al.*, 1972a).* The livers of patients with gallstones show decreased activity of the enzyme which controls the rate of bile salt synthesis—7 α-hydroxylase (Nicolau *et al.*, 1974).

Clearly, therefore, any dietary change which leads to inhibition of bile salt synthesis is a likely candidate as a cause of gallstones.

In animals, it has repeatedly been shown that semi-synthetic diets rich in refined carbohydrate suppress the liver synthesis of bile salts. This was first established by Coburn and Annegers (1950) in experiments using bile fistula dogs. In such animals, the constant drainage of bile salts stimulates the liver to synthesize new bile salt at a maximal rate. In fasting

---

* It has recently been found that small pools circulate more rapidly during digestion (Northfield and Hofmann, 1973), but whether this is cause or effect or an irrelevant side-phenomenon remains to be determined.

dogs, the output (= synthesis) of cholate could be markedly increased by feeding protein, but this effect was reduced by pre-feeding a semi-synthetic, high calorie diet, and completely abolished when the diet was rich in sucrose. In other experiments the stimulant effect of a mixed diet on cholate synthesis was abolished by adding to it 25 or 50 g sucrose per day. Similar information was obtained in rats in a more physiological setting by Portman and Murphy (1958). They used diets which were regarded as nutritionally complete but contained 68% sucrose or starch and no fibre. Rats eating such diets had a cholate pool of only 45 mg compared with 99 mg in rats eating Purina laboratory chow, which contains ground whole cereals, rich in fibre (Fig. 14.4). There was an even greater reduction in

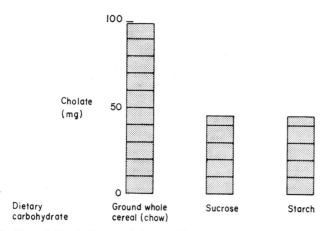

FIG. 14.4. Size of the cholate pool (comprising most of the bile salt pool) in rats fed three diets of differing carbohydrate content. Drawn from the data of Portman and Murphy (1958).

the cholate synthesis rate, from 36 mg/day on chow to 10 and 8 mg/day respectively on starch and sugar. Other studies in rats and rabbits have confirmed that bile salt synthesis is reduced on diets containing much sugar or starch and little or no fibre (Hellström et al., 1962; Lee and Herrmann, 1963; Gustafsson and Norman, 1969). In Rhesus monkeys, a fat-free sucrose-containing diet caused the bile salt pool to shrink from 1·10 to 0·50 mmol and daily bile salt synthesis to fall from 1·43 to 0·49 mmol (Redinger et al., 1973). These semi-synthetic diets are very similar to those which other investigators have used to make animals form gallstones and secrete bile supersaturated with cholesterol (Table 14.1).

At present, there is no human counterpart to these animal experiments. However, it seems reasonable to assume that, in susceptible subjects, the liver will react to a diet rich in refined carbohydrate by reducing its synthesis of bile salts and so contract the circulating bile salt pool. As to how refined diets exert this effect on the liver, there is unfortunately no evidence. Increased absorption from the colon of an inhibitory substance, possibly lithocholate, has been suggested (Heaton, 1972) but not so far confirmed.

2. Cholesterol excess

The cholesterol in gallbladder bile is cholesterol which has been secreted by the liver into the bile canaliculi and carried into the gallbladder as it fills during its post-prandial relaxation. In a given individual the liver is believed to secrete cholesterol at a rather constant rate. A minimum rate of bile salt secretion is necessary to initiate the movement of cholesterol into bile, but above quite a low rate of bile salt secretion, the movement of cholesterol seems to proceed independently (Wagner et al., 1973).

The evidence that oversecretion of cholesterol by the liver is important in the production of supersaturated bile may be summarized as follows.

(1) Direct measurement of 24 h bile lipid outputs, using a perfusion technique, has shown that women with gallstones and supersaturated bile put out nearly twice as much cholesterol as control subjects (Grundy et al., 1972a; Grundy et al., 1974). A criticism of these studies is that most of the gallstone subjects were obese and most of the controls were slim.

(2) Enrichment of the American diet with polyunsaturated fatty acids is associated with an increased incidence of gallstones (Sturdevant et al., 1973). Polyunsaturated fatty acids are believed to increase the excretion of cholesterol into the bile, and so to decrease the plasma cholesterol (Sodhi et al., 1967).

(3) The hypolipidaemic drug clofibrate increases the flux of cholesterol into bile (Grundy et al., 1972b) and makes the bile supersaturated (Pertsemlidis et al., 1974). It is under suspicion as causing more gallstones.

(4) Feeding the bile acid chenodeoxycholic acid in a dose of $1\cdot0$–$1\cdot5$ g/ day to patients with radiolucent gallstones frequently causes the stones to dissolve and almost always renders the bile undersaturated with cholesterol (Thistle and Hofmann, 1973; Mok et al., 1974). Chenodeoxycholic acid has been shown to act primarily by reducing the secretion of cholesterol into bile (Northfield et al., 1973). This suggests that an increase in cholesterol secretion was involved in the formation of these stones.

(5) Man is the only animal to develop gallstones at all commonly. The main difference in bile composition between man and other species is the much higher concentration of cholesterol in man.

3. *Diet and biliary cholesterol*

Surprisingly little is known about the effects of different diets upon the cholesterol content of bile. Studies with saturated and unsaturated fat have given conflicting results (for references see Heaton, 1972). Raising cholesterol intake has recently been shown to increase the saturation of bile with cholesterol (DenBesten *et al.*, 1973). However, the subjects in this experiment were eating a semi-synthetic diet (rich in sucrose and devoid of fibre) and the results cannot be extrapolated to normal dietary conditions. The unsaturated fat diet of Sturdevant *et al.* (1973), which seemed to cause gallstones, was a *low* cholesterol diet.

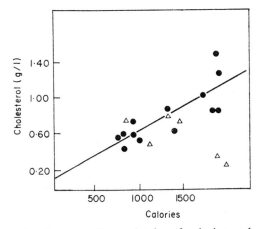

FIG. 14.5. Correlation between dietary intake of calories and concentration of cholesterol in bile. Bile samples were aspirated from a T-tube which had been placed in the common bile duct during the course of biliary surgery. In patients with gallstones, shown as closed circles, there is a significant correlation ($r = 0.81$; $P < 0.001$). From Sarles *et al.* (1968).

A link between refined carbohydrate and excess biliary cholesterol has not been proven, but it is probable on two different counts:

(1) Refined carbohydrate, especially sugar, is inherently prone to cause overnutrition, since the loss of fibre removes a natural barrier to energy intake (see Chapter 6 and Heaton, 1973b). Overnutrition undoubtedly leads to increased cholesterol secretion. In short-term experiments, Sarles *et al.* (1968) showed not only a correlation between previous calorie intake and bile cholesterol concentration (Fig. 14.5) but also a predictable rise in bile cholesterol 2 days after the calorie intake was increased. Unfortunately, these studies were done in post-cholecystectomy patients with T-tubes in their common bile ducts, and these findings need to be confirmed

in a more physiological setting. The best evidence that overnutrition causes cholesterol hyper-secrction is the strong correlation (P < 0·01) between 24 h bile cholesterol output and body weight. This has been shown by Grundy et al. (1974) in both white and Indian women. This relationship is explained by the fact that in obesity there is an increased production of cholesterol by the liver. Indeed, cholesterol production is directly related to the weight of body fat (Miettinen, 1971; Nestel et al., 1973).

Whenever cholesterol production is increased, there is an elevation of the fasting plasma triglyceride level, probably because the triglyceride-rich pre-β-lipoprotein is the major carrier of blood cholesterol (Sodhi and Kudchodkar, 1973). The association between gallstones and raised plasma triglycerides (see p. 181) is explained if both are reflections of increased cholesterol synthesis by the liver. The links between these three abnormalities and overnutrition are most satisfyingly explained by the following scheme:

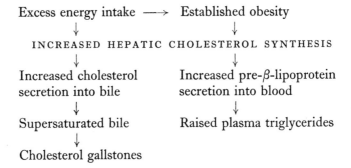

The author follows Cleave in believing that the main cause of excess energy intake in civilized societies is the consumption of fibre-depleted foods, especially sucrose. If this is so, and if the above scheme is correct, then sucrose must be considered as a major cause of oversecretion of cholesterol into bile.

(2) The second link between refined carbohydrate and cholesterol over-secretion lies in the recent discovery that the secretion of cholesterol is affected by the proportions in the bile of the two dihydroxy bile salts, chenodeoxycholate and deoxycholate. As mentioned above, feeding cheno-deoxycholate reduces cholesterol secretion and so makes bile under-saturated. Recently, two of the author's colleagues, Low-Beer and Pomare (1975), showed that feeding deoxycholate to 16 healthy volunteers made the bile *more* saturated with cholesterol. At the same time, the amount of chenodeoxycholate in the bile was markedly reduced, due to the fact that the synthesis of this bile salt was suppressed by the administered

deoxycholate (Low-Beer and Pomare, 1973). This suggests that the adverse effect of deoxycholate derives from its displacement of chenodeoxycholate.

Deoxycholate is normally present in human bile; indeed in healthy British subjects it comprises about 25% of the circulating bile salt pool. This amount of deoxycholate may not be desirable. In bile samples from Nigeria, analysed in the author's laboratory, deoxycholate comprised only 12–15% of the bile salt pool, and gallstones are uncommon in Nigeria.

Deoxycholate is a secondary bile salt, that is to say it is formed in the colon by bacterial degradation of the major bile salt cholate. The presence of deoxycholate in bile is therefore the result of two colonic events: bacterial metabolism (specifically, dehydroxylation), and absorption of a bacterial metabolite from the faecal stream. Since colonic function is so strikingly modified by dietary fibre (see Chapter 7) it would be surprising if the production and/or absorption of deoxycholate were not influenced by fibre. In fact, studies in the author's laboratory have confirmed that fibre, or at least bran, does have such an influence.

When bran, about 33 g a day, was fed to five volunteers, the proportion of deoxycholate in bile fell by about half. Studies with radioactively labelled taurocholate confirmed that bran interfered with the appearance of deoxycholate in the bile (Pomare and Heaton, 1973b). It remains to be shown whether bran acts by reducing the formation or the absorption of deoxycholate, but the latter seems more likely. Further studies showed that bran reduced the circulating deoxycholate pool by about 30% and this was matched by an increase in the pool of chenodeoxycholate, due to increased hepatic synthesis of chenodeoxycholate. Most importantly, the bran-treated liver, like the chenodeoxycholate-treated liver, secreted bile which was less saturated with cholesterol. In six women with gallstones, feeding bran in an average "dose" of 47 g daily reduced the molar percentage of cholesterol in duodenal bile samples from 14·1 to 10·6% (Pomare et al., 1974).

These studies suggest that a high-fibre diet may lessen the risk of gallstone formation. By inference, fibre-depleted foods may increase the risk of gallstones, not only by promoting surplus energy intake, but also by allowing excessive absorption of deoxycholate from the colon.

IV. Summary

Epidemiologically, cholesterol-rich gallstones are a disease of civilization, especially of modern technological societies. The disease seems to be on the increase in both developing and developed countries, and to be involving younger people. Clinically, it is associated with obesity, diabetes and raised plasma triglycerides. This points to overnutrition as a key factor. Experimentally, cholelithiasis can be produced in animals by feeding semi-synthetic diets rich in fibre-depleted carbohydrate. The essential first stage in gallstone formation is the secretion of bile supersaturated with cholesterol. Such bile has a dual origin—oversecretion of cholesterol, and underproduction of bile salts causing a shrinkage of the bile salt pool. Both biochemical abnormalities are explicable as effects of refined carbohydrates. Overnutrition, which can for the most part be blamed on refined carbohydrate, is a potent cause of excess cholesterol secretion. Cholesterol excess can also result from high levels in the circulating bile salt pool of deoxycholate, a bacterial metabolite absorbed from the colon. Bran feeding reduces this absorption and improves supersaturated bile. This suggests that the abnormal colonic function produced by a refined diet may contribute to gallstone formation. In animals refined semi-synthetic diets also depress bile salt synthesis and cause the bile salt pool to shrink. No other environmental factor apart from refined carbohydrate can explain the epidemiological, clinical, experimental and biochemical facts of cholelithiasis.

References

ADMIRAND, W. H. and SMALL, D. M. (1968). *Journal of Clinical Investigation* **47**, 1043.

ARCHAMPONG, E. Q. (1969). *Ghana Medical Journal* **8**, 134.

BECKER, J. P. and CHATGIDAKIS, C. B. (1952). *South African Journal of Clinical Science* **3**, 13.

BELL, C. C., VLAHCEVIC, Z. R., PRAZICH, J. and SWELL, L. (1973). *Surgery, Gynecology and Obstetrics* **136**, 961.

BISS, K., HO, K.-J., MIKKELSON, B., LEWIS, L. and TAYLOR, C. B. (1971). *New England Journal of Medicine* **284**, 694.

BORGMAN, R. F. and HASELDEN, F. H. (1968). *American Journal of Veterinary Research* **29**, 1287.

BOUCHIER, I. A. D. (1969). *Gut* **10**, 705.

BRAUNSTEINER, H., DI PAULI, R., SAILER, S. and SANDHOFER, F. (1966). *Schweizerische Medizinische Wochenschrift* **96**, 44.

BRENNEMAN, D. E., CONNOR, W. E., FORKER, E. L. and DENBESTEN, L. (1972). *Journal of Clinical Investigation* **51**, 1495.

BURNETT, W. (1971). *Tijdschrift voor Gastroenterologie* **14**, 79.

CARLSON, L. A. and BÖTTIGER, L. E. (1972). *Lancet* **1**, 865.

CLEAVE, T. L., CAMPBELL, G. D. and PAINTER, N. S. (1969). "Diabetes, Coronary Thrombosis and the Saccharine Disease", 2nd edition. John Wright, Bristol.

COBURN, F. F. and ANNEGERS, J. (1950). *American Journal of Physiology* **163**, 48.

COE, T. (1757). "A Treatise on Biliary Concretions." Wilson and Durham, London.

CUNNINGHAM, J. A. and HARDENBERGH, F. E. (1956). *Archives of Internal Medicine* **97**, 68.

DAM, H. and CHRISTENSEN, F. (1952). *Acta pathologica et microbiologica scandinavica* **30**, 236.

DAWSON, J. L. (1973). *Clinics in Gastroenterology* **2**, 85.

DENBESTEN, L., CONNOR, W. E. and BELL, S. (1973). *Surgery* **73**, 266.

DOOUSS, T. W. and CASTLEDEN, W. M. (1973). *New Zealand Medical Journal* **77**, 162.

DOWLING, R. H., BELL, G. D. and WHITE, J. (1973). *Gut* **14**, 415.

EDINGTON, G. M. (1957). *Transactions of the Royal Society of Tropical Medicine and Hygiene* **51**, 48.

EDLUND, Y. and OLSSON, O. (1956). *Acta chirurgica scandinavica* **111**, 481.

EHRSTRÖM, R. (1942). *Nordisk Medicin* **14**, 1559.

ENGLERT, E., HARMAN, C. G. and WALES, E. E. (1969). *Nature, London* **224**, 280.

FRIEDMAN, G. D., KANNEL, W. B. and DAWBER, T. R. (1966). *Journal of Chronic Diseases* **19**, 273.

GLENN, F. (1970). *Annals of Surgery* **171**, 163.

GROSS, D. M. B. (1929). *Journal of Pathology and Bacteriology* **32**, 503.

GRUNDY, S. M., METZGER, A. L. and ADLER, R. D. (1972a). *Journal of Clinical Investigation* **51**, 3026.

GRUNDY, S. M., AHRENS, E. H., SALEN, G., SCHREIBMAN, P. H. and NESTEL, P. J. (1972b). *Journal of Lipid Research* **13**, 531.

GRUNDY, S. M., DUANE, W. C., ADLER, R. D., ARON, J. M. and METZGER, A. L. (1974). *Metabolism* **23**, 67.

GUSTAFSSON, B. E. and NORMAN, A. (1969). *British Journal of Nutrition* **23**, 429.

HAGBERG, B., SVENNERHOLM, L. and THORÉN, L. (1962). *Acta chirurgica scandinavica* **123**, 307.

HALL, R. C. (1963). *Surgery* **53**, 621.

HEATON, K. W. (1972). "Bile Salts in Health and Disease." Churchill Livingstone, Edinburgh.

HEATON, K. W. (1973a). *Clinics in Gastroenterology* **2**, 67.

HEATON, K. W. (1973b). *Lancet* **2**, 1418.

HEATON, K. W. (1975). *In* "Topics in Gastroenterology 2" (S. C. Truelove and J. Trowell, eds). Blackwell, Oxford.

HEATON, K. W. and READ, A. E. (1969). *British Medical Journal* **3**, 494.

HELLER, F. and BOUCHIER, I. A. D. (1973). *Gut* **14**, 83.

HELLSTRÖM, K., SJÖVALL, J. and WIGAND, G. (1962). *Journal of Lipid Research* **3**, 405.

HIKASA, Y., MATSUDA, S., NAGASE, M., YOSHINAGA, M., TOBE, T., MARUYAMA, I., SHIODA, R., TANIMURA, H., MURAOKA, R., MUROYA, H. and TOGO, M. (1969). *Archiv Japanische Chirurgie* **38**, 107.

HILLS, L. L. (1971). *Medical Journal of Australia* **2**, 94.

HOLLAND, C. and HEATON, K. W. (1972). *British Medical Journal* **3**, 672.

HOLZBACH, R. T., MARSH, M. and OLSZEWSKI, M. (1972). *Gastroenterology* **62**, 850 (abstract).

HORN, G. (1956). *British Medical Journal* **2**, 732.

KAMEDA, H. (1967). *In* "Proceedings of the 3rd World Congress of Gastroenterology", Vol. 4, p. 117. Karger, Basel.

192   K. HEATON

KHOSLA, T. and LOWE, C. R. (1968). *Lancet* 1, 742.

KRAVETZ, R. E. (1964). *Gastroenterology* 46, 392.

Lancet (1968). 1, 1416.

LEE, C.-C. and HERRMANN, R. G. (1963). *Archives of International Pharmaco-dynamics* 141, 591.

LIEBER, M. M. (1952). *Annals of Surgery* 135, 394.

LOW-BEER, T. S. and POMARE, E. W. (1973). *Gastroenterology* 64, 764 (abstract).

LOW-BEER, T. S. and POMARE, E. W. (1975). *British Medical Journal*, in press.

MAKI, T. (1961). *Archives of Surgery* 82, 599.

MAKI, T., SATO, T., YAMAGUCHI, I. and SAITO, Y. (1964). *Tohoku Journal of Experimental Medicine* 84, 37.

MALHOTRA, S. L. (1968). *Gut* 9, 290.

MIETTINEN, T. A. (1971). *Circulation* 44, 842.

MIYAKE, H. and JOHNSTON, C. G. (1968). *Digestion* 1, 219.

MONTEGRIFFO, V. M. E. (1971). *Postgraduate Medical Journal* June Suppl. 418.

MOK, H. Y. I., BELL, G. D. and DOWLING, R. H. (1974). *Lancet* 2, 253.

MUNSTER, A. M. and BROWN, J. R. (1967). *American Journal of Surgery* 113, 730.

NAKAYAMA, F. and MIYAKE, H. (1970). *American Journal of Surgery* 120, 794.

NAKAYAMA, F. and VAN DER LINDEN, W. (1970). *Acta chirurgica scandinavica* 136, 605.

NAKAYAMA, F. and VAN DER LINDEN, W. (1971). *American Journal of Surgery* 122, 8.

NESTEL, P. J., SCHREIBMAN, P. H. and AHRENS, E. H. (1973). *Journal of Clinical Investigation* 52, 2389.

NEWMAN, H. F. and NORTHUP, J. D. (1959). *International Abstracts of Surgery* 109, 1.

NICOLAU, G., SHEFER, S., SALEN, G. and MOSBACH, E. H. (1974). *Journal of Lipid Research* 15, 146.

NILSSON, S. (1966). *Acta chirurgica scandinavica* 132, 275.

NILSSON, S. and SCHERSTÉN, T. (1969). *Gastroenterology* 57, 525.

NORTHFIELD, T. C. and HOFMANN, A. F. (1973). *Lancet* 1, 747.

NORTHFIELD, T. C., LaRUSSO, N. F., THISTLE, J. L. and HOFMANN, A. F. (1973). *Gastroenterology* 64, 780 (abstract).

OSLER, W. (1892). "The Principles and Practice of Medicine." Pentland, Edinburgh.

OSUGA, T. and PORTMAN, O. W. (1971). *Proceedings of the Society for Experimental Biology and Medicine* 136, 722.

OWOR, R. (1964). *East African Medical Journal* 41, 251.

PARNIS, R. O. (1964). *Transactions of the Royal Society of Tropical Medicine and Hygiene* 58, 437.

PEARSON, R. J. C., SMEDBY, B., BERFENSTAM, R., LOGAN, R. F. L., BURGESS, A. M. and PETERSON, O. L. (1968). *Lancet* 2, 558.

PERTSEMLIDIS, D., PANVELIWALLA, D. and AHRENS, E. H. (1974). *Gastroenterology* 66, 565.

PLANT, J. C. D., PERCY, I., BATES, T., GASTARD, J. and HITA DE NERCY, Y. (1973). *Lancet* 2, 249.

PLATT, B. S. (1962). *MRC Special Reports* Series No. 302. Her Majesty's Stationery Office, London.

POMARE, E. W. and HEATON, K. W. (1973a). *Gut* **14**, 885.

POMARE, E. W. and HEATON, K. W. (1973b). *British Medical Journal* **4**, 262.

POMARE, E. W., HEATON, K. W., LOW-BEER, T. S. and WHITE, C. (1974). *Gut* **15**, 824 (abstract).

PORTMAN, O. W. and MURPHY, P. (1958). *Archives of Biochemistry and Biophysics* **76**, 367.

REDINGER, R. N., HERMANN, A. H. and SMALL, D. M. (1973). *Gastroenterology* **64**, 610.

REDINGER, R. N. and SMALL, D. M. (1972). *Archives of Internal Medicine* **130**, 618.

Report from the Boston Collaborative Drug Surveillance Programme (1973). *Lancet* **1**, 1399.

SAILER, S. (1972). *In* "Nutrition and Diabetes Mellitus" (E. R. Froesch and J. Yudkin, eds). *Acta diabetologica latina*, Vol. IX, Suppl. 1, p. 147.

SAMPLINER, R. E., BENNETT, P. H., COMESS, L. J., ROSE, F. A. and BURCH, T. A. (1970). *New England Journal of Medicine* **283**, 1358.

SARLES, H., HAUTON, J., LAFONT, H., TEISSIER, N., PLANCHE, N.-E. and GÉROLAMI, A. (1968). *Clinica chimica Acta* **19**, 147.

SARLES, H., HAUTON, J., PLANCHE, N. E., LAFONT, H. and GÉROLAMI, A. (1970). *American Journal of Digestive Diseases* **15**, 251.

SCHAEFER, O. (1971). *Nutrition Today* **6**, 8.

SMALLWOOD, R. A., JABLONSKI, P. and McK. WATTS, J. (1972). *British Medical Journal* **4**, 263.

SODHI, H. S. and KUDCHODKAR, B. J. (1973). *Lancet* **1**, 513.

SODHI, H. S., WOOD, P. D. S., SCHLIERF, G. and KINSELL, L. W. (1967). *Metabolism* **16**, 334.

STERNBY, N. H. (1968). *Acta pathologica et microbiologica scandinavica*, Supplement 194.

STOKES, T. and WYNN, V. (1971). *Lancet* **2**, 677.

STURDEVANT, R. A. L., PEARCE, M. L. and DAYTON, S. (1973). *New England Journal of Medicine* **288**, 24.

SUTOR, D. J. and WOOLEY, S. E. (1971). *Gut* **12**, 55.

TEPPERMAN, J., CALDWELL, F. T. and TEPPERMAN, H. M. (1964). *American Journal of Physiology* **206**, 628.

THISTLE, J. L. and HOFMANN, A. F. (1973). *New England Journal of Medicine* **289**, 655.

THUDICHUM, J. L. W. (1863). "A Treatise on Gallstones." Churchill, London.

TROTMAN, B. W. and SOLOWAY, R. D. (1973). *Gastroenterology* **65**, 573 (abstract).

VAN DER LINDEN, W. and RENTZHOG, U. (1960). *Acta chirurgica scandinavica* **119**, 489.

VLAHCEVIC, Z. R., BELL, C. C., BUHAC, I., FARRAR, J. T. and SWELL, L. (1970). *Gastroenterology* **59**, 165.

VLAHCEVIC, Z. R., BELL, C. C., GREGORY, D. H., BUKER, G., JUTTIJUDATA, P. and SWELL, L. (1972). *Gastroenterology* **62**, 73.

WAGNER, C. I., SOLOWAY, R. D., TROTMAN, B. W. and SCHOENFIELD, L. J. (1973). *Gastroenterology* **65**, 575 (abstract).

WALKER, A. R. P. and RICHARDSON, B. D. (1971). *Lancet* **2**, 1146.

WATKINSON, G. (1967). *In* "Proceedings of 3rd World Congress of Gastro-enterology", Vol. 4, p. 125. Karger, Basel.

WHEELER, M., HILLS, L. L. and LABY, B. (1970). *Gut* **11**, 430.

YAGI, T. (1960). *Tohoku Journal of Experimental Medicine* **72**, 117.

Chapter 15

Ischaemic heart disease, atheroma and fibrinolysis

HUGH TROWELL

I. Ischaemic heart disease 195
   A. Recognized risk factors. 195
   B. Epidemiology 197
   C. Association with diverticular disease 202
II. Atherosclerosis. 203
   A. Experimental studies in animals 204
   B. Experimental studies in man 207
   C. Metabolic mechanisms 209
   D. Triglycerides 211
   E. Attempts to assess the role of dietary fibre in ischaemic heart
      disease 214
III. Fibrinolysis 217
   A. Thrombosis and fibrinolysis 217
   B. Fat intakes 218
   C. Fibre intakes 219
IV. Summary of dietary fibre hypothesis concerning ischaemic heart
    disease 221
References 222

I. Ischaemic heart disease

A. Recognized risk factors

1. The western world

In the western world high levels of plasma cholesterol and triglyceride, smoking and high blood pressure have been established as some of the risk factors involved in ischaemic heart disease (IHD) which is more common in men than in women, especially in those aged 40–60 years. Diabetes and hypertension markedly, but not invariably, increase the risk of IHD, and obesity is sometimes a factor. Diets rich in fat, especially saturated fat, raise plasma cholesterol levels, and are often regarded as increasing the risk of IHD. The role of physical activity is less clearly defined. Increased activity is considered by many workers to confer some degree of protection, although the world's highest prevalence of IHD is found among manual workers in East Finland. As will be discussed later, increased physical activity is usually coupled with the consumption of large amounts of starchy carbohydrate foods, which, if only lightly processed, provide much fibre. In Ireland, where potatoes, rich in fibre, are the staple diet, there is a low prevalence of IHD (Brown *et al.*, 1970). Hyperuricaemia and soft drinking water have been incriminated as possibly contributing to the prevalence of IHD. Psychological factors also may operate, for IHD has been reported as being more common in those who have a tense driving personality.

Attempts to assess risk factors have been made in primary prevention IHD trials. One risk factor was decreased in one of several pairs of groups, while the other group acted as a control. The prevalence of any manifestation of IHD was noted and calculated in the two groups. Thus in primary trials, those who stopped smoking soon showed a definite decreased IHD prevalence. In other trials those who ate less fat, especially saturated fat, soon showed lower serum cholesterol levels and there is some evidence that these persons developed less IHD.

In secondary prevention trials, the effects of single or multiple factors in persons who had developed a definite manifestation of IHD were assessed. When smoking was discontinued the manifestations of IHD decreased but the elimination or reduction of other risk factors had less effect on the prognosis of survivors of an initial attack of coronary thrombosis (Jones, 1970).

There have been very few attempts in primary or secondary prevention trials to assess the effects of fibre-depleted starchy carbohydrate foods as an IHD risk factor. Conversely, fibre-rich starchy foods might be a protective IHD factor. (See the summary of the dietary fibre hypothesis, p. 221.)

2. *Africa and Asia*

The position with regard to recognized risk factors appears to be somewhat different among Africans and Asians. Thus in Africa cigarette smoking, obesity, hypertension, even diabetes, do not appear to increase the prevalence of IHD to any marked degree (Shaper, 1972). Serum cholesterol levels, which are usually an excellent indicator of increased IHD risk in the western world, may be high in certain African groups but are not associated with increased manifestations of IHD (Lee *et al.*, 1962).

In India statistics supplied by different doctors in the railway service must be considered with reservation. These suggested that there was less IHD among North Indian railroad sweepers who smoked many cigarettes and ate more saturated fat than among South Indian sweepers who smoked fewer cigarettes and ate less saturated fat (Malhotra, 1971). In Japan, diabetic autopsies displayed far less IHD than that encountered in diabetic autopsies of comparable age and sex in Britain or the U.S.A. (Okamoto *et al.*, 1971). It is therefore important to consider what other protective factors may diminish a disease which has been described as "potentially the greatest epidemic mankind has faced" (World Health Organization, 1969).

B. Epidemiology

1. Geographical aspects

(*a*) *The western world.* In many of the advanced countries of the west, IHD causes four out of ten deaths in men and two out of ten deaths in women. The high prevalence of IHD, assessed by ECG evidence, is now fairly similar in office workers of various northern European cities as far apart as Brussels and Moscow. A striking difference may, however, be seen in the lower prevalence in certain south-eastern European countries. Age-standardized average yearly deaths per 10,000 men aged 40–59 years were 111 in the Netherlands, 36 in Greece, 75 in Yugoslavia and 95 in Italy (Keys, 1970). It is generally considered that environmental factors predominate, although genetic factors also operate. For instance, home-based Italians have significantly less IHD than those who have emigrated to Australia. It has been asserted that third and fourth generation Italians, who lived in one town in the U.S.A. and who were said to have retained their traditional food habits, had less than half the standard American IHD mortality although they consumed as much fat as other Americans (Stout *et al.*, 1964). In the U.S.A. the prevalence of IHD is high and remains steady although the consumption of saturated fat has declined slightly since 1950. In other western nations IHD prevalence is still said to be rising but it is difficult to say which factors, apart from smoking, may be responsible. More information is required concerning IHD death rates in age- and sex-groups, for the proportion of older persons has increased in western countries. It is not possible to agree with those who have associated the continued rise in IHD mortality in all western nations with an alleged increasing consumption of sugar (Cleave *et al.*, 1969), for the consumption of this commodity has actually fallen since 1924 in the U.S.A. and since 1958 in Britain, while there has been an increased number of coronary heart deaths in both of these countries since these dates. Other dietary factors, such as fibre-rich carbohydrate foods, should be considered as being possibly protective against this disease. The diet of south and south-east European countries contains more fibre-rich carbohydrate foods, such as leguminous seeds and lightly processed cereal flours, than that of North America and northern European countries. For example, a southern Italian-type hospital diet contained crude fibre 18·8 g/day, whereas a typical U.S.A. hospital diet contained crude fibre 8·7 g/day (Keys et al., 1960).

Ireland–Massachusetts heart study. The varied incidence of IHD in different countries of the western world has been studied in the Ireland–Massachusetts heart study (Brown et al., 1970). It had already been ascertained that 29% of all deaths in Ireland in men aged 45–64 years were due to IHD, compared with 42% of all deaths in the same age-group in second generation American men in Massachusetts. In Ireland and Boston, autopsy studies of coronary arteries and aortae had revealed that atheromatous changes were less severe and occurred later in men in Ireland. In their study, Brown and his colleagues examined 1154 aged-matched Irish brothers who had grown up together in Ireland. Subsequently one brother had emigrated to Massachusetts, U.S.A., the other remaining in Ireland. This minimized the role of inheritance and permitted a more accurate assessment of environmental factors. A comprehensive clinical survey demonstrated electrocardiographic evidence of IHD in only 2·1% of the Irish brothers in Ireland compared with 4·0% in those in Massachusetts, which meant that the latter had 90% more IHD. The Irish-based brothers ate more animal fat, but surprisingly had lower mean serum cholesterol levels than the Massachusetts-based brothers (Table 15.1). The two groups had a similar intake of sugar, protein, cholesterol and alcohol, and the same smoking habits. Blood pressures were also similar. The main dietary difference was in their consumption of carbohydrate foods. The brothers in Ireland ate large amounts of potatoes and more whole grain cereals and bread and 6·4 g/day of crude fibre, while their counterparts in the U.S.A. ate crude fibre 3·6 g/day, mostly derived from fruit and vegetables. (There are no precise figures for the extraction rate of the cereal products: F. J. Stare, p.c. 1973.) It is not generally recognized that in proportion to their energy (calorie) content potatoes contain almost as much crude fibre as wheat wholemeal bread, which may explain why those who stayed in Ireland developed less IHD.

(b) *Africa.* Shaper (1972) emphasized the rarity of IHD among Africans in all countries south of the Sahara. Its infrequency in South African Bantu is particularly well documented (Schrire, 1971). Even in the largest cities of South Africa hospital records demonstrate the rarity of IHD in Bantu. The Baragwanath Hospital, Johannesburg, admitting 40,000 Bantu patients a year, recorded IHD in only 30 patients during 1960–72, most of which had occurred in the last two years. Many of these Bantu IHD patients had eaten western diets (Seftel *et al.*, 1970, 1973). In South Africa the most popular maize meal is 80% extraction, crude fibre 1·4 g/100 g (Metz *et al.*, 1970) and this is still consumed in large amounts even in the towns. It appears probable that South African urban Bantu consume more high-fibre cereal products than any other group of city dwellers in the world. In most Africans serum cholesterol levels are low and these levels may rise only very slightly with age in certain African groups (Truswell and Mann, 1972). On the other hand wealthy East Africans have serum

TABLE 15.1. Ischaemic heart disease in Irish brothers living in Ireland and Massachusetts; data concerning dietary intakes of fat, carbohydrate and fibre, serum cholesterol level and incidence of IHD

	Ireland	Massachusetts
Fat intake	159 g/day	135 g/day
% animal	90	84
Serum cholesterol	213±44 mg/100 ml	219±39 mg/100 ml
Carbohydrate	267 g/day	116 g/day
Crude fibre	6·4 g/day	3·6 g/day
IHD—demonstrated by ECG	2·1%	4·0%

It will be seen that the brothers in Ireland ate 78% more crude fibre than those in Massachusetts who had 90% more heart disease; this suggests that fibre-rich starchy foods provide some protection against it (Trowell, 1973a).

lipid levels that rise with age to a height which resembles that of U.S. Americans (Lee *et al.*, 1962). In spite of this, coronary heart disease is rarely diagnosed clinically or at autopsy in East Africa (Lee *et al.*, 1964).

(c) *The Indian sub-continent.* This covers a vast area and comprises India, Pakistan and Bangladesh, within which there are so many differences among the social classes and between urban and rural areas that generalizations are not possible.

In India, milled polished low-fibre white rice has been the traditional carbohydrate food, especially in the urban areas of the southern and eastern states. Less refined medium-fibre rice is still consumed in the rural areas. In Pakistan, high-fibre wheat wholemeal bread, chupatties and fibre-rich leguminous seeds were formerly eaten, but in recent years refined low-fibre white bread is being eaten in increasing amounts, especially in the urban areas.

In all parts of the Indian sub-continent IHD has been reported more commonly in towns than in the countryside, and it is more prevalent in the upper socio-economic groups. Serum cholesterol levels are usually lower in Indian groups than in comparable western groups, but have risen markedly in some cities in recent years (Pinto et al., 1970). A large survey in an industrial city in India during 1967 revealed a prevalence of abnormal electrocardiograms, suggestive of coronary heart disease, that was almost comparable to that in the U.S.A. (Sarvotham and Berry, 1968). More clinical studies and autopsy data are required before a balanced judgement of the incidence of IHD in the Indian sub-continent can be made.

It has already been indicated that some reservations are made concerning the data of the morbidity and mortality of Indian railway workers in many different parts of that vast sub-continent (Malhotra, 1967a, b, c, 1971). Greater weight is given to the more detailed smaller study of two specific groups of railway sweepers; one group worked in Udaipur, a town in northern India, and the other group lived in Madras in southern India (Malhotra, 1968, 1971). During the years of observation, 1958–1962, a lower mortality (20/100,000 men) occurred in Udaipur and contrasted markedly with a higher figure (135/100,000) in Madras. The north Indian diet was based on chupatties made from high-extraction flour 440 g/day, supplemented by fibre-rich legumes 60 g/day. These two foods probably provided crude fibre 6–12 g/day, but no dietary details were given other than that the north Indian "diet is rich in cellulose and vegetable fibres, while the Madras diet lacks these" (Malhotra, 1968). This diet was in fact based on low-fibre white rice and "lacked" fibre. It should be noted that the high-fibre wheat diets of north Indian railway workers produced an average stool weight in the region of 230 g/day, whereas on the low-fibre rice diets of the south Indians the average stool weight was only 135 g/day (Malhotra, 1971). This, incidentally, is more than the English average stool weight. Among the north Indian workers the mean clotting time was longer and clot lysis was more rapid than in the south Indians (Malhotra, 1968, 1972). As discussed later (p. 217), both of these factors might reduce the frequency and severity of thrombosis in atheromatous coronary arteries. North Indian sweepers were also reported to have less varicose veins than those of south India (Malhotra, 1972).

(d) Israel. The incidence of IHD varies markedly among the various ethnic groups in Israel. IHD prevalence appears to have been much lower in Jewish immigrants from the Middle East, Iran, Iraq and the Negev desert. One survey demonstrated that men of this group had an IHD prevalence, age-adjusted, of 0·9/100,000 compared to 3·2/100,000 in men born in Central and Eastern Europe. It was postulated that the low serum cholesterol of Yemenite Jews prior to emigration to Israel could be explained by diets which had been low in fats (Groen et al., 1964). Attention should, however, also be directed to their consumption of stone-ground, often unsieved, wheat wholemeal bread, with crude fibre 2·0 g/100 g.

(e) *Conclusion.* As far as it is known, every one of the 25 groups cited by Lowenstein (1964) as having low serum cholesterol levels and low IHD prevalence, were those who ate a diet which contained a large amount of lightly processed high-fibre carbohydrate foods. This survey ranged through Belgian Trappist monks who consumed much wholemeal bread, North Indians in Pakistan who ate large amounts of wheat wholemeal chupatties and leguminous seeds, plantain-eating tropical Africans, and those who consumed lightly processed maize meal or millet meal in Rhodesia and South Africa, or a similar diet eaten in the highlands of the Andes and parts of Central America. These groups all performed hard manual work throughout the course of their lives and energy (calorie) intakes would be high in proportion to body size. It is probable that many of these groups ate only a moderate amount of fat, in which case the carbohydrate content of the diet would be high and the crude fibre intake would be very high.

2. *Historical aspects*

(a) *Classifications of the disease: angina pectoris and coronary thrombosis.* Ischaemic heart disease can manifest itself in different ways, the distinctive pain of angina pectoris being the first of these to have been recognized, and it was clearly described for the first time in the middle of the seventeenth century (Leibowitz, 1970a). Subsequently it was given the status of a clinical entity, and named "angina pectoris" by Heberden in 1768 (Leibowitz, 1970b). Cases were diagnosed with increasing frequency in Britain during the nineteenth century, but the crude mortality rate, as then reported, remained stationary at 20–22 per million, all persons, from 1880 to 1904. During this period the consumption of potatoes and bread decreased and the fibre content of the flour diminished (Chapter 5). After 1904 angina mortality crude death rates rose steadily from 22 per million to 35 per million in 1915, 47 per million in 1925 and 148 per million, all persons, in 1930. After that date a new classification of disease, as will be discussed later, obscured the course of the rising morality rates.

In the second half of the nineteenth century a broad group of diseases, recorded as a single category by the Registrar-General, was collectively designed "degenerative heart disease". This included not only fatty heart, fibroid heart and chronic myocarditis, but probably also cases of coronary thrombosis and other varieties of IHD. The recognition of coronary thrombosis was delayed until Pardee (1920) in the U.S.A. reported the distinctive electrocardiographic changes which were confirmed in Britain by Parkinson and Bedford (1928). It then became possible for well informed doctors to report deaths due specifically to coronary thrombosis. Reclassification of the diseases in Britain during 1939 allowed the notification of a new category: "diseases of the coronary artery and angina pectoris". New terminology and regrouping occurred from time to time, with a further reclassification in 1945. In 1967 ischaemic heart disease (IHD) was listed with five sub-headings: (*a*) mycardial infarction, (*b*) acute and subacute IHD, (*c*) chronic IHD, (*d*) angina pectoris, (*e*) asymptomatic IHD.

(*b*) *Increased IHD incidence 1930–70.* During this period the total crude death rates from all varieties of heart disease rose markedly except for rheumatic heart disease, which decreased. Since IHD now accounts for approximately half of all cardiac deaths in England and Wales, and rheumatic heart disease, formerly very common, has decreased, it is agreed that there has been a marked rise in the number of IHD deaths in this period of 40 years. In England and Wales in 1931 the recorded crude death rate, all persons, from diseases of the coronary arteries and angina pectoris was 166/million, and in 1969 from IHD (all varieties), all persons, the crude death rate was 2856/million. This is partly explained by a high incidence of disease among an increased number of older men and women, but death rates have risen in middle-aged and elderly groups of both sexes (Registrar-General, 1931–70). In the United States IHD recorded crude death rate rose from 79/million persons in 1930 to 2900/million persons in 1963, a true and marked increase (Friedberg, 1966). Most workers consider that IHD mortality was underestimated in the 1930s and even in the 1940s, for not all cases of the disease were diagnosed correctly, but the prevalence has truly increased in a spectacular manner in all advanced western nations during the present century.

The modest decline in IHD in England and Wales during the Second World War 1939–45 can best be studied in Table 15.2, which sets out (A) annual figures for the men and women in the 45–64 years group (which bears the brunt of IHD deaths) alongside (B) the approximate mean annual content of crude fibre in the flour and the mean yearly intakes of sugar and fat. No conclusion can be reached about the relationship between A and B since factors such as other dietetic changes and a decrease in smoking occurred at that time. After 1945 IHD mortality rose markedly and steadily in men aged 45–64 years, but altered little in women; during 1945 the crude fibre content of the flour fell and rose only moderately 1946–54, the years during which the National flour continued to be eaten (see Table 16.1).

C. Association with diverticular disease

1. In communities

Although it is difficult to imagine two diseases less similar than ischaemic heart disease and diverticular disease of the colon (DD), their epidemiology has much in common (Trowell *et al.*, 1974). The emergence of these diseases on the clinical scene in different situations seems to have occurred simultaneously. Both appear to be extremely rare in communities little influenced by modern civilization, who still eat large amounts of unprocessed or lightly processed carbohydrate foods. The geographical distribution of DD has been discussed in Chapter 9. It can be noted here that

TABLE 15.2. (A) Ischaemic heart disease age-specific mortality rates per 100,000 men and women aged 45–64 years, England and Wales 1939–1945; (B) crude fibre, approximate mean yearly content in the flour, and mean yearly intakes of sugar and fat

	A		B		
Year	Men 45–64 years	Women 45–64 years	Flour crude fibre g/100 g	Sugar lb/head/year	Fat lb/head/year
1939	351	176	0·10	106	47
1940	311	160	0·10	80	43
1941	269	137	0·15	72	42
1942	253	123	0·68	72	41
1943	257	122	0·55	72	39
1944	277	120	0·45	77	41
1945	276	125	0·21	74	38

Source: Registrar-General (1931–70) and Table 16.1.

some Jewish immigrants to Israel from Middle East countries where IHD and DD were still rare, had low serum cholesterol levels, and subsequently developed less IHD than other immigrant groups from Europe (Medalie *et al.*, 1968).

2. *In individuals*

In the western world IHD and severe atheroma and DD often occur in the same individual, as was demonstrated in 840 autopsies of American whites and non-whites (Schowengerdt *et al.*, 1969) and post mortems of Australian whites (Hughes, 1969).

The evidence that a low intake of fibre-rich carbohydrate foods is a cause of DD strengthens the case for the possibility that such foods are protective against IHD (Trowell *et al.*, 1974).

II. Atherosclerosis

Severe progressive atheromatous disease of the coronary arteries develops rarely except in man, some non-human primates and in pigs. Even western man, when he was following his traditional outdoor pursuits and satisfying his hunger with his customary, very largely whole cereal food, rarely suffered from diseases of the coronary arteries. Some atheroma of the aorta may have been present from the age of the Pharaohs, but severe atheroma and myocardial infarction, as a common condition, is a pheno-menon of modern times. Primates which used to range in the forest are now more confined; when captured they are restricted to enclosures and subjected to changes of diet and environment. Pigs no longer roam afield or root up their traditional tough fibrous food. Among wild animals coronary atherosclerosis as a severe, possibly fatal, condition is very rare.

A. Experimental studies in animals

In most animals maintained in a laboratory it is difficult to produce any condition resembling coronary atherosclerosis in man unless usually a large amount of cholesterol is added to the diet. In this and various other ways experimental atherosclerosis has been produced in a variety of animals. Efforts have been made to study in animals possible risk factors, such as the amount of cholesterol, the amount and type of fat, the kinds of starchy carbohydrate and the amount of sucrose in the diet. There has been little study of any possible protective factors, since it has been assumed that if all the risk factors could be eliminated disease would be prevented. In laboratory animals much research has been conducted in cholesterol metabolism and this aspect dominates the following discussion. High plasma triglyceride levels are a risk factor in IHD in men and triglyceride metabolism is linked with carbohydrate in the diet and so possibly with dietary fibre. Discussion of this is deferred until p. 211.

In India clinical workers commented on the low prevalence of IHD among peasant communities who ate large amounts of starchy foods and fair amounts of leguminous seeds. Laboratory workers therefore began to study experimental atherosclerosis in animals fed these foods. It was found that cholesterol metabolism and blood glucose levels responded differently to various carbohydrate foods and leguminous seeds, and there was some speculation concerning which portion of the food was responsible (Vijayagopalan and Kurup, 1970). It was therefore suggested that the fibre content of the starchy foods, which had not been reported, might explain the anomalous results (Table 15.3) (Trowell, 1972b). Subsequent analysis of the starchy foods and leguminous seeds appeared to demonstrate a correlation between the crude fibre content of the various laboratory diets and the hypolipidaemic and hypoglycaemic effect in the cholesterol-fed rats (Vijayagopal et al., 1973). No statistical analysis of the correlation, however, was made.

Further work led to the isolation of a polysaccharide fraction from

TABLE 15.3. Effect of various carbohydrates on cholesterol metabolism and blood sugar levels in rats fed high-cholesterol, high-fat diets (Vijayagopalan and Kurup, 1970; Trowell, 1972b).

	Carbohydrate			Cholesterol		Blood glucose
Starch	Rice %	Bran %	Fibre g/100 g of starchy food	Serum mg/100 ml	Aorta mg/g	1 h mg/100 ml
Rice starch	56	—	0·2	348	14	140
Rice starch	40	16	4·0	256	11	121
Whole ground rice	56	—	2·0	166	6	103
Tapioca starch	56	—	1·5	205	8	115
Tapioca starch	40	16	5·3	130	4	94

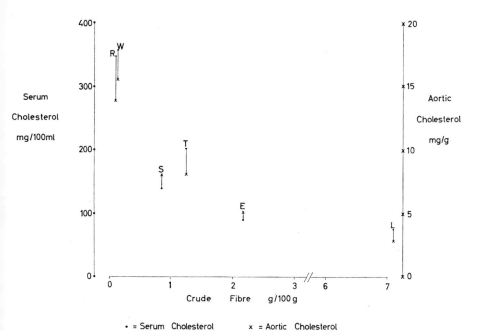

• = Serum Cholesterol   x = Aortic Cholesterol

FIG. 15.1. Effect of various starchy foods of different crude fibre content on serum cholesterol and aortic cholesterol levels in cholesterol-fed rats (Vijayagopal et al., 1973).
R = polished rice,   W = white wheat flour,
S = sorghum,   T = tapioca,
E = eleusine millet, L = leguminous seed (*Phaseolus mungo*) polysaccharide.

defatted rice bran (crude fibre 13 g/100 g) which even at the very low dose of 0·56 mg/day has proved to be strongly hypolipidaemic in cholesterol-fed rats (Vijayagopalan and Kurup, 1972a). This polysaccharide fraction contained nitrogen and uronic acid and is comparable in many respects to a polysaccharide fraction obtained from a leguminous seed (*Phaseolus mungo*) (crude fibre 4·5 g/100 g) (Devi and Kurup, 1972). Active investigation of the hypolipidaemic polysaccharide fractions continues at Trivandrum, South India (Vijayagopalan and Kurup, 1972b; Vijayagopal *et al.* 1973).

It is desirable, even at this stage, to set out some of the probable implications of these Indian laboratory studies of cholesterol-fed rats. It should be noted that serum cholesterol levels in the rats were reduced much more by whole ground rice than by a combination of refined rice flour and bran, although this mixture contained twice as much crude fibre as did the ground whole rice (Table 15.3). In other words, whole ground rice, in which dietary fibre and starch are still in close physical relationship, was about four times as hypolipidaemic and hypoglycaemic as an equal amount of the fibre of rice bran when this was mixed again with the refined rice flour from which it had been removed. When this mixture was given and rice bran contributed 16% of the daily calories, its hypolipidaemic and hypoglycaemic action was poor (Vijayagopalan and Kurup, 1970; Table 15.3). A comparable amount for a daily human western-type diet would be 120 g (about 4 oz). Few people would agree to take this amount of bran, which in any case might prove less effective in reducing serum cholesterol levels than would the whole cereal, whether wheat wholemeal or brown rice. Merely adding modest amounts of bran to human diets may have little effect on cholesterol metabolism. No change in serum cholesterol levels were observed by Eastwood *et al.* (1973) in eight healthy men who added wheat bran 8 g twice daily to their food, nor by Heaton and Pomare (1974) who added wheat bran 38 g daily, although they noted that serum triglyceride levels fell (p. 213).

In Japan research has demonstrated that various foodstuffs eaten in certain parts of the country reduced serum cholesterol levels in cholesterol-fed rats. These foods included mushrooms and a tuber, konnyaku (*Amorphophalus konjac*). Konnyaku powder contains much glucomannan, which is a hemicellulose. Like other hemicelluloses it is not hydrolysed by the alimentary enzymes of man, but is probably degraded by bacteria in the colon. In Japan other chemical polysaccharides, celluloses, carboxymethylcellulose, pectin, agar-agar, and gum arabic, have been found to reduce serum cholesterol levels in cholesterol-fed rats (Kiriyama *et al.*, 1969). Moreover, certain seaweeds and spinach, also eaten in Japan, have a similar effect, and in addition increase faecal excretion of cholesterol and coprostanol (Iritani and Nogi, 1972).

Experiments performed largely in Britain and the U.S.A. demonstrated that a wide variety of substances obtained from plants reduced serum cholesterol levels in animals fed atherogenic diets. These substances include wheat straw and peat (Moore, 1967), ground whole cereals such as wheat, barley and particularly oats, also oat hulls (Fisher and Griminger, 1967). Wheat wholemeal bread, barley, and especially rolled oats, reduced serum cholesterol levels in cholesterol-fed rats (de Groot et al., 1963). It was not apparently recognized that all these substances are rich sources of fibre. Oat hulls are almost the richest natural source of crude fibre, containing as much as 36 g/100 g. Purina chow, a common laboratory foodstuff, derived from ground cereals and bran (crude fibre 4·5 g/100 g) protected squirrel monkeys against an atherogenic diet (Maruffo and Portman, 1968). Butter-fed rabbits were also similarly protected against atheroma, but not if the crude fibre of the chow was replaced by an equal weight of chemical cellulose, which had previously been considered to be an adequate replacement for the fibre content of the chow (Kritchevsky and Tepper, 1968; Kritchevsky et al., 1968).

Increasingly, pure chemical polysaccharides have been used in experiments in both animals and man. Pectin, which proved hypolipidaemic in animals eating an atherogenic diet, was hypolipidaemic in man when given in enormous doses amounting to 6–10 g/day (Palmer and Dixon, 1966), or 15 g/day (Keys et al., 1961). Pure chemical cellulose was not hypolipidaemic in man if 15 g/day were eaten (Keys et al., 1961), but a hypocholesterolaemic effect was demonstrated and faecal excretion of bile acids was increased when volunteers ate 100 g/day (Shurpalekar et al., 1971).

A wide variety of mucilaginous polysaccharides, such as carrageenan, salep root, guar gum and many other gums, have displayed hypocholesterolaemic properties in cockerels (Fahrenbach et al., 1966), likewise scleroglucan in chicken (Griminger and Fisher, 1966). These discoveries have tended to remain uncoordinated, and there has been little to suggest that the fibre in plant cell-walls might reduce serum cholesterol level in man, largely because it was considered that no one ate sufficient cellulose, i.e. 15 g/day, to prove effective (Keys et al., 1961). Moreover, many workers erroneously regarded fibre in all its complexity as identical to chemically pure cellulose (Keys et al., 1961; Griminger and Fisher, 1966).

B. Experimental studies in man

I. Cereals and potatoes

Experiments have demonstrated that certain cereal products, if rich in fibre and taken in large amounts, can reduce high serum cholesterol levels in human volunteers. Twenty-one Dutch male volunteers first ate white bread, 300 g daily for 3 weeks, and then rolled oats, 140 g daily (crude fibre 1·2 g/day) were substituted for an equal amount of the bread during a second period of 3 weeks, during which time their mean serum cholesterol levels dropped from 258 mg/100 ml to 226 mg/100 ml (Luyken et al., 1962). Maize meal 350 g/day (crude fibre 5·0 g/day) given to ten male white South African volunteers for 28 days had a similar effect (Booyen et al., 1966).

Normally, western man eats little rice, but in the Kempner diet for the treatment of hypertension, 400–500 g/day of rice was often consumed, while fats were much reduced. The marked fall of serum cholesterol levels noted in patients taking this therapeutic diet (Kempner, 1948) exceeded that anticipated as a result of reducing dietary fat (Olson et al., 1958). Although a critical review of the influence of dietary carbohydrate foods on serum cholesterol levels considered that both cereals and potatoes were hypolipidaemic, it made no attempt to assess whether or not the effect was proportional to the crude fibre content, and moreover most of the experimental diets had been consumed for only a few weeks (McGandy et al., 1966). In proportion to their calories, potatoes contain as much fibre as wholemeal bread. Most communities who eat lightly processed carbohydrate foods do so all their lives.

2. Leguminous seeds

These are eaten regularly in large quantities in northern India and adjacent countries of the Middle East, particularly by the poorer inhabitants who have low serum cholesterol levels and little IHD. Numerous experiments in animals and man have substantiated the hypocholesterolaemic effect of such foods (Mathur et al., 1968). Other investigations in Holland (Luyken et al., 1962) and America have confirmed this hypolipidaemic effect and linked this experimental observation to the fact that southern Italian-type diets contain large amounts of mature leguminous seeds and that the inhabitants have a very low rate of IHD. Both in the U.S.A. (Grande et al., 1965) and in India (Mathur et al., 1968) large amounts of beans, 100–400 g/day, eaten in dietary experiments, have demonstrated their effect on serum cholesterol levels. For maximum effectiveness the experiments should be continued for 20 weeks or more. When this was done the excretion of bile salts increased while serum cholesterol levels fell (Mathur et al., 1968). All attempts to explain this phenomenon in terms of the protein content of the leguminous seeds have proved misleading. These mature seeds are the richest source of fibre, containing 2–3 times as much as an equal weight of whole cereals. Among westernised nations leguminous seeds (once eaten fairly regularly in Lent) are now seldom eaten in large amounts except by Trappist monks, who also take large amounts of wholemeal bread and have low serum cholesterol levels (Groen *et al.*, 1962).

C. Metabolic mechanisms

1. Unidentified factors

There has been considerable investigation of possible metabolic mechanisms involved in the various dietary risk factors in IHD. Firstly fat has been extensively investigated and the role of certain saturated fatty acids has been clearly established. Secondly the role of dietary cholesterol has been examined. A third factor, dietary fibre, has until recently received almost no consideration, yet Keys (1968), after mentioning the first two dietary factors, suggested that a third factor must exist, because "with the same calories, protein, fatty acid and cholesterol composition, diets containing large amounts of legumes, fruit and leafy vegetables tend to produce serum cholesterol levels somewhat lower than otherwise". Later Keys *et al.* (1972) again suggested that some unidentified dietary factor was operating in IHD. It has been suggested that this third unidentified factor may be dietary fibre, which is not restricted to legumes, fruit and leafy vegetables (Trowell, 1972a, b, c). In the Boston–Ireland heart study (p. 198), the Irish brothers who lived in Massachusetts consumed far more fruit and vegetables than did their brothers in Ireland, but the latter ate much more potato undepleted of fibre (Trowell, 1973a). Similarly, South African urban Venda Bantu men who consumed much fibre-rich maize meal but very little fruit and green vegetables (Lubbe, 1971) would develop scarcely any IHD.

Serum cholesterol levels appear to be a poor indicator of increased susceptibility to develop IHD in any group who eat a large amount of fibre-rich starchy carbohydrate (p. 199). The Irish brothers who lived in Massachusetts had a mean serum cholesterol level of 219 mg/100 ml, yet subsequently many developed more IHD than their brothers who lived in Ireland and had a comparable mean serum cholesterol level of 213 mg/ 100 ml. Both groups of Irish brothers developed much more IHD than did the urban Bantu men who had a higher mean serum cholesterol level of 231 mg/100 ml (Nel *et al.*, 1971). While not denying that dietary fibre may influence cholesterol metabolism, other metabolic mechanisms such as serum triglycerides (p. 211) and fibrinolysis (p. 217) must be explored.

2. Enterohepatic circulation of bile salts

Cholesterol is converted in the liver into bile salts, which are passed into the intestines in the bile and, on western diets, are largely reabsorbed mainly from the ileum into the enterohepatic circulation. Only a small proportion is excreted in the stool. Bile salts, reabsorbed in the entero-hepatic circulation, influence the formation of cholesterol in the liver. Faecal cholesterol is derived from cholesterol secreted into the bile, from un-absorbed dietary cholesterol and, to a small extent, from cholesterol excreted by the mucosal cells.

Heaton (1972) has recently reviewed the substantial amount of evidence indicating that fibre-depleted carbohydrate foods decrease the faecal excretion of bile salts. Rats fed on a fibre-rich cereal diet of chow had a greater excretion of bile salts than rats fed a synthetic fibre-free diet (Portman et al., 1955; Portman and Murphy, 1958; Portman, 1960). In cholesterol-fed rats those fed Purina chow (crude fibre 4·5 g/100 g) excreted more cholic acid, dihydroxycholanic acid and total bile acids than did those fed synthetic fibre-free diets (Portman and Mann, 1955). Other workers have confirmed these results, which indicate that fibre influences bile salt metabolism (Chapter 14). Dietary fibre contains hemicellulose molecules which contain uronic acids which could act as weak ion ex-changers and might bind bile salts (Southgate, 1973).

There have been no comparable experiments in man to test the relative effect on bile salt metabolism of fibre-rich natural carbohydrate foods and synthetic fibre-free diets. It has, however, been demonstrated that fibre-rich leguminous seeds can increase the faecal excretion of bile salts. In one experiment 30 Indian men had an isocaloric dietary switch from wheat and other cereals to Bengal gram (Cicer arietinum) 400 g/day, crude fibre 16 g (Fig. 15.2). This was followed by a significantly increased faecal excretion of total bile acids, of cholic acid and of deoxycholic acid, and by a large reduction of serum cholesterol levels. The diets both before and after the switch contained much saturated fat in the form of butter 156 g/day. On the high-fibre diet some 20 weeks passed before the maximal effect on faecal bile acid excretion was noted (Mathur et al., 1968).

In another large experiment in South Africa, white and Bantu men ate over long periods of time eight diets, each of which differed considerably in its fibre and fat content. Usually at each dietary switch both the fibre and the fat content was altered, but on one occasion, in the switch from diet 7 to diet 8, only the fibre content was altered, from low-fibre refined flours of diet 7 to high-fibre cereal whole meals of diet 8. Following this dietary switch the excretion of faecal bile acids and faecal sterols signifi-cantly increased, but serum cholesterol levels were not reduced, the mean serum cholesterol levels in both white and Bantu men still being between 165 and 177 mg/100 ml (Antonis and Bersohn, 1962a, b). These low levels probably reflected the low intakes of fat, 14% of the daily calories, in both diet 7 and diet 8. It seems most unfortunate that this experiment in South Africa, in which two dietary factors, fibre and fat, were both altered at seven out of the eight dietary switches, was interpreted as demonstrating that even large amounts of fibre-rich starchy carbohydrate foods did not influence serum cholesterol levels (Ancel Keys, p.c. 1972).

In another experimental study in which serum cholesterol levels were raised in human volunteers who ate cholesterol 4 g/day, the consumption of a large amount of cellulose, 100 g/day in the diet, both reduced serum lipids and increased bile acid excretion (Shurpalekar *et al.*, 1971). Similarly,

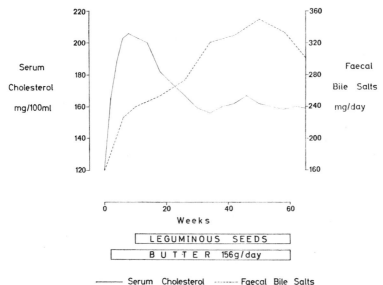

FIG. 15.2. Effect of leguminous seeds on serum cholesterol levels and faecal bile salt excretion in Indian men eating a diet supplemented by much butter (Mathur *et al.*, 1968).

large quantities of pectin, 6-10 g/day, have been shown both to reduce serum cholesterol levels and to increase bile acid excretion in man (Palmer and Dixon, 1966).

3. *Cholesterol absorption*

Most of the dietary cholesterol in the small intestine is present in the undissolved state and some of it is presumably trapped in the meshes of the dietary fibre. This may explain why pectin reduced cholesterol absorption in cholesterol-fed rats (Coleman and Baumann, 1959; Shuhachi *et al.*, 1961; Kiriyama *et al.*, 1969).

D. *Triglycerides*

Triglyceride metabolism is clearly implicated in the pathogenesis of IHD, but comparatively little attention has so far been paid to this aspect of the problem, far more research having been done on cholesterol metabolism. This is partly because the estimation of plasma triglycerides is both technically difficult and time-consuming. Numerous IHD surveys have reported plasma cholesterol levels in relationship to the diet, and in many animal experiments, in which large amounts of cholesterol and fat have been added to various carbohydrate foods, the production of atherosclerosis has been studied. It has therefore been possible to examine a hypothesis concerning the influence of starchy foods and fibre on the prevalence of IHD in man, and on cholesterol metabolism in experimental animals; this theme has run like a thread through the preceding pages, but it is not possible to pursue a similar enquiry in respect of triglyceride metabolism. Until recently IHD-dietary surveys seldom reported plasma triglyceride levels and comparatively few animal experiments have studied the production of atherosclerosis in relationship to triglyceride metabolism. Yet many diabetics, likewise obese persons, have high plasma triglyceride levels and an increased IHD risk.

There is considerable uncertainty about the upper limit of the normal range of plasma triglyceride and plasma cholesterol levels. The upper limit of normal plasma cholesterol in the western world has been defined as the 95th percentile, but if a lower of 275 mg/100 ml is considered it has been demonstrated that 20%, not a mere 5% (Harlan et al., 1967), of American ex-servicemen exceed this level and have an increased IHD risk. Lewis (1972) drew attention to this point in his review of the plasma lipoproteins and considered therefore that both abnormally high plasma cholesterol and triglyceride levels "may well be the commonest metabolic lesion in industrialised communities".

In all parts of the world plasma lipids rise throughout childhood and, in western society, continue to rise during adult life, at least until the age of 50–59 years. This state of affairs is considered "normal". In many African communities there is no rise in plasma triglyceride levels throughout adult life; this was noted in South African Bantu males (Antonis and Bersohn, 1960) and in East African males (Lee et al., 1962). Both these groups ate much high-fibre starchy carbohydrate foods. Serum triglyceride levels were low and did not rise during adult life in New Guineans who ate high-fibre carbohydrate foods (Goldrick et al., 1970). In western society, however, a high consumption of low-fibre refined starchy foods is often accompanied by high plasma triglyceride levels in adults.

In the western world there appears to be an association between high plasma triglyceride levels and the prevalence of IHD. In Sweden a large IHD prospective study observed 3168 men during a period of 9 years, to detect any new manifestation of the disease. It was ascertained that the IHD risk rate increased linearly with rising plasma triglyceride levels and likewise with rising cholesterol levels, but that the former gave a better indicator of increased IHD risk. It was considered that both these risk factors were acting either independently or in association to increase the prevalence of the disease (Carlson and Böttiger, 1972). This was confirmed in a study of 500 U.S.A. persons who survived myocardial infarction for 3 months. Among survivors only those over 60 years were examined and the results were compared with those obtained in 950 healthy controls, matched in age and sex. The survivors of myocardial infarction had three times more hypertriglyceridaemia than the control group and elevation of serum triglyceride levels was commoner than that of serum cholesterol (Goldstein et al., 1973).

Plasma triglyceride levels are much influenced by diet, especially the carbohydrate portion. Among 16 normal British subjects who ate high-carbohydrate diets of which 86% was largely derived from refined carbohydrate foods—white flour and sugar—some 15 subjects showed a significant rise of plasma triglyceride levels (Mancini et al., 1973). These investigators considered plasma triglyceride levels in excess of 160 mg/100 ml to be "abnormal" in western man. Possibly even this is too high a level of division between healthy and unhealthy, for many western men having serum triglyceride levels below 160 mg/100 ml are regarded as "normal" but they develop ischaemic heart disease. Bantu mine workers, who consumed high-fibre maize meal diets, had mean serum triglyceride levels of 66 ± 17 mg/100 ml when aged 41–50 years and 68 ± 12 mg/100 ml when aged 51–60 years, and very rarely developed IHD (Antonis and Bersohn, 1960).

It is therefore important to ascertain whether the high plasma triglyceride levels of western man fall if the predominantly low-fibre refined white flour of their diets is replaced by high-fibre wholemeal, or their diets are supplemented with high-fibre bran. With this in view Heaton and Pomare (1974) gave wheat bran in a median dosage of 38 g/day for 5 weeks to 14 adults, among whom there was no change in serum cholesterol levels although three of them had values exceeding 325 mg/100 ml. On the other hand serum triglyceride levels fell in 12 out of the 14 subjects, and there was a significant reduction in the level of the group ($P < 0.01$). It is interesting to note that plasma triglycerides fell in all six subjects in whom plasma triglyceride levels were initially in the range of 100–150 mg/100 ml and would be considered "normal" in western man. Plasma triglyceride levels fell significantly also in a group of monks who ate fibre-rich bran biscuits but not in a control group who ate white bread (Eastwood, 1969) (p. 215).

If carbohydrate foods and dietary fibre influence IHD this is more likely to operate mainly through triglyceride metabolism than through cholesterol metabolism. Since dietary factors seldom act alone in the pathogenesis of disease, the intake of all varieties of fat must also be studied in triglyceride metabolism as in cholesterol metabolism. Of particular interest also is the possible effect on the coagulation–fibrinolysis mechanism which is known to be altered in the hypertriglyceridaemia induced by carbohydrate or by fat.

E. Attempts to assess the role of dietary fibre in ischaemic heart disease

1. Difficulties in assessment

It is impossible to obtain dietary fibre by itself for experimental purposes, and in any case since little is known about its complex physical and chemical composition it is difficult to carry out experiments with fibre-rich starchy carbohydrate foods. In dietary fibre there are many different physical varieties of celluloses, many different groups of complex polysaccharides formerly called the hemicelluloses, different varieties of lignin, probably unavailable fat, nitrogen and trace elements. It is possible, if not probable, that many of these do not act as single chemical substances, but in groups and in various combinations. In the natural state they are always in very close physical association, not only with one another but also with starch granules and other dietary constituents. The situation is totally different when fibre-rich bran is added to refined fibre-depleted white flour or white rice. Of great importance was the observation that rolled oats, 140 g/day, rapidly reduced serum cholesterol levels in hyperlipidaemic men (p. 208) and that leguminous seeds, 400 g/day, slowly reduced serum cholesterol levels in men rendered hyperlipidaemic by butter (p. 208). The difficulty in assessing the hypolipidaemic effect of dietary fibre was demonstrated by Mathur et al. (1968), who reported that 14 weeks were required to obtain the maximal hypocholesterolaemic effect of the leguminous seed Bengal gram, although a significant reduction of serum cholesterol levels could be demonstrated after other beans had been given in very large amounts for only 3 weeks (Grande et al., 1965).

2. Dietary fibre—not identical to cellulose

Previous mistakes which have impeded assessment of the role of dietary fibre arose largely because fibre was erroneously equated with cellulose (Grande, 1967) and, in addition, that one physical variety of cellulose, say that prepared by a chemist from cotton or wood, had the same physical structure and action as some other variety such as, for example, that contained in rolled oats or Purina chow. Further, when it was ascertained that chemical cellulose, 15 g/day, which is in excess of that present in any human diet, had no hypocholesterolaemic effect in man, and that a similar amount of pectin was only slightly effective, it was concluded that the natural fibre, regarded as cellulose, was without effect (Keys *et al.*, 1961).

Since fibre has been equated with cellulose this substance has been given to animals to provide "bulk" in various atherogenic diets (Ershoff and Wells, 1962; Fisher *et al.*, 1967; Kritchevsky and Tepper, 1968). Other investigators have used carboxymethyl cellulose (Antar *et al.*, 1970) or other relatively pure polysaccharides such as agar, alphacel or celluflour. The anomalous results of these experiments frequently puzzled the investigators, none of whom apparently asked whether the complex group of substances in the fibre derived from the vegetable cell-wall could in fact be adequately replaced by a single polysaccharide, different also in its physical structure.

3. *Fibre and cholesterol metabolism*

Experiments in cholesterol-fed rats have demonstrated that rice bran was hypocholesterolaemic when it contributed 16% of the daily calories, but that it was far less effective than an equal amount of crude fibre in whole ground rice (p. 205). This suggests that the hypocholesterolaemic effect depends both on the quantity of fibre and also its physical state in relation to the granules of starch and other food normally contained within the vegetable cell-wall. A comparable amount of bran for a man is 120–150 g/day, 16% of the daily calories.

Attempts have been made to ascertain if wheat bran is hypocholesterolaemic in man. Eastwood (1969) tested wheat bran biscuits on 28 monks of a Cistercian Trappist monastery. All monks gave up their customary staple food of wholemeal bread 300 g/day; half took fibre-rich wheat bran biscuits and the other half ate low-fibre white bread. At the end of the 12 week experiment the mean serum cholesterol levels of the two groups of monks did not differ significantly, but the mean serum triglyceride levels had fallen more in the younger monks, those under 40 years of age, who had eaten the fibre-rich biscuits ($P < 0.05$). In an experiment by Eastwood *et al.* (1973), wheat bran 16 g/day was added to the western-type diet of eight healthy men aged 25–43 years for a period of 3 weeks. There was no change in the mean serum cholesterol levels or in total faecal bile acid excretion during this short period of observation. Unfortunately, serum triglyceride levels were not observed. Serum cholesterol levels did not change when during a period of 5 weeks wheat bran 38 g/day was added to the western-type diet of 14 men, five of whom had severe hypercholesterolaemia (Heaton and Pomare, 1974).

From the foregoing it would appear that moderate amounts of fibre-rich wheat bran do not alter serum cholesterol levels in man, at least in short-term experiments. No attempts to confirm the reported hypocholesterolaemic effect of large amounts of whole unprocessed seeds, rolled oats (de Groot *et al.*, 1963) or mature leguminous seeds (Mathur *et al.*, 1968) have been traced.

4. The dietary fibre hypothesis

Walker and Arvidsson (1954) were the first to suggest that crude fibre might protect against IHD, which was very rare among South African Bantu who consumed much fibre-rich maize meal. In numerous publications Walker (1955, 1956, 1961, 1968) amplified this hypothesis, pointing out that many diseases, common in western man, were rare among the Bantu: constipation, obesity, diabetes, peptic ulcer, gallstones, and IHD, but little supporting experimental data could be produced. Two mistakes unfortunately delayed the development of this fibre hypothesis of IHD, because, as has been mentioned: (1) crude fibre was equated with cellulose (Walker, 1956); and also (2) a dietary experiment in South African white and Bantu people appeared to show that crude-fibre intakes did not influence serum cholesterol levels. However, Cleave *et al.* (1969) ascribed IHD solely to the consumption of refined carbohydrate foods, and to the excessive consumption of sugar in particular, and they stressed the association of IHD and diabetes mellitus.

The work of Southgate (1969) on the estimation of the unavailable carbohydrates and lignin emphasized the fact that fibre could not be equated with cellulose. It then became possible to re-define fibre with greater precision. The term and concept of dietary fibre as the remnants of vegetable cell-walls unhydrolysed by human alimentary enzymes was set forth by Trowell (1972a, b, c), who postulated that it might be a protective factor against IHD. Previously Trowell (1960), having learned about fibre from Dr A. R. P. Walker, had suggested that fibre might protect Africans not only against constipation but against many other diseases of the colon, such as diverticular disease, cancer and ulcerative colitis.

Criticisms of dietary fibre fall under two headings: (1) those of nutritionalists concerning a new definition of fibre; (2) those which concern the dietary fibre hypothesis of IHD (summary, p. 221).

(1) Nutritionalists began to clarify their ideas concerning fibre at a meeting of the Nutrition Society held during 1973 (Proceedings of Nutrition Society, 1973). Subsequently Southgate (1973) concluded an article entitled "Dietary Fibre" with the statement that "the present position with regard to dietary fibre seems to be that there is some quite strong epidemiological evidence of the association of some diseases with a low fibre intake". He accepted the term dietary fibre as synonymous, in the present state of knowledge, with the unavailable carbohydrates and

lignin. Cummings (1973) concluded his review entitled "Dietary Fibre" in a gastroenterological journal by stating that "dietary fibre is an important component of our food. Its role in the gut has been underestimated."

(2) Some data which were considered to support the dietary fibre hypothesis of IHD have provoked criticism and have also stimulated experimental studies. Cummings (1973) criticized certain supporting data by drawing attention to the fact that in South Africa "serum cholesterol levels do not always show the expected difference between rural and urban Bantu". He referred to the recent study of Venda Bantu among whom no significant difference was demonstrated between the mean serum cholesterol levels in urban men 231 mg/100 ml and in rural men 219 mg/100 ml (Nel *et al.*, 1971). He omitted to state that among these Venda males "all age-groups of urban subjects had higher intakes of animal fat (mean 106·4 g/day) than rural subjects (mean 18·7 g/day)" (Lubbe, 1971), but the reported similarity of serum cholesterol levels in urban and rural Bantu is still partially unexplained. Animal fats certainly raise serum cholesterol levels; dietary fibre in large amounts may lower these levels. This requires further investigation. It should be noted that IHD would still be a very rare disease even among urban Venda Bantu who ate carbohydrate 559 g/day, mainly derived from maize meal called "baker's cones" (Lubbe, 1971), which contained crude fibre 0·8 g/100 g (Metz *et al.*, 1970), thus providing crude fibre 4 g/day from starchy foods, compared to 1·1 g/day of crude fibre derived from all starchy foods by people in Britain in 1970 (Trowell, 1973b).

It should be noted also that similar serum cholesterol levels in various countries carry a different significance as indicators of the risk of development of IHD. There is an increased IHD risk if in India serum cholesterol levels exceed 195 mg/100 ml, in Italy 203 mg/100 ml, in Norway 270 mg/100 ml, and in the U.S.A. 265 mg/100 ml (Walker, 1973).

III. Fibrinolysis

A. Thrombosis and fibrinolysis

If thrombosis never occurred in an atheromatous coronary artery, then myocardial infarction would be rare. If thrombosis never formed in the deep veins of the leg, then post-operative pulmonary embolism would seldom be seen. Both of these conditions are very rare in Africans and in the inhabitants of certain islands of the Pacific, such as New Guinea. Although in these widely separated areas the groups who had less IHD and less post-operative pulmonary embolism ate more fibre-rich starchy food, it remains uncertain to what extent, if at all, this altered thrombosis and fibrinolysis.

It is probable that minute thrombi are often forming on the roughened surface of an atheromatous artery. One theory concerning the pathogenesis of atheroma postulates that minute thrombi form on the intima of the arterial wall and are transformed into atheromatous plaques. These thrombi, however formed, are not static and provide an interface at which dynamic processes occur. Thrombosis can extend and clot accumulate, or fibrinolysis can decrease the size of the clot.

B. Fat intakes

There is evidence to suggest that diet influences the incidence and severity of thrombosis, even though mechanisms are little understood. In Germany serum cholesterol levels fell and pulmonary embolism decreased to approximately a quarter of its previous level during the period of severe war-time food restrictions, 1940–48. The incidence of fatal pulmonary embolism was lowest in 1948, following a period of a few years when fat consumption was reduced to 5–10 g/day (Schettler, 1970).

Blood fibrinolysis activity is inhibited and blood coagulation is accelerated by high-fat feeding. This has been demonstrated in three racial groups, Scotsmen in Glasgow, and in both Asian and African medical students in Nairobi, Kenya. These were tested by the same investigators (Mackay et al., 1970). Half of each racial group ate a very high-fat (95 g) breakfast; the other half had only a trace of fat (0·6 g) in their meal. In the Scots alone, after the high-fat breakfast, fibrinolysis was inhibited (shown as euglobulin clot-lysis time increased and urokinase sensitivity reduced) and platelet aggression time was prolonged. Neither of these features occurred in the Asians and Africans. In all groups blood coagulation was accelerated after the high-fat breakfast (shown as increased fibrin formation, measured by Stypven time—Russell's viper venom). No reason could be suggested for the differences in fibrinolysis and blood coagulation.

In elderly Danes the incidence of thrombo-embolism appeared to be influenced by the fat intake of the diet. One group who had a reduced fat intake (40 g/day), largely derived from unsaturated vegetable oils, had much less thrombo-embolism than a control group who continued to eat their previous diet of high fat content (80 g/day), largely derived from saturated fats (Hansen et al., 1962).

The possible role of dietary fibre in promoting brisk fibrinolysis in man has never been investigated. It has, however, been shown that rats fed an atherogenic diet were protected against thrombosis when their diet was based on fibre-rich Purina chow; nevertheless thrombosis did occur if their diet was synthetic and contained cellulose in place of fibre (Gresham and Howard, 1960; Howard et al., 1968).

C. Fibre intakes

1. Africa

In Africans fibrinolysis is brisk when compared to Asians or Europeans resident in the same area of the country. South African rural Bantu men, aged 41–50 years, were shown to have a mean clot-lysis time of 5·6 h compared with 10·4 h in South African white men of comparable age (Merskey et al., 1960). The diets of these two groups were very different. The Bantu ate fibre-rich starchy carbohydrate food but took little fat (18% of the daily calories), whereas the whites ate fibre-depleted starchy food and much fat (43% of the daily calories). No differences were noted in the women of the same two groups. It should also be recognized that the laboratory methods of examination were, by modern standards, insensitive. Other observers have confirmed the brisk fibrinolysis of Africans in Nigeria (Howell, 1965) and in East Africa (Barr et al., 1973).

Not only is fibrinolytic activity brisker in Africans than in Asians and Europeans domiciled in the same country but this activity does not decrease significantly with age, as it does in other racial groups (Shaper et al., 1966). This may explain the low prevalence of all forms of thrombo-embolism which become increasingly common in older western age-groups. Thrombo-embolism at any site was detected in only 2·4% of 1427 Ugandan autopsies of subjects aged over 40 years, whereas in a comparable group in the United States the incidence was 52% (Thomas et al., 1960). In South Africa fibrinolytic activity was brisker in rural than in urban Bantu males, and in both Bantu groups was more active than in South African white males. No difference, however, was detected between rural or urban Bantu women and South African white women (Walker, 1961).

Recently a careful study of the blood coagulation and fibrinolytic systems has been undertaken in Nairobi. Fifty Kenyan Africans (25 males, 25 females) aged 19–39 years, and a similar number of European men and women of comparable age were examined (Barr et al., 1973). The results suggested relative hypercoagulability in European males compared to the African males. These results, set out in Table 15.4, showed that European males had decreased fibrinolytic activity, less plasminogen and plasminogen activator than did the African males. No such differences were demonstrated between European and African females.

2. New Guinea and Malaysia

Brisk fibrinolysis has been detected also in New Guineans (Goldrick, 1961; Grace et al., 1970).

All of these indigenous groups in Africa and New Guinea ate a similar

TABLE 15.4. Blood coagulation and fibrinolytic enzyme systems in healthy adult African males and European males (Barr et al., 1973)

Index	African male (AM)	European male (EM)	Ratio AM:EM
Euglobulin lysis times (min)	76–557 (median 193)	73–810 (median 380)	$P < 0.025$
Plasminogen (casein units)	3.9 ± 1.5	3.4 ± 2.0	$P < 0.02$
Urokinase sensitivity test (s)	287 ± 66	370 ± 185	$P < 0.001$
One stage prothrombin time (s)	16 ± 2	15 ± 2.5	$P < 0.01$
Thrombin clotting time (s)	9.5 ± 2.5	8 ± 1	$P < 0.005$
Factor VIII (%)	42–213 (median 100)	37–173 (median 80)	$P < 0.005$

diet in which unprocessed or lightly processed fibre-rich carbohydrate foods contributed 70–85%, and fat 5–20%, of the daily energy intake. Brisk fibrinolysis has also been found in Malaysians (Loncin et al., 1968), but few particulars concerning their diet were reported.

3. India

Little study of fibrinolysis and blood coagulation has been done in India and Pakistan. In many urban Indians fibrinolysis times appear comparable to those regarded as normal in Europe and North America. Fibrinolysis was, however, found to be much less active in Indians suffering from ischaemic heart disease (Sikka et al., 1968; Basu et al., 1971), especially if this was associated with diabetes, and in these patients improvement followed tolbutamide therapy (Gupta, 1969). No reference has been traced to investigations in India concerning any variation in fibrinolysis in different groups consuming different diets, apart from the observations of Malhotra (1972) who studied railway sweepers from two different areas. Fibrinolysis was much brisker and blood coagulation was slower in one group of North Indians, who ate a large amount of coarse flour milled from wheat or millet, fibre-rich legumes, and a moderate amount of fat, than it was in another group of South Indians, who ate a large amount of white rice of low fibre content, a small amount of legumes, and a minimal amount of fat. These results suggest that fibre might play an important role in producing brisk fibrinolysis.

4. Europe and America

It is premature to compare any observations concerning fibrinolysis in Africa and Asia with those made in Europe and America. Briefly it may be noted, however, that in western man there is a highly significant inverse relationship between all estimates of fibrinolytic activity and body fatness in men and women (Grace and Goldrick, 1968). Fibrinolytic activity decreased from its former normal level in male survivors of myocardial infarction (Chakrabort *et al.*, 1968) and also in diabetes, especially if it was associated with IHD (Fearnley *et al.*, 1963). In Europe and America more information is needed concerning the relationship of fibrinolysis and blood coagulation to the diet, and especially to its content of starchy carbohydrate foods, fibre and fat, and the prevalence of IHD, diabetes and thrombo-embolism.

IV. Summary of dietary fibre hypothesis concerning ischaemic heart disease

A high consumption of starchy carbohydrate foods containing their full complement of dietary fibre appears to protect against IHD; starches partially depleted of dietary fibre appear to offer only partial protection. Conversely, a high consumption of fibre-depleted starchy carbohydrate foods appears to be a risk factor in IHD.

Although a high consumption of fat, especially saturated fat, has been recognized to be a risk factor in IHD, the possible significance of the fact that its increased consumption is almost invariably accompanied by a decreased intake of starchy food, and consequently of fibre, has been overlooked. Sugar if eaten in large quantities also expels other starchy foods, richer in fibre, from the customary diet. Large amounts of fibre-rich starchy carbohydrate foods have been shown to reduce plasma cholesterol levels and to increase bile salt excretion in both animals and man. Populations who eat large quantities of starchy foods, undepleted of dietary fibre, not only have low plasma triglyceride and low cholesterol levels but also rapid fibrinolysis throughout adult life. These factors may contribute to their low IHD prevalence.

Smoking, high blood pressure, diseases such as diabetes mellitus and obesity, likewise heredity, sex, and many other factors, also influence the IHD prevalence.

This hypothesis is part of the larger one, namely that man has adapted well to traditional food eaten for many millennia, which was largely unprocessed carbohydrate foods. Special ethnic groups, like the Eskimos for example, adapted many millennia ago to special diets, which in other groups, not adapted to these diets, might induce disease. Eskimos consume plant fibre during the short Arctic summer; they also eat fibre in the plankton of the intestines of fish, which are consumed. Nothing is known concerning the action of this small and variable seasonal intake of dietary fibre.

222   H. TROWELL

References

ANTAR, M. A., LITTLE, J. A., LUCAS, C., BUCKLEY, G. C. and CSIMA, A. (1970). *Atherosclerosis* **11**, 191.
ANTONIS, A. and BERSOHN, I. (1960). *Lancet* **1**, 998.
ANTONIS, A. and BERSOHN, I. (1962a). *American Journal of Clinical Nutrition* **10**, 484.
ANTONIS, A. and BERSOHN, I. (1962b). *American Journal of Clinical Nutrition* **11**, 142.
BARR, R. D., OUMA, N. and KENDALL, A. G. (1973). *Scottish Medical Journal* **18**, 93.
BASU, H. N., HUSSAIN, Q., MITTAL, M. M. and SHARMA, M. L. (1971). *Journal of the Indian Medical Association* **57**, 135.
BOOYEN, J., DE WAAL, V. M., RADEMAYER, L. J. and CALITZ, F. (1966). *South African Medical Journal* **40**, 237.
BROWN, J., BOURKE, G. J., GEARTY, G. F., FINNEGAN, A., HILL, M., HEFFERNAN-FOX, F. C., FITZGERALD, D. E., KENNEDY, J., CHILDERS, R. W., JESSOP, W. J. E., TRULSON, M. F., LATHAM, M. C., CRONIN, S., MCCANN, M. B., CLANCY, R. E., GORE, I., STOUDT, H. W., HEGSTED, D. M. and STARE, F. J. (1970). *World Review of Nutrition and Dietetics* **12**, 1.
CARLSON, L. A. and BÖTTIGER, L. E. (1972). *Lancet* **1**, 865.
CHAKRABORT, R., HOCKING, E. D., FEARNLEY, G. R., MANN, R. D., ATWELL, T. M. and JACKSON, D. (1968). *Lancet* **1**, 987.
CLEAVE, T. L., CAMPBELL, G. D. and PAINTER, N. S. (1969). "Diabetes, Coronary Thrombosis and the Saccharine Disease", pp. 113–127. John Wright, Bristol.
COLEMAN, D. L. and BAUMANN, C. A. (1959). *Archives of Biochemistry and Biophysics* **66**, 226.
CUMMINGS, J. H. (1973). *Gut* **14**, 69.
DE GROOT, A. P., LUYKEN, R. and PIKAAR, N. A. (1963). *Lancet* **2**, 303.
DEVI, K. S. and KURUP, P. A. (1972). *Atherosclerosis* **15**, 223.
EASTWOOD, M. (1969). *Lancet* **2**, 1222.
EASTWOOD, M. A., KIRKPATRICK, J. R., MITCHELL, W. D., BONE, A. and HAMILTON, T. (1973). *British Medical Journal* **2**, 392.
ERSHOFF, B. H. and WELLS, A. F. (1962). *Proceedings of the Society for Experimental Biology and Medicine* **110**, 580.
FAHRENBACH, M. J., RICCARDI, B. A. and GRANT, W. C. (1966). *Proceedings of the Society for Experimental Biology and Medicine* **123**, 321.
FEARNLEY, G., CHAKRABORT, R. and AVIS, P. R. D. (1963). *British Medical Journal* **1**, 921.
FISHER, H. and GRIMINGER, P. (1967). *Proceedings of the Society for Experimental Biology and Medicine* **126**, 108.
FISHER, H., GRIMINGER, P. and SILBER, W. G. (1967). *Journal of Atherosclerosis Research* **7**, 381.
FRIEDBERG, C. K. (1966). "Diseases of the Heart", 3rd edition, p. 771. W. B. Saunders, Philadelphia.
GOLDRICK, R. B. (1961). *Australasian Annals of Medicine* **10**, 20.

GOLDRICK, R. B., SINNETT, P. H. and WHYTE, H. M. (1970). "Atherosclerosis, Proceedings of the Second International Symposium" (R. J. Jones, ed.), pp. 336–338. Springer-Verlag, Berlin.

GOLDSTEIN, J. L., HAZZARD, W. B., SCHROTT, H. G., BIERMAN, E. L. and MOTULSKY, A. G. (1973). *Journal of Clinical Investigation* 52, 1533.

GRACE, C. S. and GOLDRICK, R. B. (1968). *Journal of Atherosclerosis Research* 8, 705.

GRACE, C. S., SINNETT, P. and WHYTE, H. M. (1970). *Australasian Annals of Medicine* 19, 329.

GRANDE, F. (1967). *American Journal of Clinical Nutrition* 20, 176.

GRANDE, F., ANDERSON, J. T. and KEYS, A. (1965). *Journal of Nutrition* 86, 313.

GRESHAM, G. A. and HOWARD, A. N. (1960). *British Journal of Experimental Pathology* 41, 395.

GRIMINGER, P. and FISHER, H. (1966). *Proceedings of the Society for Experimental Biology and Medicine* 122, 551.

GROEN, J. J., BALOGH, M., LEVY, M. and YARON, E. (1964). *American Journal of Clinical Nutrition* 14, 37.

GROEN, J. J., TIJONG, K. B., KOSTER, M., WILLEBRANDS, A. F., VERDONCK, G. and PIERLOOT, M. (1962). *American Journal of Clinical Nutrition* 10, 456.

GUPTA, K. K. (1969). *Journal of the Association of Physicians of India* 17, 323.

HANSEN, P. F., GEILL, T. and LUND, E. (1962). *Lancet* 2, 1193.

HARLAN, W. R., OBERMAN, A., MITCHELL, R. E. and GRAYBIEL, A. (1967). *Annals Internal Medicine* 66, 540.

HEATON, K. W. (1972). "Bile Salts in Health and Disease", p. 191. Churchill Livingstone, Edinburgh.

HEATON, K. W. and POMARE, E. W. (1974). *Lancet* 1, 49.

HOWARD, A. N., GRESHAM, G. A. and LINDGREN, F. T. (1968). *Journal of Atherosclerosis Research* 8, 739.

HOWELL, M. (1965). *Journal of Atherosclerosis Research* 5, 80.

HUGHES, L. E. (1969). *Gut* 10, 336.

IRITANI, N. and NOGI, J. (1972). *Atherosclerosis* 15, 87.

JONES, A. M. (1970). *British Heart Journal* 32, 583.

KEMPNER, W. (1948). *American Journal of Medicine* 4, 545.

KEYS, A. (1968). *In* "Dietary Studies and Epidemiology of Heart Diseases" (C. D. Hartog, K. Buzina, F. Fidanya, A. Keys and P. Roine, eds), p. 23. Voedingsgebied, The Hague.

KEYS, A. (1970). "Coronary Heart Disease in Seven Countries", American Heart Association Monograph No. 29, Supplement to *Circulation* 40, 186.

KEYS, A., ANDERSON, J. T. and GRANDE, F. (1960). *Journal of Nutrition* 70, 257.

KEYS, A., ARAVANIS, C., BLACKBURN, H., VAN BUCHEM, F. S. P., BUZINA, R., DJORDJEVIK, B. S., FIDANYA, F. and KAROVER, J., (1972). *Circulation* 45, 815.

KEYS, A., GRANDE, F. and ANDERSON, J. T. (1961). *Proceedings of the Society for Experimental Biology and Medicine* 106, 555.

KIRIYAMA, S., OKAZAKI, Y. and YOSHIDA, A. (1969). *Journal of Nutrition* 97, 382.

KRITCHEVSKY, D. and TEPPER, S. A. (1968). *Journal of Atherosclerosis Research* 8, 357.

KRITCHEVSKY, D., SALLATA, P. and TEPPER, S. A. (1968). *Journal of Atherosclerosis Research* **8**, 697.

LEE, K. T., GOODALE, F., SCOTT, R. F. and SNELL, E. S. (1964). *American Journal of Cardiology* **13**, 30.

LEE, K. T., SHAPER, A. G., SCOTT, R. F., GOODALE, F. and THOMAS, W. A. (1962). *Archives of Pathology* **74**, 481.

LEIBOWITZ, J. O. (1970). "The History of Coronary Heart Disease." Wellcome Institute of the History of Medicine, London. (a) p. 63; (b) p. 83.

LEWIS, B. (1972). "The Scientific Basis of Medicine Annual Reviews" (I. Gilliland and J. Francis, eds), pp. 118–144. Athlone Press, London.

LONCIN, H., GURIAN, J. M. and LONCIN, M. E. (1968). *Journal of Atherosclerosis Research* **8**, 471.

LOWENSTEIN, F. W. (1964). *American Journal of Clinical Nutrition* **15**, 175.

LUBBE, A. M. (1971). *South African Medical Journal* **45**, 1289.

LUYKEN, R., PIKAAR, N., POLMAN, H. and SHIPPERS, F. A. (1962). *Voeding* **23**, 447.

MCGANDY, R. B. D., HEGSTED, D. M., MYERS, M. L. and STARE, F. J. (1966). *American Journal of Clinical Nutrition* **18**, 237.

MACKAY, N., FERGUSON, J. C. and MCNICOL, G. P. (1970). *Journal of Clinical Pathology* **23**, 580.

MALHOTRA, S. L. (1967). *British Heart Journal* **29**, (a) 337; (b) 895.

MALHOTRA, S. L. (1967c). *American Journal of Clinical Nutrition* **20**, 462.

MALHOTRA, S. L. (1968). *British Heart Journal* **30**, 303.

MALHOTRA, S. L. (1971). *American Journal of Clinical Nutrition* **24**, 1195.

MALHOTRA, S. L. (1972). *International Journal of Epidemiology* **1**, 177.

MANCINI, M., MATTOCK, M., RUBAYA, E., CHAIT, A. and LEWIS, B. (1973). *Atherosclerosis* **17**, 445.

MARUFFO, C. A. and PORTMAN, O. W. (1968). *Journal of Atherosclerosis Research* **8**, 237.

MATHUR, K. S., KHAN, M. A. and SHARMA, R. D. (1968). *British Medical Journal* **1**, 30.

MEDALIE, J. H., RISS, E., GROEN, J. J., KAHN, H. A. and BACHRACH, C. A. (1968). *Israel Journal of Medical Science* **4**, 775.

MERSKEY, C., GORDON, H. and LACKNER, H. (1960). *British Medical Journal* **1**, 219.

METZ, J., LURIE, A. and KONIDARIS, M. (1970). *South African Medical Journal* **44**, 539.

MOORE, J. H. (1967). *British Journal of Nutrition* **21**, 297.

NEL, A., DU PLESSIS, J. P. and FELLINGHAM, S. A. (1971). *South African Medical Journal* **45**, 1315.

OKAMOTO, K., HAZAMA, F. and YAMASAKI, Y. (1971). *In* "Diabetes in Asia, 1970" (S. Tsuji and M. Wada, eds), pp. 106–119. Excerpta Medica, Amsterdam.

OLSON, R. E., VESTER, J. W., GURSEY, D., DAVIS, N. and LONGMAN, D. (1958). *American Journal of Clinical Nutrition* **6**, 310.

PALMER, G. H. and DIXON, D. G. (1966). *American Journal of Clinical Nutrition* **18**, 437.

PARDEE, H. E. B. (1920). *Archives of Internal Medicine* **26**, 244.

PARKINSON, J. and BEDFORD, D. E. (1928). *Lancet* **1**, 4.

PINTO, I. J., THOMAS, P., COLACO, F. and DATEY, K. K. (1970). *In* "Atherosclerosis, Proceedings of the Second International Symposium" (R. J. Jones, ed.), pp. 328–335. Springer-Verlag, Berlin.

PORTMAN, O. W. (1960). *American Journal of Clinical Nutrition* **8**, 462.

PORTMAN, O. W. and MANN, G. V. (1955). *Journal of Biology and Chemistry* **213**, 732.

PORTMAN, O. W., MANN, G. V. and WYSOCKI, A. P. (1955). *Archives of Biochemistry and Biophysics* **59**, 224.

PORTMAN, O. W. and MURPHY, P. (1958). *Archives of Biochemistry and Biophysics* **76**, 367.

Proceedings of the Nutrition Society (1973). **32**, 123.

Registrar-General's Statistical Review of England and Wales, 1931–1970, Part 1, Tables, Medical. Her Majesty's Stationery Office, London.

SARVOTHAM, S. G. and BERRY, J. N. (1968). *Circulation* **37**, 939.

SCHETTLER, G. (1970). *In* "Atherosclerosis" (R. J. Jones, ed.), p. xxviii. Springer-Verlag, Berlin.

SCHOWENGERDT, C. G., HEDGES, G. R., YAW, P. B. and ALTEMEIER, W. A. (1969). *Archives of Surgery* **98**, 500.

SCHRIRE, V. (1971). *South African Medical Journal* **45**, 634.

SEFTEL, H. C., KEW, M. C. and BERSOHN, I. (1970). *South African Medical Journal* **44**, 8.

SEFTEL, H. C., SPITZ, M. G., BERSOHN, I., GOLDIN, A. R., JAFFE, B. I., RUBINSTEIN, A. H. and METZGER, B. E. (1973). *South African Medical Journal* **47**, 1571.

SHAPER, A. G. (1972). *British Medical Journal* **4**, 32.

SHAPER, A. G., KYOBE, J. and JONES, M. (1966). *Journal of Atherosclerosis Research* **6**, 313.

SHUHACHI, K., OKAZAKI, Y. and YOSHIDA, A. (1969). *Journal of Nutrition* **97**, 382.

SHURPALEKAR, K. S., DORAISWAMY, T. R., SUNDARAVALLI, O. E. and RAO, N. M. (1971). *Nature* **232**, 554.

SIKKA, K. K., NAVANI, H. H., TIAGI, G. K. and NIGAM, D. N. (1968). *Indian Journal of Medical Research* **56**, 411.

SOUTHGATE, D. A. T. (1969). *Journal of Science of Food and Agriculture* **20**, 331.

SOUTHGATE, D. A. T. (1973). *Plant Foods for Man* **1**, 45.

STOUT, C., MORROW, J., BRANDT, E. N. and WOLF, S. (1964). *Journal of the American Medical Association* **188**, 845.

THOMAS, W. A., DAVIES, J. N. P., NEAL, R. M. O. and DIMAKULANGAN, A. A. (1960). *American Journal of Cardiology* **5**, 41.

TROWELL, H. (1960). "Non-infective Disease in Africa", pp. 217–220. Edward Arnold, London.

TROWELL, H. (1972a). *European Journal of Clinical and Biological Research* **17**, 345.

TROWELL, H. (1972b). *Atherosclerosis* **16**, 138.

TROWELL, H. (1972c). *American Journal of Clinical Nutrition* **25**, 926.

TROWELL, H. (1973a). *Proceedings of the Nutrition Society* **32**, 150.

TROWELL, H. (1973b). *Plant Foods for Man* **1**, 11.

TROWELL, H., PAINTER, N. and BURKITT, D. (1974). *American Journal of Digestive Diseases* **19**, 864.

TRUSWELL, A. S. and MANN, J. I. (1972). *Atherosclerosis* **16**, 15.

VIJAYAGOPALAN, P. and KURUP, P. A. (1970). *Atherosclerosis* **11**, 257.

VIJAYAGOPALAN, P. and KURUP, P. A. (1972a). *Atherosclerosis* **15**, 215.

VIJAYAGOPALAN, P. and KURUP, P. A. (1972b). *Atherosclerosis* **16**, 247.

VIJAYAGOPAL, P., DEVI, K. S. and KURUP, P. A. (1973). *Atherosclerosis* **17**, 156.

WALKER, A. R. P. and ARVIDSSON, U. B. (1954). *Journal of Clinical Investigation* **33**, 1358.

WALKER, A. R. P. (1955). *Lancet* **1**, 565.

WALKER, A. R. P. (1956). *South African Medical Journal* **30**, 411.

WALKER, A. R. P. (1961). *South African Medical Journal* **35**, 114.

WALKER, A. R. P. (1968). *South African Medical Journal* **42**, 944.

WALKER, A. R. P. (1973). *South African Medical Journal* **47**, 85.

WORLD HEALTH ORGANIZATION (1969). *Bulletin of the International Society of Cardiology* **1**, 1.

Chapter 16

Diabetes mellitus and obesity

HUGH TROWELL

I. Diabetes mellitus 227
  A. Normal homeostatic control of blood glucose 227
  B. History of diabetes mellitus 228
  C. Prevalence in modern times 229
  D. Experimental studies 238
  E. Sugar. 239
II. Obesity 240
  A. Definition and prevalence 240
  B. History of obesity and diet 241
  C. Experimental studies 242
  D. Evolution and obesity 245
III. Summary of fibre-depleted starchy carbohydrate foods hypothesis
  concerning diabetes and/or obesity 245
References 246

I. Diabetes mellitus

A. Normal homeostatic control of blood glucose

The homeostatic control of the blood glucose level is very important. If its concentration falls too low the central nervous system is deprived of the large amounts of energy it requires. Hyperglycaemia is prevented partially by the kidney, the renal threshold for reabsorption being usually about 180 mg/100 ml. The most important factor tending to reduce a high blood glucose level is the insulin secreted by the β-cells of the pancreatic islets. The most important organ in regulating blood glucose is the liver: if blood glucose is high, it stores glucose as glycogen; if blood glucose is low, glucose is passed from the liver into the blood stream. A number of other factors affect blood glucose levels; thus adrenalin, cortisol, growth hormone and glucagon raise the level. Diabetes mellitus represents a breakdown of this fundamental homeostasis, with a tendency to develop progressively more severe hyperglycaemia.

B. *History of diabetes mellitus*

"Urine exceeding sweet . . . resembling the juice of the sugar cane" which attracted ants, was described in India by Charaka and Sushruta about 2000 years ago; the former even advocated treatment by fibre-rich leguminous seeds (Tulloch, 1962a). The actual date remains uncertain; some place it as early as the sixth century B.C., others in the second or first centuries B.C. (Major, 1954a). Inheritance, obesity and a possible relationship to the consumption of sugar were all mentioned. Change-Ke is said to have been the first to describe sweet urine attracting dogs in China, possibly as early as the third century (Barach, 1928) and certainly in the seventh century A.D. (Gwei-Djen and Needham, 1967).

Because the name "diabetes" is derived from a Greek word, many have considered it to be a disease known in the Mediterranean cultures of antiquity. This is doubtful. The Ebers papyrus of ancient Egypt in the sixteenth century B.C. described undue thirst, as did Aretaeus (A.D. 120–200), who mentioned the "unquenchable thirst, excessive drinking . . . one cannot stop them from drinking or making urine" (Major, 1954b). Neither Aretaeus nor Galen, who recorded only two cases of diabetes in some 36 years of medical practice in the Roman empire (A.D. 164–200), saw many patients who had this disease, which was probably diabetes insipidus (Henschen, 1966); no mention was made of a sugary urine. Avicenna (A.D. 980–1027), an Islamic physician of Persia, was dealing with diabetes mellitus, for he noted that the urine had a residue like honey. Obesity, which will be discussed later in this chapter, was rare in Rome, Greece and Egypt. The two conditions usually appear together in any community.

Willis (1621–1675) was the first physician of modern Europe to note in 1673 that the diabetic urine was "wonderfully sweet as if it were imbued with Honey or Sugar" (Major, 1954c). The physicians of Britain in Tudor times (Copeman, 1960) made a habit of inspecting the urine in a flask; it was almost the main part of the clinical examination. If diabetes mellitus had been present in Britain at that time no doubt the attraction of flies would have been noted. Willis (1679) was indeed correct when he stated that "Diabetes was a Disease so rare among the Ancients that many physicians make no mention of it". Willis effected for the first time the differentiation of diabetes mellitus from diabetes insipidus. Matthew Dobson in 1776 demonstrated sugar in the urine by fermentation. These earlier writers on diabetes mellitus all stressed that the disease was common in the more wealthy social classes but rare among the poor, and more common in towns than in rural areas. At the beginning of the twentieth century the same points were made concerning wealthy Hindu men (Bose, 1907), Cingalese (Fernando, 1907) and Egyptians (Sandwith, 1907). At that time in all these countries diabetes was reported to be commoner in men than in women; this was the situation in Britain during the period 1861–1923 after which the disease became common in women (Stocks, 1944).

C. Prevalence in modern times

1. Among underdeveloped communities

Whenever a community has been examined under conditions of its natural habitat, manner of life and traditional diet, diabetes mellitus has appeared to be virtually absent, as among pure Laplanders, pure-bred Eskimos, Australian Aborigines, South African Bushmen or Hottentots (Jackson, 1971). Indeed this was the author's own experience for the 5 years 1930–34 among all African tribes in Nairobi hospital. When certain developing groups, such as Yemenite Jews, South African Bantu and New Zealand Maoris, all of whom ate large amounts of lightly processed carbohydrate foods, adopted western patterns of living in towns, the prevalence of diabetes increased markedly (Jackson, 1971). In the process of this change many food habits altered, but the largest dietary change involved the consumption of refined carbohydrate foods. Diabetes is still considered to be uncommon in West Africa (Tulloch, 1962b) but it is now common among American negroes in whom the age-adjusted death rate, 21·1 per 100,000 persons, is much higher than that of American whites, 12·6 per 100,000 persons (Joslin, 1971a).

2. Among western nations

There are two main sources of evidence concerning the occurrence of diabetes in the developed countries of the western world: mortality data and prevalence surveys. If mortality data are compared either between one country and another at the same period of time, or within one country during a long period of time, there would appear to be considerable truth in the statement of Joslin and his colleagues (1940) that the highest incidence of diabetes occurs where (1) the average age is highest, (2) women predominate, (3) obesity is most frequent, (4) medical supervision is excellent and (5) deaths are accurately recorded. These conditions occur to a most marked degree in the most technologically advanced countries of the western world, but many facts still remain unexplained by these criteria, as will be discussed later.

(a) *England and Wales.* The apparent rise of diabetes mortality (Stocks, 1944) might be explained in terms of Joslin's five points, but these do not

explain the fall in female diabetes mortality which occurred during the
food restrictions of both World Wars (1914–18, 1939–45):

Crude mortality rates—female diabetes per million

1861–70	1915	1918	1919	1940	1941	1945	1954
21	120	90	100	153	141	122	86

The fall to 90/million in 1918 has been attributed to the wartime
rationing of 1916–18. In the Second World War food rationing began in
1940, and the year 1941 saw the largest reduction in diabetic mortality
since the First World War. In 9 of the subsequent 14 years 1941–54 the
rate declined, and was at its lowest in 1954, 86/million (see Table 16.1,
Fig. 16.1).

Similar change occurred in male diabetes mortality 1940–70, but
interpretation is uncertain, at least during the period of the 1939–45 War.
Two facts should be borne in mind. Firstly, most diabetic persons die
from some vascular complication. Thus the causes of death among
diabetics in England and Wales April–June 1955 included general arteriosclerosis and/or gangrene 31%, arteriosclerotic heart disease 29%, cerebral
vascular disease 15%, a total of 75% (Joslin, 1971b). Secondly, since 1940
in England and Wales diabetes death signified death due to diabetes, not
death of a diabetic. Stocks (1944) ascribed the decreasing diabetes mortality
to wartime food restrictions, especially that of sugar. Himsworth (1949)
linked female diabetes mortality, England and Wales 1940–47 with the
official food consumption levels of calories, fat, protein and carbohydrate.
He reported also a decreased number of applications for diabetes rations
1945–47 and considered that the number of new cases of diabetes had
been diminishing. He suggested that the falling female diabetes mortality
1941–47 was due to decreased consumption of fat or some related factor
such as calories.

Cleave et al. (1969a) produced a graph of sugar consumption and
presented this with the mortality data of Himsworth (1949). They suggested
that the falling female diabetes mortality 1941–47 was due largely to decreased consumption of sugar and partly to increased consumption of less-
refined flour.

None of these investigators had access to the comprehensive data on
food supplies pre-war, and 1940–66 (Ministry of Agriculture, Fisheries
and Food, 1968). It is difficult to explain why death rates fell so much in
1941 if supplies of energy (calories) decreased only 5%, fat only 12% and
sugar only 25% during 1940–41. Comparable decreases have not influenced
either diabetes or ischaemic heart disease in experiments in animals or in
man. It is difficult to explain why diabetes death rates stopped falling in
1954 for all varieties of food and the supply of energy (calories) had reached

TABLE 16.1. Female diabetes mortality, crude rates, England and Wales, 1939–57, and the diet. Mean yearly food supplies (lb/head) and mean yearly crude fibre content of wheat flour, white and National

	1939	1940	1941	1942	1943	1944	1945	1946	1947	1948	1949	1950	1951	1952	1953	1954	1955	1956	1957
Female diabetes mortality/million	152	153	141	130	129	122	122	111	107	98	104	109	109	98	93	86	96	92	91
Wheat flour crude fibre g/100 g	0·10	(0·15)		0·68	0·55	0·45	0·20	0·61	0·51	0·48	0·44	0·42	0·32	0·28	0·30	(0·18)	(0·12)	(0·12)	0·10
Fat lb/head/year	47	43	42	41	39	41	38	37	36	41	47	48	50	45	46	49	48	48	49
Sugar lb/head/year	106	80	72	72	72	77	74	82	87	88	98	90	99	94	105	112	115	116	118
Protein lb/head/year	79	80	83	87	85	86	90	88	89	87	86	87	83	82	82	82	82	84	83
Carbohydrate lb/head/year	414	390	409	403	411	429	427	421	433	438	446	419	429	424	425	431	425	422	422
Calories kcal/day	3050	2890	2900	2930	2920	3060	3010	2940	3000	3120	3120	3120	3080	3030	3100	3190	3170	3170	3180

Sources: Registrar-General, 1939–57; Fraser, 1951, 1958; Ministry of Agriculture, Fisheries and Food, 1968; Robertson, 1972; Trowell, 1974a, b, c.

Figures within parentheses represent assessments during years of transition during which National flour was not obligatory, and was consumed by a minority: the majority ate white flour and a negligible minority ate brown bread or wholemeal bread.

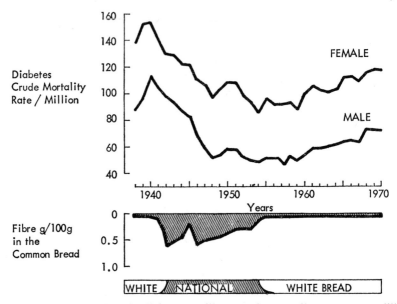

FIG. 16.1. Female and male diabetes mellitus crude mortality rates per million persons and the mean yearly crude fibre content of the flour, white and/or National, used in the common bread.

pre-war levels many years before that date (Table 16.1). The largest change in the diet was the intake of crude fibre in the National flour. Cereal crude fibre increased 100–600% all years of the compulsory National flour 1942–53, but less during 1941 and 1954–56 when it was optional (Trowell, 1973, 1974a, b, c).

It is proposed to examine a hypothesis, stated fully at the end of this chapter, that fibre-depleted starchy carbohydrate foods, such as low extraction white flour, are diabetogenic in susceptible genotypes and, conversely, that fibre-rich starchy foods, such as the National flour, are protective (Trowell, 1973, 1974a, b, c). It is postulated that (1) dietary changes could begin to influence diabetes and/or its complications within a few months of their occurrence and this effect might be detected in the changing mortality rates of the same year; (2) a falling diabetes mortality rate reflects either a prolongation of life of existing diabetics, largely on account of the delayed development of cardiac and vascular complications, and/or a decrease in the number of persons who develop clinically diagnosed diabetes, and/or a decrease in the severity of diabetes mellitus in persons who had already developed the disease.

In 1941 National flour was milled as a voluntary measure; from April 1942 to September 1953 it was the only flour milled in Britain and therefore compulsory. From 1953, 70% extraction white flour was again permitted and this proved so popular that the sales of the subsidized National flour dwindled rapidly until in September 1956 it was discontinued. During 1941–56 the extraction rate of the National flour was altered many times, with corresponding changes in the crude fibre content. Figures for the crude fibre content of the National flour were published (Ministry of Food, 1941–46; Fraser, 1951, 1958) and the dates of the alterations of the extraction rates were recorded (Horder *et al.*, 1954). These provided firm data for the calculation of the annual average crude fibre content of the National flour, the only variety available 1942–53 in Britain (Kent, 1970a). During 1941 the average crude fibre of the two flours, National flour and white flour, was at least half as much as that of 1940 (Trowell, 1973). It is interesting to note that during the period of compulsory National flour 1942–53 female diabetes mortality fell from 130/million to 93/million, and the largest annual decreases during this period were during 1942 and 1946, when the annual average crude fibre of the National flour was at its highest level. On the other hand, when the annual crude fibre of the National flour was at its lowest level, as in 1945, female diabetes mortality remained stationary. In 1954, the first year in which the average crude fibre of the two flours, National and white, approximated to that of the white flour (Table 16.1) (Trowell, 1973), female diabetes mortality stopped falling. All these data strongly support the hypothesis that fibre-depleted starchy carbohydrate foods are diabetogenic and fibre-rich starchy foods are protective.

Those who are conversant with modern statistical procedures will recognize the limitations of the preceding sections. Diabetes deaths as recorded by the Registrar-General considerably underestimate the number of persons who are known diabetics but who die of some associated disease such as ischaemic heart disease. The proportion of older persons has increased considerably during the present century, and the rising crude mortality rates reflect this change in the age-structure of the population. The only satisfactory answer to this difficulty is to compare yearly death rates at various ages and in both sexes 1920–70. This involves the presentation of enormous tables. Suffice it to say that this data, also comparative mortality indices, and standardized mortality ratios indicate that diabetes deaths decreased in men by approximately 55% and in women by about 54% from 1941 until 1954–57, perhaps 1959 (Trowell, 1974b, c).

(*b*) *United States.* Although it is not possible to present comprehensive data on so vast a country and among both whites and non-whites, a few examples will be cited. In New York City in 1866, when the inhabitants were predominantly white, the recorded crude diabetes mortality was 15/million all persons. It had risen to 17/million by 1876, 56/million by 1886, 110/million by 1896, 150/million by 1906, and 210/million by 1916

(Emerson and Larimore, 1924). During 1917–18 the latter part of the First World War, the extraction rate of flour was raised, and other cereals were mixed with it, further increasing its fibre content. Diabetes mortality fell moderately in 1918 to 184/million and to 171/million in 1919, and thereafter it rose almost every year (Emerson and Larimore, 1924; Joslin, 1971c; Joslin *et al.*, 1933) until it reached a plateau in about 1950. There are many sources of error in these statistics and even more in a facile interpretation. It should be noted that the change from stone-ground flour to more refined roller-milled flour occurred some 10 years earlier in the U.S.A. than in Britain, say 1875–95, during which time there was a 5-fold increase in recorded diabetes deaths in New York City. The rising mortality was halted only when the fibre in the flour rose during the period towards the end of the First World War.

3. *Prevalence assessed by community surveys in western nations*

These have been numerous in advanced countries. The number of new cases revealed as a result of the glucose tolerance test (GTT) (discovered diabetics) is greater than the number of patients already under treatment (known diabetics) (Table 16.2).

TABLE 16.2. Estimated percentage prevalence of normal and abnormal glucose tolerance in the general population of England (after Malins, 1968)

	Aged under 50 %	Aged over 50 %	Total %
Known diabetics	0·2	1·6	0·6
"Diabetic" abnormality	1·4	14·5	5·6
Lag storage	5·2	17·9	9·3
Normal GTT	75·7	41·5	64·8
Unclassified	17·5	24·5	19·7

In addition to the 0·6% of known diabetics, such surveys have revealed hitherto unrecognized diabetics 5·6%. The total prevalence in advanced western nations is about 6·2–6·4%. Varying methods of sampling, screening, testing, and also increasing prevalence with age, have made comparisons between communities difficult.

No firm line divides the apparently normal population from those whose glucose tolerance test (GTT) is considered hyperglycaemic. Fasting blood glucose, and blood glucose levels 1 h after 50 g glucose, tend to be considerably higher in older age-groups in western society. A comparable rise does not occur in other parts of the world where diet is based on large amounts of natural or lightly processed carbohydrate foods (Walker, 1966; Sinnett, 1972).

4. *Prevalence surveys in ethnic groups undergoing dietary changes*

(*a*) *India.* In recent years there have been many reports concerning the frequency of diabetes in India, but most of these have involved urban populations attending hospitals. Jackson (1971) commented in his review that "none of these reports can be considered to yield accurate information about prevalence". Subsequently a survey of 2006 adults, men and women over 20 years of age, who lived in a rural area near the city of Hyderabad, showed that men 2·9% and women 2·0% had glycosuria in the morning urine, passed while still fasting. All of these had a diabetic-type glucose tolerance test (GTT). Prevalence increased with age and in persons over 50 years old, men 4·0% and women 5·4% had glycosuria (Rao *et al.*, 1972). Jackson (1971) approved of the more accurate data from a diabetes prevalence survey in the Cuttack area, of rural Indians who had a known diabetes rate of 0·2% and discovered hyperglycaemia 0·7%, compared to urban Indians, known diabetes rate 1·0%, discovered hyperglycaemia 10·5% (B. B. Tripathy *et al.*, p.c. 1969 to Jackson). These investigators subsequently reported their investigation of the urban group in the city of Cuttack in considerable detail. A random sample of 592 subjects (311 male and 281 female) aged 10 years and over, were tested by sophisticated modern methods. Seventy-five had blood sugar levels above 130 mg/100 ml 2 h after glucose 50 g, a total incidence of 12·7%; 12 of these had frank diabetes, 11 had suggestive signs of diabetes and 52 were considered to have asymptomatic (latent) diabetes. Glycosuria, detected either in the fasting urine or in the sample collected 2 h after 50 g of glucose, was 4·4% (Tripathy *et al.*, 1970). Figures obtained from this survey were very similar to those obtained in the Bedford Survey (Sharp *et al.*, 1964). It is hoped that other diabetes surveys will be carried out and details offered of the diet, including the fibre content of the cereals. It is probable that the prevalence of diabetes in urban Indians is comparable to that in many countries in Europe and North America, but that prevalence in certain rural groups is definitely lower.

In many parts of India rice is the main cereal. At the beginning of the present century the social groups in rural areas who tended to eat rough paddy rice (fibre up to 9·0%), brown rice (fibre 1·1%) (Kent, 1970b) or parboiled rice (fibre 0·5%) (Platt, 1962) were said to have less diabetes than those living in the urban areas (Bose, 1907). Polished rice (fibre 0·2%), which was always popular among the upper classes, is being eaten increasingly by all classes.

(b) *Pakistan.* Unrefined or lightly milled wheat flour is often the main cereal and fat consumption is often low (7% of calories). Diabetes mellitus is stated to be less common among these chupatti-eating Pakistanis than among the Indians (Bose, 1907; Cleave *et al.*, 1969a). Glucose tolerance tests have revealed a very low prevalence (1·5%) of diabetic-type curves, lower than in any of the other nine Asian and American countries tested by the same investigators (West and Kalbfleisch, 1970, 1971). Prevalence is usually lower in the rural than in the urban areas of Pakistan, such as Ahmedabad, where consumption of refined white flour is increasing, and where the prevalence of diabetes has risen, especially in the higher income groups (4·9%) compared with the lower income groups (2·7%) (Gupta *et al.*, 1971).

(c) *Japan.* Until recently rice contributed 80% of all grain eaten in Japan, and carbohydrate foods supplied some 75–80% of calories, fats 9–14% and protein 13–14%. In recent decades, especially in urban areas, more white wheat flour and bread and less rice has been eaten. During the period 1955–67 fat consumption more than doubled but protein intake and total calories (2500 kcal/day) have remained almost stationary (Oiso, 1971). Along with these dietary changes there has been a marked increase in the crude death rate from diabetes, which in Japanese men rose from 2·5/ 100,000 in 1950 to 6·3/100,000 in 1968 (Kuzuya and Kosaka, 1971). In Hiroshima a careful diabetes mellitus prevalence survey, employing a standard GTT on 25,574 men and 41,785 women, has shown that in this city the prevalence of the disease doubled in both sexes in the period 1963–69 (Kawate, 1971) which, even allowing for the increased age of the group studied, represents a definite rise in prevalence. Moreover, diabetes autopsy studies in Japan have shown that cardiovascular complications have been less common than in western countries. They caused only 15·5% of the deaths in one *post mortem* series, four-fifths of whom were over 50 years of age (Okamoto *et al.*, 1971), whereas in the U.S.A. cardiovascular complications caused 44% of the deaths of diabetics of all ages (Joslin, 1971d).

(d) *Ethnic groups in South Africa.* Table 16.3 (Swanpoel *et al.*, 1971) presents data on diabetes prevalence in different South African ethnic groups, together with certain aspects of their diet (Lubbe, 1971; Walker *et al.*, 1971, 1973).

South African Bantu in their rural homelands, among whom diabetes is very low, still eat their traditional home-pounded maize, home-ground millet, beans, vegetables and a little meat. A hardworking rural Bantu eats a high-calorie diet (nearly 4000 kcal/day) containing much carbohydrate (580 g/day) and therefore much crude fibre (25 g/day); the intake of protein is moderate (60 g/day), that of fat is low (55 g/day) (Lubbe, 1971). Sugar consumption is moderate (30–60 g/day) in rural areas; it rises rapidly, up to 85 g/day when westernization of the diets commences (Walker *et al.*, 1971). Certain workers in South Africa have therefore thrown doubt on the role of sugar in the pathogenesis of diabetes (Walker *et al.*, 1971).

When Indians emigrate from India to South Africa their prevalence of diabetes increases greatly. This has been ascribed by Cleave *et al.* (1969a) largely to the increased consumption of sugar. Others maintain that, despite this increased consumption of sugar, it is still less than that of the South African whites who have a lower incidence of diabetes (Table 16.3) (Walker *et al.*, 1971). The very high prevalence of diabetes in South African

TABLE 16.3. South Africa Diabetes Prevalence Surveys and Food Intakes

Group	Number	Known %	Diabetes discovered %	Total %	Crude fibre mean g/day	Sugar mean g/day	Fat mean g/day
Transvaal Bantu	2015	—	1 case only	—	24·0	30–60	65
Cape Bantu	1027	0·9	2·7	3·3	6·5	55–85	85
Cape White	1650	0·8	2·4	3·2	4·3	80–140	110
Cape Indian	1520	4·3	4·2	8·5	4·0	70–90	80

Indians may be partly due to inheritance displaying itself in ethnic variations; for instance, hyperinsulaemia has been detected in many of their children. Data concerning the fibre content of their starchy carbohydrate food are lacking, though it has been estimated that their daily total intake of crude fibre is the lowest of any ethnic group in South Africa (Table 16.3).

(e) *Rhodesia.* Investigators report a rarity of diabetes in non-westernized Africans in Rhodesia, and consider that this may be due to their diet of lightly processed carbohydrate foods (Wicks and Jones, 1973). The disease is still very rare in rural areas (Wicks *et al.*, 1972). Fasting blood glucose concentration and oral glucose-tolerance curves were significantly lower in Africans who ate lightly processed maize (270 g/day) and little fat (35 g/day) than in African students who ate their starch largely as white bread (120 g/day) and had more sugar and more fat (Wapnick *et al.*, 1972). The body weight of these African groups did not differ significantly; both were thinner than a comparable group of Rhodesian whites who had higher GTT curves.

(f) *Israel.* Among western nations, whose staple carbohydrate food is wheat, only Yemenite and Kurd Jews have been clearly identified as recognized sub-groups having a low diabetes prevalence. Some 15,000 immigrants were tested on their arrival in Israel, and all who were glycosuric after the morning meal were examined by means of GTT. It was found that those coming from Europe had the expected figure of most European nations, some 2·5%, but those coming from the Yemen had the extremely low figure of 0·06% (Cohen, 1961). After 25 years' residence in Israel the prevalence was approximately the same in the two groups. Jews in the Yemen consumed large amounts of stone-ground flour milled from wheat, barley or millet; flour was sieved of its bran only once a week for the sabbath cake-bread (Groen *et al.*, 1966). Their diet was stated to have been low in sugar but to contain as much, if not more, fat, and especially animal fat, than that taken in Israel. In recent years white bread with a low fibre content has been increasingly eaten in Israel (A. Reshef, p.c. 1973). Quantitative data on these items of diet have not been published.

D. Experimental studies

A prolonged search of the literature on the experimental production of diabetes has not revealed a single experiment designed to test the possible effect of fibre in the pathogenesis of diabetes mellitus in animals or in man. This is surprising, seeing that diabetes is a disease of carbohydrate metabolism, and that starch and sugar are associated with fibre in all natural foods. The word fibre has not been traced in any volume of the journal *Diabetes* and only four times in the volumes of *Diabetologia*.

Diabetes mellitus appears to be a rare condition in animals living in their natural habitat even when feeding *ad libitum* on their traditional diets. It is commoner in domesticated animals and particularly in dogs, in which the prevalence may reach 0·5% (Meier, 1961). Diabetes mellitus does not occur in the sand rat (*Psammomys obesus*) when it lives in its natural habitat, the hot salty marsh areas of Egyptian deserts, wherein grow special salt-loving plants of the family Chenopodiacae; this desert vegetation presumably has a high fibre/calorie ratio. When captured, confined to a cage and fed *ad libitum* a mixed vegetable diet of spinach, carrot, beet leaves and a little beetroot (crude fibre about 2·5 g/100 kcal/370 g), they ate 40 kcal/day and did not develop diabetes. When fed *ad libitum* on a starchy laboratory food, Purina chow (crude fibre 1·3 g/100 kcal/27 g), they ate 53 kcal/day and frequently developed diabetes and obesity (Hackel *et al.*, 1966). When other sand rats were fed *ad libitum* on a synthetic diet of dextrin, casein and corn oil, agar 8% (fibre nil/100 kcal/20 g), but no natural fibre, their calorie intake increased from 30 kcal/day on the fibre-rich mixed vegetable diet to 62 kcal/day. Their weight increased at once, plasma insulin rose and glucose tolerance decreased. In fact, one died with hyperglycaemia in a condition resembling diabetes. On restricting this synthetic fibre-free diet to 30 kcal/day, which was the level of the mixed vegetable diet, weight and plasma insulin decreased and glucose tolerance improved, but none of these reverted to a normal level (Hackel *et al.*, 1966, 1967). Interpretation of this phenomenon was in terms of calorie intakes. If these were high, as on the fibre-free synthetic diet consumed *ad libitum*, then hyperglycaemia and diabetes occurred. If the calorie intakes of this diet were reduced to the normal level, then hyperglycaemia became more normal (Hackel *et al.*, 1967). The low-fibre high-calorie laboratory cereal Purina chow also caused increased weight, hyperglycaemia and a diabetic-type GTT. No fat was added to any of these diabetogenic diets; the main change was in the fibre/calorie ratio (Haines *et al.*, 1965).

In another study, Gleason *et al.* (1967) fed two different cereal laboratory foods to mice. They developed hyperglycaemia on a low-fibre (2%) moderate-fat (11%) diet, but not on a high-fibre (5%) low-fat (3%) diet. Other examples of comparable dietary changes could be cited (Wise *et al.*, 1968; Kramer *et al.*, 1969; Miki *et al.*, 1967).

It remains to be proved whether or not the different amount of fibre consumed was in fact responsible for these changes, but the fundamental question has not yet been answered: Why did the sand rats on the concentrated fibre-free diet consume more calories than those fed on the high-fibre mixed vegetable diet, both fed *ad libitum*? The answer may well lie in fibre. No animal experiment has been traced in which diabetes developed when the diet was altered only in respect of fat, protein or sugar content.

Human diabetes mellitus may develop in a similar manner. As long as man fed mainly on his traditional diet of fibre-rich cereals he contracted little diabetes, but on a diet of low-fibre modern cereal products—white wheat flour and white polished rice—the disease became common. Maturity-onset diabetes, often accompanied by obesity, usually improves dramatically when refined starchy carbohydrate food is restricted (Wall *et al.*, 1973).

E. Sugar

In conclusion, it is desirable to say something about the possibility of sucrose being diabetogenic in man. At least two aspects can be evisaged: a direct diabetogenic action on susceptible genotypes and an indirect action due to the possible production of obesity, a recognized risk in maturity-onset diabetes, to be discussed in the second part of this chapter. Any direct diabetogenic action of sugar may be summarized thus:

1. There has been an apparent association between increasing crude diabetes mortality rates and a rising consumption of sugar in western nations (Cleave *et al.*, 1969a) but there is also an apparent association with an increased consumption of fat (Himsworth, 1949) and of fibre-depleted starchy cereal foods (Trowell, 1973). The detailed study of mortality at various ages reveals that English diabetes death rates have remained almost stationary in younger age-groups in men and women since the advent of insulin in 1925, but death rates have increased in the older age-groups, those over 55 years, more in men than in women (Trowell, 1974b).

2. Animal experiments have not demonstrated that either sugar (20% of the daily calories) or fat (40% of the daily calories) is diabetogenic in susceptible animals, but have suggested that attention should be paid to fibre-depleted starchy carbohydrate foods (pp. 238–239).

3. It may prove impossible to assess the diabetogenic action of sucrose in man until there is more information about dietary fibre. For instance, is sucrose free of diabetogenic risk when taken with its natural complement of dietary fibre in dates, figs and beetroot, but does an equal portion of sucrose become a risk factor if taken as the pure refined product, even if this is diluted in other foods or in fluid to the same degree as it was when it occurred in its natural state? Or is it only the *level* of sucrose consumption which is important, whether from natural sources such as sugar cane and beetroot, or as the refined product?

These questions await investigation.

II. Obesity

A. Definition and prevalence

Most authorities define obesity as occurring when a person's weight is at least 10% in excess of the normal desirable weight; excessive obesity occurs when normal weight is exceeded by 20% (Craddock, 1973a).

The Metropolitan Life Insurance Company of New York has published an authoritative table of "desirable weights" for men and women aged 25 years and over, according to whether the individual frame is small, medium or large (Craddock, 1973b). In all advanced countries many men and women are obese and the percentage increases with age. In the U.S.A. 30% of men aged 20–29 years and 60% of those aged 40–49 years are obese; in women the figures are higher. By comparison, obesity in English women is similar but in men it is lower than in the U.S.A.

In eastern and central countries of Africa, excessive obesity was rarely seen until after the Second World War; it is now commonly seen among upper socio-economic groups in urban areas (Trowell, 1975). A comparable change occurred in South African Bantu earlier in the present century: excessive obesity became commonly seen, especially in Bantu women. It is impossible to generalize about obesity in the countries of Asia, except to note that country peasants tend to remain thin throughout adult life but town dwellers are often obese and upper socio-economic groups have a fair proportion of excessive obesity.

It is accepted that healthy adult weight should not increase after the age of 25 years. Body weight does not increase in healthy Africans in rural areas (Slome *et al.*, 1960; Nurse, 1968).

B. History of obesity and diet

Severe obesity occurring in many members of a community is largely a modern phenomenon. The Venus of Willendorf, dating from about 20,000 B.C. and located in Austria, is one of the rare examples of obesity seen in ancient art and probably reflected some magico-religious symbol of fertility. The belly and breasts are obese, but the arms and legs are slender, which does not occur in simple obesity. Cave-men drawings invariably depict scraggy limbs, as did temple reliefs of Egypt and Assyria, and statues of Greece, Rome and mediaeval Europe. The British National Portrai͘ Gallery has portraits dating from the fourteenth century, and obesity was rarely depicted before the end of the seventeenth century. Thereafter the aristocracy had double chins and prominent abdomens (Trowell, 1975).

In the eighteenth century the agricultural revolution, which was slowly gathering momentum, provided more meat, butter and milk for those who could afford it. At the same time the high-grinding system of milling flour provided flours of more than one quality for different social classes (Kent, 1970c). Sugar began to be taken in coffee and tea, but the amount consumed was probably moderate until it entered newly concocted dishes, cakes and confectionery.

Less is known about the history of obesity and diet in Asian countries (Trowell, 1975). Sugar reached India from the islands of the Pacific about A.D. 300 (Chapter 4), but its cultivation increased slowly. Slight obesity is clearly seen in Indian statues as early as A.D. 100, at about the same time as sugary diabetic urine was described. In China obesity and diabetes appeared together about the seventh century A.D.

Few scientists in recent centuries have described the physique of food-gathering hunters, but in 1836 Charles Darwin described the slender limbs of the Australian aborigine (Moorehead, 1968). Early travellers in the New World depicted slim figures of the Red Indian hunters; eventually they began to cultivate maize, which was eaten on the cob (Sinclair, 1953). This was replaced in recent decades by white wheat flour and sugar. Pima

Indians now exhibit much obesity and 50% of those over the age of 35 years have diabetes (Bennett *et al.*, 1971).

C. Experimental studies

1. Appetite centre and energy balance

How far does the appetite centre in the hypothalamus solve the problem of obesity? Margen (1969) stated, "There is a breakdown in this system for obesity to occur . . . the control mechanism tends to break down in the affluent society. . . . No one has yet explained what type of precise 'stat' operates with such regulation." The problem has usually been simplified by explaining that obesity is caused when calorie intake exceeds calorie expenditure in physical activity and basal metabolism. This entirely over-looks the role of dietary fibre, which decreases the absorption of energy (calories) (Trowell, 1975). Certainly the "stat" that controls calorie balance is extremely sensitive; if 1% of the daily calorie intake (30 kcal) were in excess and were cumulatively stored in the body during 40 years of life, then the excess adipose tissue would amount to 45 kg. Built-in safety mechanisms exist: as individual body weight increases, so the output of energy increases, both as basal metabolism, and to perform an identical amount of physical activity. There is more weight to be moved with every step. This tends to re-establish calorie balance in persons who become over-weight, but benefit may be offset by decreased physical activity and decreased thermal loss, both of which are features of those who are obese (Anderson, 1972). Individuals may differ as much as 80–140 kcal/day in the digestion and absorption of food (Lees and Turner, 1963), but the reason for this variation is seldom stated, and the effect of fibre on absorp-tion is not mentioned in conventional nutrition texts.

2. Intestinal absorption of energy and nutrients

The effect of dietary fibre has been studied in different experimental British diets. On a low-fibre diet of white bread, potatoes, butter, meat, milk, fruit and vegetables, containing approximately 5 g/day of crude fibre, 93% of the total energy intake (calories) was absorbed from the food. Another diet substituted brown bread for white and more fruit and vegetables were added; the crude fibre content was nearly doubled and the energy absorbed (calories) decreased to 91% (Durnin, 1961). A recent experiment showed that the dietary fibre of wholemeal bread, fruit and vegetables apparently decreased the absorption of energy by 2%, of fat by 2%, and of protein by 3% (Southgate and Durnin, 1970). Starch and sugar appear to be completely digested and absorbed, whether dietary fibre is present in large or small amounts.

3. Experimental production of obesity

The experiments carried out to produce diabetes in small rodents (pp. 238–239) throw some light on the pathogenesis of obesity, for the two conditions are often associated both in animals and in man. Most of the animals selected for these studies have been small rodents from hot, arid desert regions, where vegetation is scarce, tough and fibrous. Their traditional foodstuffs have a very high fibre/calorie ratio. Some of these animals appear to have difficulty in adapting to whole cereal foods such as Purina chow, never encountered in their natural habitat. Thus Egyptian sand rats, accustomed to the fibrous vegetation of the desert, cannot adapt to moderate-fibre laboratory chow; mice, accustomed to whole cereals, cannot adapt to fibre-depleted laboratory foodstuffs.

Other experiments to produce obesity or even diabetes in animals should be reviewed in the light of a possible role of dietary fibre. Monkeys (*Macaca mulatta*) in their natural habitat eat much fibrous food, leaves, shoots and fruit; they may develop obesity and diabetes when fed Purina chow (Hamilton et al., 1972). This cereal food has a high energy/fibre ratio. Rabbits feeding on their natural diet of vegetation rich in fibre and low in calories do not develop obesity, but when fed for 4 months on an experimental diet of white bread, butter, milk and eggs, containing almost no fibre, mean body weight almost doubled and diverticula could be demonstrated in the colon (Hodgson, 1972). An association of obesity, diabetes and diverticulosis has been seen in autopsies in the U.S.A. (Schowengerdt et al., 1969).

Another approach to this complex problem, at least in man, may lie in a consideration of the satiety/calorie ratio of foods (Heaton 1973a, b). Sugar is a concentrated food which is rapidly absorbed and probably produces only transient satiety. On the other hand it is difficult to measure satiety, except perhaps to record energy (calorie) intake if food is consumed *ad libitum*. Persons often take a snack if they feel "empty" and dietary fibre is the only portion of the diet completely unabsorbed in stomach and small intestine. Further, any dietary change which leads to increased consumption of food taken *ad libitum* might lead to obesity. The role of fat, which is said to increase palatability, and therefore intake, cannot be ignored. Thus whereas a low-fat (3%) high-fibre (5%) laboratory cereal diet did not produce obesity in mice fed *ad libitum*, obesity did appear when the same mice fed *ad libitum* on a moderate-fat (11%) low-fibre (2%) laboratory cereal diet (Gleason et al., 1967; Miki et al., 1967). Both the fat and the fibre content were varied at a single dietary switch, and the two factors may have acted in unison.

4. Foods supplied for consumption in Britain 1939–66

The supplies of fat and sugar during the years of food rationing do not correlate well with the energy (calorie) content of the diet. Both fat and sugar supplies exceeded the 1939 pre-war levels during most of the years 1950–57 (Table 16.1), but energy (calorie) intakes exceeded the 1939 pre-war level only when white bread was consumed in large amounts during 1954 and in all subsequent years. Young men and middle-aged men in Britain are nowadays on average 15 lb heavier than men of the same height and age during the pre-war period (Khosla and Rowe, 1968). Doubtless other factors, such as rapid growth in childhood, have influenced the weight of adults, but the role of dietary fibre at all ages requires critical assessment.

5. Energy/fibre ratio

A mixed diet has a certain energy/fibre ratio; this may be called the E/F ratio of the diet. It is postulated that many ethnic groups, such as western man, Asians and Africans have inherited an appetite centre adjusted to consume *ad libitum* traditional foods of low E/F ratio, but that certain susceptible persons, that is certain genotypes, will slowly become obese if the diet has a high E/F ratio. In other words, as clinicians have noted, foods having a high E/F ratio are considered to be fattening: sugar, refined starchy carbohydrate foods, fats, milk and alcohol. Foods having a low E/F ratio are prescribed in slimming diets: leafy vegetables, and fruit, also whole cereal crispbreads and wafers. Two recent studies of diet and body weight support this suggestion (Table 16.4). The first study concerned 1154 Irish brothers: both grew up in Ireland, then one emigrated to Massachusetts, U.S.A., and ate fewer calories in a low-fibre diet; the other brother stayed in Ireland and ate much fibre-rich potato but consumed more calories (Brown *et al.*, 1970). The second study from South Africa concerned 248 Venda Bantu urban men who ate more calories in refined low-fibre maize meal compared with 260 Venda Bantu rural men who ate unrefined high-fibre maize meal (Lubbe, 1971; Loots and Lambrecht, 1971).

Mean body weight remained stationary (56·8 kg) throughout life in Venda rural men, but increased slightly in Venda urban men from 60·1 kg at the age of 20–29 years to 64·6 kg at 40–44 years. Doubtless many factors influence body weight, but it is suggested that the E/F ratio of any diet, consumed *ad libitum*, is an important factor in men and in animals.

TABLE 16.4. Energy/fibre ratio of diet and body weight

| | Irish brothers | | Venda men | |
| | Massachusetts | Ireland | Urban | Rural |
		(mean values in all groups)		
DIETS				
Energy (kcal/day)	3075	3768	3976	3664
Crude fibre (g/day)	3·6	6·4	5·7	24·8
Ratio (energy/fibre)	854:1	588:1	697:1	148:1
BODY WEIGHT				
Triceps skinfold (mm)	10·0	7·5	8·2	6·7
At age (years)	20–39	20–39	30–39	30–39
Body weight (kg)	78·5	76·0	60·1	56·8
Obesity in group	common	less common	uncommon	rare

D. Evolution and obesity

One of the most brilliant seminal concepts of Cleave et al. (1969b) was the appreciation of the role of evolution in the prevention of obesity. The present study recognizes that fat is stored in a wild animal's body only if it is beneficial; it is seldom gross unless it is an asset because the animal feeds only at certain seasons, such as the seal during the short arctic summer. Cleave et al. (1969c) considered that the great concentration both of sugar from sugar beet and refined white flour "deceived the appetite" and thus led to overconsumption. They contended that flour was less important than sugar, the latter being concentrated eight times more than the former.

Obesity would have been a problem to hunter food–gatherer men, also to peasants growing their own crops, and it is still a disability today in modern man who has not only reduced his intake of carbohydrate foods but has also decreased the fibre content. At the same time he has increased the intake of foods that have little or no fibre—sugar, meat, milk and fats— and these are completely or almost completely absorbed. Modern man often complains of an empty feeling in the abdomen, thus stating the problem correctly and succinctly.

III. Summary of fibre-depleted starchy carbohydrate foods hypothesis concerning diabetes and/or obesity

Fibre-depleted starchy carbohydrate foods appear to be a risk factor in the pathogenesis of diabetes mellitus and/or obesity. Both of these diseases are very rare in communities accustomed to eating large amounts of starchy foods undepleted of dietary fibre.

Diabetes mellitus and/or obesity increase markedly in prevalence in such a community when a complex set of dietary changes occur:

(1) processed fibre-depleted starchy foods replace natural high-fibre carbohydrate foods;
(2) less starchy food is eaten;
(3) more sugar and fat are consumed, also protein; none of these foods contains fibre;
(4) energy (calorie) intakes increase;
(5) the energy/fibre ratio of the total diet increases.

At the same time physical activity and energy requirements decrease. It is possible that increased intakes of sugar, fat, protein and energy (calories) may also be risk factors in the pathogenesis of diabetes mellitus and/or obesity.

Inheritance, hormonal factors, sex, psychological and social factors, also influence the development of obesity and/or diabetes mellitus.

References

ANDERSON, T. (1972). *British Medical Journal* 1, 560.

BARACH, J. (1928). *Annals of Medical History* 10, 387.

BENNETT, P. H., BURCH, T. A. and MILLER, M. (1971). *Lancet* 1, 125.

BOSE, R. K. C. (1907). *British Medical Journal* 2, 1053.

BROWN, J., BOURKE, G. J., GEARTY, G. F. *et al.* (1970). *World Review of Nutrition and Dietetics* 12, 1.

CLEAVE, T. L., CAMPBELL, G. D. and PAINTER, N. S. (1969). "Diabetes, Coronary Thrombosis and the Saccharine Disease", 2nd edition. John Wright, Bristol. (a) p. 15; (b) p. 60; (c) p. 8.

COHEN, A. M. (1961). *Metabolism* 10, 50.

COPEMAN, W. S. C. (1960). "Doctors and Disease in Tudor Times", p. 118. Dobson, London.

CRADDOCK, D. (1973) "Obesity and its Management", 2nd edition. Churchill Livingstone, Edinburgh. (a) p. 1; (b) p. 180.

DURNIN, J. V. G. A. (1961). *Proceedings of the Nutrition Society* 10, 2.

EMERSON, H. and LARIMORE, L. D. (1924). *Archives of Internal Medicine* 34, 587.

FERNANDO, H. M. (1907). *British Medical Journal* 2, 1060.

FRASER, J. R. (1951). *Journal of the Science of Food and Agriculture* 2, 193.

FRASER, J. R. (1958). *Journal of the Science of Food and Agriculture* 9, 125.

GLEASON, R. E., LAURIS, V. and SOELDNER, J. S. (1967). *Diabetologia* 3, 175.

GROEN, J. J., BALOGH, M. and YARRON, E. (1966). *Israel Journal of Medical Sciences* 2, 202.

GUPTA, O. P., DAVE, D. M., RAWAL, M. L., SUTARIA, V. M., BODIWALA, N. K., PARIKH, H. K., PARIKH, N. K., SHAH, B. S., GUPTA, P. S., JOSHI, M. N. and

AGRAWAL, S. B. (1971). *In* "Diabetes Mellitus in Asia, 1970" (S. Tsuji and M. Wada, eds), p. 6. Excerpta Medica, Amsterdam.

GWEI-DJEN, L. and NEEDHAM, J. (1967). *In* "Diseases of Antiquity" (D. Brothwell and A. T. Sandison, eds), p. 235. Thomas, Springfield.

HACKEL, D. B., FROHMAN, L. A., MIKAT, E., LEBOVITZ, H. E., SCHMIDT-NIELSEN, K. and KINNEY, T. D. (1966). *Diabetes* **15**, 105.

HACKEL, D. B., LEBOVITZ, H. E., FROHMAN, L. A., MIKAT, E. and SCHMIDT-NIELSEN, K. (1967). *Metabolism* **16**, 1133.

HAINES, H. B., HACKEL, D. B. and SCHMIDT-NIELSEN, K. (1965). *American Journal of Physiology* **208**, 297.

HAMILTON, C. L., KUO, P. T. and FENG, L. Y. (1972). *Proceedings of the Society for Experimental Biology and Medicine* **140**, 1005.

HEATON, K. W. (1973a). *Nutrition, London* **27**, 170.

HEATON, K. W. (1973b). *Lancet* **2**, 1418.

HENSCHEN, F. (1966). "The History of Diseases", p. 195. Longmans, London.

HIMSWORTH, H. P. (1949). *Proceedings of the Royal Society of Medicine* **42**, 323.

HODGSON, W. J. B. (1972). *Gut* **13**, 802.

HORDER, T., DODDS, E. C. and MORAN, LORD (1954). "Bread", p. 170. Constable, London.

JACKSON, W. P. U. (1971). *Acta diabetologica latina* **7**, 361.

JOSLIN, E. P. (1971). "Diabetes Mellitus" (A. Marble, P. White, R. F. Bradley, and L. P. Krall, eds), 11th edition. Lea and Febiger, Philadelphia. (a) p. 238; (b) p. 231; (c) p. 247; (d) p. 230.

JOSLIN, E. P., DUBLIN, L. I. and MARKS, H. H. (1933). *American Journal of Medical Science* **186**, 753.

JOSLIN, E. P., DUBLIN, L. I. and MARKS, H. H. (1940). *Journal of the American Medical Association* **115**, 2033.

KAWATE, R. (1971). *In* "Diabetes Mellitus in Asia, 1970" (S. Tsuji and M. Wada, eds), p. 76. Excerpta Medica, Amsterdam.

KENT, N. L. (1970). "Technology of Cereals." Pergamon, Oxford. (a) p. 163; (b) p. 37; (c) p. 115.

KHOSLA, T. and ROWE, C. R. (1968). *Lancet* **1**, 742.

KRAMER, M. W., LIBERMAN, D. F., SOELDNER, J. S. and GLEASON, R. E. (1969). *Diabetologia* **5**, 353.

KUZUYA, N. and KOSAKA, K. (1971). *In* "Diabetes Mellitus in Asia, 1970" (S. Tsuji and M. Wada, eds), p. 11. Excerpta Medica, Amsterdam.

LEES, F. and TURNER, J. W. A. (1963). *British Medical Journal* **2**, 1607.

LOOTS, J. M. and LAMBRECHT, DE V. (1971). *South African Medical Journal* **45**, 1284.

LUBBE, A. M. (1971). *South African Medical Journal* **45**, 1289.

MAJOR, R. H. (1954). "A History of Medicine", Volume 1. Thomas, Springfield. (a) p. 75; (b) p. 181; (c) p. 524.

MALINS, J. (1968). "Diabetes Mellitus", p. 46. Eyre and Spottiswoode, London.

MARGEN, S. (1969). *In* "Obesity" (N. L. Wilson, ed.), p. 77. Davis, Philadelphia.

MEIER, H. (1961). *American Journal of Medicine,* **31**, 868.

MIKI, E., LIKE, A. A., STEINKE, J. and SOELDNER, J. S. (1967). *Diabetologia* **3**, 135.

MINISTRY OF AGRICULTURE, FISHERIES AND FOOD (1968). *Board of Trade Journal* **194**, 753.

MINISTRY OF FOOD Fibre Figures (1941–46). Published in *Nature* (1941) **148**, 599; (1942) **149**, 460; **150**, 538; (1943) **151**, 629; **153**, 154; (1944) **154**, 582, 788; (1945) **155**, 717; (1946) **157**, 181.

MOOREHEAD, A. (1968). "The Fatal Impact", p. 160. Penguin, Harmondsworth.

NURSE, G. T. (1968). *Central African Journal of Medicine* **14**, 122.

OISO, T. (1971). *In* "Diabetes Mellitus in Asia, 1970" (S. Tsuji and M. Wada, eds), p. 234. Excerpta Medica, Amsterdam.

OKAMOTO, K., HAZAMA, F. and YAMASAKI, Y. (1971). *In* "Diabetes Mellitus in Asia, 1970" (S. Tsuji and M. Wada, eds), p. 106. Excerpta Medica, Amsterdam.

PLATT, B. S. (1962). "Tables of Representative Values of Foods Commonly Used in Tropical Countries." Her Majesty's Stationery Office, London.

RAO, K. S. J., MUKERJEE, N. R., and RAO, K. V. (1972). *Diabetes* **21**, 1192.

REGISTRAR GENERAL (1939–57). Statistical Review of England and Wales, Part I, Tables, Medical, 1861–1970.

ROBERTSON, J. (1972). *Nature* **238**, 290.

SANDWITH, F. M. (1907). *British Medical Journal* **2**, 1059.

SCHOWENGERDT, C. G., HEDGES, G. R., YAW, P. B. and ALTEMEIER, W. A. (1969). *Archives of Surgery* **98**, 500.

SHARP, C. L., BUTTERFIELD, W. J. H. and KEEN, H. (1964). *Proceedings of the Royal Society of Medicine* **57**, 193.

SINCLAIR, H. M. (1953). *Proceedings of the Nutrition Society* **12**, 69.

SINNETT, P. (1972). *Human Biology Oceania* **1**, 299.

SLOME, C., GAMPEL, B., ABRAMSON, J. M. and SCOTCH, N. (1960). *South African Medical Journal* **34**, 505.

SOUTHGATE, D. A. T. and DURNIN, J. V. G. A. (1970). *British Journal of Nutrition* **24**, 517.

STOCKS, P. (1944). *Journal of Hygiene* **43**, 242.

SWANPOEL, H., CAMPBELL, G. D., GOLDBERG, M. and JACKSON, W. P. U. (1971). *In* "Diabetes Mellitus in Asia, 1970" (S. Tsuji and M. Wada, eds), p. 3. Excerpta Medica, Amsterdam.

TRIPATHY, B. B., KAR, B. C., PANDA, N. C., PAIRAH, N. and TEJ, S. C. (1970). *Journal of the Indian Medical Association* **54**, 55.

TROWELL, H. (1973). *Proceedings of the Nutrition Society* **32**, 150.

TROWELL, H. (1974a). *Plant Foods for Man*, **1**, 91.

TROWELL, H. (1974b). *Lancet* **2**, 998.

TROWELL, H. (1974c). *Lancet* **2**, 1510.

TROWELL, H. (1975). *Plant Foods for Man* (in press).

TULLOCH, J. A. (1962). "Diabetes Mellitus in the Tropics." Livingstone, Edinburgh. (a) p. 1; (b) p. 48.

WALKER, A. R. P. (1966). *South African Medical Journal* **40**, 814.

WALKER, A. R. P., HOLDSWORTH, C. M. and WALKER, E. J. (1971). *South African Medical Journal* **45**, 516.

WALKER, A. R. P., WALKER, B. F., RICHARDSON, B. D. and WOOLFORD, A. (1973). *Postgraduate Medical Journal* **49**, 243.

WALL, J. R., PYKE, D. A. and OAKLEY, W. G. (1973). *British Medical Journal* 1, 577.

WAPNICK, S., WICKS, A. C. B., KANENGONI, E. and JONES, J. J. (1972). *Lancet* 2, 300.

WEST, K. M. and KALBFLEISCH, J. M. (1970). *Diabetes* 19, 656.

WEST, K. M. and KALBFLEISCH, J. M. (1971). *Diabetes* 20, 99.

WICKS, A. C. B. and JONES, J. J. (1973). *British Medical Journal* 1, 773.

WICKS, A. C. B., CASTLE, W. M. and GELFAND, M. (1972). *Diabetes* 22, 733.

WILLIS, T. (1679). "Pharmaceutice Rationalis or an Excitation of the Operations of Medicines in Human Bodies", p. 79. London.

WISE, P. H., WEIR, B. J., HIME, J. M. and FORREST, E. (1968). *Nature* 219, 1374.

Chapter 17

Dental caries and periodontal disease

ABDUL ADATIA

I. Introduction 251
II. Dental caries and periodontal disease in the western world . . 252
III. Historical emergence 253
    A. Dental caries 253
    B. Periodontal disease 254
IV. Prevalence of dental caries and periodontal disease in contemporary
    traditional environment 254
    A. Dental caries 254
    B. Periodontal disease 255
V. Pathogenesis of dental caries and periodontal disease . . . 255
    A. General considerations 255
    B. Oral microorganisms 256
    C. Host resistance 258
    D. Diet 259
VI. Dental caries, periodontal disease and refined carbohydrate foods. 259
    A. Dental caries 259
    B. Periodontal disease 262
VII. Unrefined foods and resistance of teeth against dental caries and
    periodontal disease 263
    A. Dental caries 263
    B. Periodontal disease 264
VIII. Possible natural mechanism of resistance of teeth against dental caries
    and periodontal disease 265
IX. Preventive measures against dental caries and periodontal disease . 269
References 270

I. Introduction

The universal occurrence of dental caries and periodontal disease is well
documented (Mummery, 1869; Wallace, 1900; Klatsky and Klatell, 1943;

251

Russell, 1963; Brabant, 1967; Marthaler, 1967). Nevertheless the prevalence of these diseases is not uniform throughout the world, and in certain populations it has apparently been markedly different at different periods. In the western world the prevalence of dental caries and periodontal disease is now substantially higher than it was some centuries ago (Begg, 1954; Brothwell, 1959; Hardwick, 1960; Alexandersen, 1967; Brabant, 1967; Miles, 1969; James and Miller, 1970; Moore and Corbett, 1971). Indeed it is increasingly apparent that even in populations which were, until recently, relatively free of these diseases the prevalence of dental caries and periodontal disease has greatly increased within one or two decades of adopting foods characteristic of western civilization (Friel and Shaw, 1931; Pedersen, 1947; Gamblen, 1953; Russell et al., 1961a; Holloway et al., 1963; Adatia, 1974).

The purpose of this paper is 3-fold. Firstly, to discuss the significance of refined carbohydrate foods in the aetiology of dental caries and periodontal disease; to this end a brief account of the epidemiology of these diseases will be given and some recent literature on their pathogenesis will be reviewed. Secondly, to assess the evidence concerning the local influence of unrefined foods on the resistance of teeth to dental caries and periodontal disease. Thirdly, to consider a possible natural mechanism of resistance against these diseases and to suggest preventive measures.

II. Dental caries and periodontal disease in the western world

It is generally accepted that the prevalence of dental caries and periodontal disease is high in modern western countries (Mummery, 1869; Wallace, 1900; Davies, 1963; Russell, 1963; Marthaler, 1967). In Great Britain, for example, Goose (1967) examined 309 infants aged 1–2 years and found that over 6% had dental caries. This rate rose to include a quarter of all 4-year-old children in the study by Winter et al. (1971). Other recent studies in England suggest that of children aged 5 years, only one in four is free from dental caries (Beal and James, 1971; Timmis, 1971). Unless preventive measures were taken, e.g. fluoridation of community water supply, Beal and James (1971) found that on average every child of 5 years in their study had five decayed, missing or filled (DMF) teeth. A large study by Sheiham and Hobdell (1969) suggests that this number of DMF teeth may be doubled by the time a child in Britain becomes a late teenager, and trebled in a further 10 years.

In a survey of 2004 subjects, Sheiham (1969) found that only 13·3% were relatively free of periodontal disease. Even at the early age of 15–19 years 58% showed signs of this disease; 2·2% of these young adults had marked periodontal disease, a percentage which increased 15 times in those who were 35 years old. Indeed advanced periodontal disease affected no less than three-quarters of the subjects aged 50 years.

A study of 5000 persons aged 25–35 years (Gould, 1965) showed that only 7% had all their teeth. On average 24% of teeth were missing in each individual. Another study (Hobdell et al., 1969) suggests that in England most persons lose at least half, and approximately one in two lose all their teeth by the age of 50. A high incidence of dental caries and widespread prevalence of periodontal disease have been reported in Europe, and in those parts of the United States of America, Canada, Australia, New Zealand and South America where the western way of life predominates (Healey and Cheyne, 1942; Pedersen, 1947; Barnard, 1956; Russell, 1957, 1963, 1966; Lawrence, 1958; Russell et al., 1961a; Davies, 1963; Harris, 1963; Lilienthal et al., 1965; Hennon et al., 1969; Töth, 1970; Bagramian and Russell, 1971; Wegner, 1971; Hankin et al., 1973).

III. Historical emergence

A. Dental caries

In Great Britain, the prevalence of dental caries and periodontal disease was very low in ancient times. Lunt (1972) examined 83 deciduous molars of 22 children from approximately 3000 B.C. to A.D. 1000, and found not a single carious tooth. Miles (1969) noted dental caries in only 3·6% of 193 deciduous teeth dating from A.D. 600–800. Moore and Corbett (1971) reported dental caries in only 13 out of 370 deciduous teeth from the Anglo-Saxon period, and Hardwick (1960) detected only 82 carious lesions in 1014 teeth in Anglo-Saxon skulls. Brothwell (1959) gave the following percentages of carious teeth at different periods in Britain:

Neolithic	4%
Roman (first century A.D.)	12%
Saxon	5%

Although there was a rise in the prevalence of dental caries during Roman times, when, incidentally, "fine-ground flour and sweet-tasting delicacies would be available" (Hardwick, 1960), it fell during the Anglo-Saxon period and rose again in the sixteenth century, as did the consumption of refined carbohydrate foods. Sugar was then expensive, and dental caries was probably commoner among those who were relatively affluent (Hardwick, 1960; James and Miller, 1970). In Britain the continuing rise in the prevalence of dental caries has been related to the widespread consumption of sugar (Hardwick, 1960).

In America, Leigh (1929) found only 187 carious teeth in 75 out of 300 skulls of the ancient Californians. Rabkin (1942) found dental caries in 1·9% of 736 skulls dated A.D. 1000 and earlier, and in 6·5% of 596 skulls dated A.D. 1500–1600. Parfitt (1959) has reported a rising incidence of dental caries among the Navajo Indians in North America as they increasingly adopt a modern western type of diet. Thus the pattern of historical emergence of dental caries in America is similar to that in Britain.

It is interesting that in Anglo-Saxon and similar American material carious lesions appear to have started at the gingival margins, both interstitially and buccally. Dental caries starting near the points of contact between adjacent teeth, now so common in the western world, was extremely rare in ancient peoples. Moreover dental caries, now so common in children, was rare in the young Anglo-Saxon (Leigh, 1929; Rabkin, 1942, 1943; Klatsky and Klatell, 1943; Brothwell, 1959; Hardwick, 1960; Brabant, 1967; Miles, 1969; Moore and Corbett, 1971).

B. Periodontal disease

Examination of ancient material suggests that although periodontal disease occurred it was "less frequently encountered then than at present" (Brabant, 1967). "Pyorrhoea is hardly ever present in stone age man" (Begg, 1954), and "alveoloclasia in these skulls is rare about anterior teeth. This is in contrast with the condition of modern people" (Leigh, 1929). Brothwell (1959), however, found some degree of alveolar recession in at least 74% of 130 skulls dating between Neolithic and Saxon periods. Such cases may have been related to extreme attrition leading to food impaction (Leigh, 1929; Brothwell, 1959; Alexandersen, 1967), but faulty nutrition may have been partly responsible (Brothwell, 1959). However, Moore and Corbett (1971) state that alveolar recession was generally of equal severity in all parts of Anglo-Saxon jaws they examined and that it increased with age. Lavelle and Moore (1969) found significantly greater resorption of alveolar bone in the mandibles of the seventeenth century than in those of the Anglo-Saxon period. It would thus seem that in ancient times periodontal disease, like dental caries, appeared in later life and that periodontal tissues were resistant to disease in populations whose diet contained much firm and unrefined foodstuffs.

IV. Prevalence of dental caries and periodontal disease in contemporary traditional environment

A. Dental caries

It is evident that the prevalence of dental caries is low among people living in a traditional environment (Klatsky, 1948; Davies, 1963; Russell, 1963;

Marthaler, 1967). For example, a very low incidence of dental caries has been reported in rural Alaska (Russell *et al.*, 1961a), China (Afonsky, 1951), Egypt (Dawson, 1948), Greenland (Pedersen, 1947), India (Marshall-Day, 1944), Kenya (Schwartz, 1946), Kuria Muria islands of the Middle East (Rugg-Gunn, 1968), Mexico and Peru (Neumann and DiSalvo, 1958), Morocco (Poulsen *et al.*, 1972), North America (Parfitt, 1959), Sudan (Emslie, 1966), Tristan da Cunha (Sampson, 1932) and Uganda (Akpabio, 1970; Møller *et al.*, 1972). In many cases the mean rate of decayed, missing or filled (DMF) teeth was less than two teeth per person compared with 16 DMF teeth per person in the adult population in Britain (Sheiham and Hobdell, 1969) or 10–11 DMF teeth per person in urban United States of America (Healey and Cheyne, 1942; Bagramian and Russell, 1971).

B. Periodontal disease

While the prevalence of dental caries in rural communities living on natural foods is universally low, the prevalence of periodontal disease in such communities varies. Those who include firm fibrous foods in their regular diet have good periodontal health (Sampson, 1932; Schwartz, 1946; Pedersen, 1947; Neumann and DiSalvo, 1958; Parfitt, 1959; Russell *et al.*, 1961b; Rugg-Gunn, 1968). Indeed, some North American Indian children in rural areas had better gingival health than the children of European extraction in Alabama (Parfitt, 1959). On the other hand a high prevalence of periodontal disease has been recorded in several rural populations (Greene, 1960; Akpabio, 1966; Emslie, 1966; Skougaard *et al.*, 1969). These surveys show a positive correlation between calculus, standard of oral cleanliness and periodontal disease. Although accumulation of calculus may be related to inadequate oral hygiene, and extensive nutritional deficiencies may predispose some communities to destructive periodontal disease (Mann *et al.*, 1947; Dawson, 1948; Russell, 1963), periodontal disease is apparently more marked among people consuming largely soft foods than among those eating mostly firm fibrous foods.

V. Pathogenesis of dental caries and periodontal disease

A. General considerations

1. Dental caries

Aristotle suspected that stagnation of food, particularly of sweet foods, around the teeth caused dental disease (Hardwick, 1960). Nearly three and a half centuries ago it was recognized in Britain that dental pain might be prevented by "keeping cleane your teeth when as you feede" (Kanner,

1928). In 1890 Miller suggested that acids produced by bacterial fermentation of foods were responsible for the causation of dental caries, a hypothesis subsequently well substantiated (Bowen, 1965; Darling, 1970; Jenkins, 1972).

2. Periodontal disease

There is much evidence to suggest that periodontal disease, like dental caries, is initiated by the formation of dental plaque (McHugh, 1970). Dental plaque may be defined as densely packed colonies of bacteria in an adherent film of gelatinous polysaccharides and proteins which accumulates on teeth. Inflammatory periodontal disease is believed to be due to effects on the periodontal tissues of plaque microorganisms and/or their metabolites either acting directly, through immunological reactions, or in both ways (Gibbons, 1964; Sussman et al., 1969; Genco, 1970; Ivanyi and Lehner, 1970; Löe, 1970; Nisengard and Beutner, 1970; Rizzo, 1970; Schroeder, 1970). In a study on conventional and germ-free rats, Rovin et al. (1966) have suggested that a source of local irritant, such as calculus, together with microbial flora are necessary for the initiation of periodontal disease. If the gingiva is denuded of its epithelial covering, even very low concentrations of antigen can apparently produce marked local reactions (Rizzo, 1970). The gingival area most likely to become denuded of epithelial cover soon after eruption of teeth is the area between two adjacent teeth (Cohen, 1959). This adds significance to the positive correlation between high prevalence of interproximal calculus and plaque and inflammation of the interdental gingival tissue reported by Alexander (1971).

The pathogenesis of dental caries and periodontal disease therefore involves three interacting factors: the oral microorganisms, host resistance, and diet, the last providing the substrate for the plaque flora.

B. Oral microorganisms

The mouth is colonized by microorganisms shortly after birth (Carlsson et al., 1970; Cornick and Bowen, 1971). Lactobacilli, streptococci (particularly Strep. mutans), actinomyces and veillonella are believed to be implicated in the causation of dental caries (Bowen, 1965; Jenkins, 1972; Loesche and Syed, 1973). The microorganisms commonly associated with periodontal disease are cocci, bacteroides, fusiformes, spirochaetes and other filamentous bacteria (Gibbons et al., 1963; Socransky et al., 1963; Gibbons, 1964; Howell et al., 1965; Theilade et al., 1966; Loesche, 1968).

The relative population density of any microbial species in dental plaque is governed by the local environment in different areas of the mouth and on different surfaces of the same tooth (Krasse, 1970; Schroeder and de

Boever, 1970). Although the microorganisms in dental plaque readily metabolize sucrose they can also utilize starch (Grenby, 1965, 1967a; Green and Hartles, 1967a, b; Frostell and Baer, 1971; Shaw and Ivimey, 1972). The cariogenic microorganisms can also utilize extracellular polysaccharides formed from starch by other oral microorganisms (Leach et al., 1969; Parker and Creamer, 1971). Moreover, the cariogenicity of an organism may be influenced by the presence or absence of other microorganisms (Green et al., 1972).

Dental caries and periodontal disease are not the result of the activity of any single organism. Indeed, in caries-susceptible individuals Lehner et al. (1970) found antibodies to all seven cariogenic organisms tested. Everhart et al. (1972), in a study of dental caries and salivary immunoglobulins, showed that more than one microorganism could cause dental caries and that protection against one microorganism would not protect against another of a different antigenic specificity. Several studies indicate that periodontal disease is also associated with a complex microbial flora (Gibbons et al., 1963; Socransky et al., 1963; Gibbons, 1964; Krasse, 1970). Thus arbitrary reduction in the numbers of any particular group of organisms by the use of antibiotics or antibodies would not appear to be of lasting benefit to the host. The emergence of resistant strains of organisms and sensitivity in the host to drugs used is well known. Moreover, the presence of certain bacteria in a healthy mouth may be beneficial in that they could exclude others more liable to cause acute infections.

Addition of sucrose to plaque reduces the plaque pH very rapidly in man and in animals (Stephan, 1940; Bowen et al., 1966; Mühlemann and de Boever, 1970). Microorganisms which can survive low pH may therefore be found in larger numbers where sucrose is a constant source of energy (Drucker, 1970; Poole and Newman, 1971). A change in the sucrose content of the diet would not only lead to an alteration in the total microbial population but increased sucrose content would also lead to a relative increase in acidogenic organisms, as demonstrated by Bowen and Cornick (1967), Fitzgerald and Fitzgerald (1972) and Loesche et al. (1972). Higher pH in the gingival sulcus due to the presence of other cellular metabolites may encourage a different microbial species to flourish; a readily metabolizable substrate such as sucrose may nevertheless promote multiplication.

Dental caries and periodontal disease may be partly due to excessive accumulation of products of normal bacterial metabolism. Duany et al. (1972a) found no significant difference in the prevalence of potentially cariogenic streptococcal types AHT, BHT, GS–5 and HHT on two specific tooth regions in 138 caries-free and 114 caries-active students. Bowen (1963) reported that the salivary flora of caries-free monkeys (*Macaca irus*) included microorganisms "which, given suitable conditions, could take part in the initiation and development of oral disease similar to that occurring in man". It would thus appear that the severity of microbial injury leading to dental caries and periodontal disease largely depends upon host resistance and diet. Host resistance determines the susceptibility of the tissues to attack from, and response to, microorganisms and the products of their metabolism. Diet may favour or hinder the metabolism of particular organisms.

C. Host resistance

The factors which commonly influence host resistance to dental caries and periodontal disease are largely those fostering optimum growth and maturation of tissues and minimizing stagnation areas in the mouth. Genetic factors also play a part.

Enamel is completely formed before a tooth erupts. Although it has been suggested that hypoplasia of enamel makes teeth more susceptible to dental caries (Mellanby, 1923, 1927; Mansbridge, 1959a), an invariable relationship between these two disorders has not been established (Shafer et al., 1967; Darling, 1970; Shaw, 1970). A balanced diet including adequate vitamins and minerals is, however, necessary for optimum development of teeth and for the post-eruptive resistance of dental tissues to caries and periodontal disease (Mellanby, 1923; Nikiforuk, 1970; Shaw, 1970; Waerhaug, 1971). It is generally accepted that adequate intake of fluoride, during the period of odontogenesis and following eruption of teeth, increases resistance to dental caries (Brudevold et al., 1960; Darling, 1970; Nikiforuk, 1970; Shaw, 1970). Indeed, fluoridation of public water supply has been shown to be one of the most effective and safest public health measures against dental caries (Beal and James, 1971; Timmis, 1971; Marthaler, 1972a). The solubility of enamel in acid is reduced by factors in some unrefined foods (Osborn et al., 1937; Jenkins et al., 1959a, b; Andlaw, 1960; Jenkins and Smales, 1966; Grenby, 1967a, b). Although nutritional deficiencies apparently may not initiate periodontal disease, they would seem to predispose to and increase its severity (Bradford, 1959; Stahl, 1970). Thus host resistance may be impaired, not only by such deficiency diseases as scurvy but also by a reduction in immune factors resulting from protein deficiency (Walter and Israel, 1970).

In rats the enamel becomes more resistant to caries with age (Hodge, 1943; Fanning et al., 1954; Larson and Fitzgerald, 1964; Fitzgerald and Larson, 1967; Larson and Keyes, 1967), and the hypomineralized areas in molars become fully mature in about 15 days in the presence of saliva (Speirs, 1967). Using human teeth in vitro Poole and Silverstone (1973) showed that salivary calcium and phosphate ions may be reprecipitated into areas of decalcification in very early carious lesions or in small fractures in enamel. Nevertheless the work of Hodge (1943) and Larson and Keyes

(1967) demonstrates that although the occurrence of dental caries may depend on the age of the tooth, the extent and the number of lesions seem to depend upon the strength and duration of the cariogenic challenge.

Adequate oral hygiene is readily maintained when the teeth are regularly aligned or spaced. Genetic factors determining the dento-alveolar proportions and tooth morphology may therefore indirectly influence resistance of the teeth to dental caries and periodontal disease, since overcrowding and occurrence of deep pits and fissures result in increased food stagnation on and around the teeth. The host resistance to dental caries and periodontal disease may certainly be raised by efficient oral hygiene and dental prophylaxis (Fosdick, 1950; Mansbridge, 1960; Koch and Lindhe, 1965; Theilade *et al.*, 1966; Zaki and Stallard, 1969; Sheiham, 1970; Gilmore and Russell, 1972; Hamp *et al.*, 1972; Listgarten and Ellegaard, 1972; Marthaler, 1972b). Topical application of fluorides to teeth appears to increase the resistance of the host against dental caries (Marthaler, 1972a, b; Koch, 1973).

D. Diet

When increased dietary sucrose lowers the Net Dietary Protein Calorie percentage below the level recommended for a weanling rat, degenerative changes occur in the liver and salivary glands and serum protein levels are altered. The total effect, in the rat, may contribute to an oral environment favouring dental caries (Bunyard, 1970a, b). It is, however, not certain whether an excessive intake of refined carbohydrate foods during the period of odontogenesis affects the caries susceptibility of developing teeth in their post-eruptive period (Shaw, 1970). Nevertheless much evidence suggests that consumption of refined carbohydrate foods after the eruption of teeth is a major aetiological factor in dental caries and periodontal disease in man and animals.

VI. Dental caries, periodontal disease and refined carbohydrate foods

A. Dental caries

Many human and animal studies have shown that refined carbohydrate foods are the most cariogenic of all foods (Davies, 1963; Marthaler, 1967; Winter, 1968; Darling, 1970; Nikiforuk, 1970; Mäkinen, 1972). Although starch, especially when cooked, is cariogenic, it is far less so than sucrose (Gustafson *et al.*, 1959; Green and Hartles, 1967a, b; Grenby, 1969; Shaw and Ivimey, 1972). Sucrose appears to be the most cariogenic of all sugars (Frostell *et al.*, 1967; Marthaler, 1967; Grenby, 1967c, 1969; Grenby and

Hutchinson, 1969; Green and Hartles, 1969; Larje and Larson, 1970; Fitzgerald and Fitzgerald, 1972). In an experimental study in monkeys (*Macaca irus*) Cohen and Bowen (1966) have demonstrated that dietary items such as sweet biscuits, white bread, jam, etc., as normally sold for human consumption, are highly cariogenic. In 1968 Larson *et al.* reported that rats which were previously supposed to be of a caries-resistant strain developed as many carious lesions as rats of a caries-susceptible strain when their diet was changed from coarse to fine particle and the sucrose content was increased from 25 to 56%. Kite *et al.* (1950) have shown that feeding high sucrose diet via stomach tube does not cause dental caries in caries-susceptible rats, which suggests that the cariogenic effect of sucrose is exerted locally.

Although King *et al.* (1955) suggested that there was no correlation between the incidence of dental caries and the total amount of sugar consumed, they stated that their study did not "throw any direct light on whether a more prolonged high local concentration of sugar on the tooth surface influences the carious process", nor did it "prove that the sugar content of the diet, *however distributed and however eaten*, never affects the teeth". Much evidence suggests that in man, at any age, the effect of cariogenic foods increases when they remain in the mouth for a prolonged time, e.g. if such foods form a large part of regular diet, if they are eaten between meals, or if oral hygiene habits are unrelated to mealtimes.

1. Studies in children

Studies in Britain (Mansbridge, 1960; Bradford and Crabb, 1961; Stephen and Sutherland, 1971; Winter *et al.*, 1971) have shown that dental caries is more prevalent in children who regularly consume beverages and/or confectionery containing sugar and refined carbohydrates than in those who do not, or who are restricted from eating such foods at bed-time or between meals. A recent study of caries-free and caries-active school children in the U.S.A. (Duany *et al.*, 1972b) clearly showed that caries-free children, in distinct contrast to caries-active children, either did not have sugar-containing foods or had them very infrequently. Similarly Afonsky (1951) observed in China that infants developed rampant caries when they were given "candy pacifiers".

2. Studies in adults

The Vipeholm study (Gustafsson *et al.*, 1954) emphasized the association in man of dental caries and the consumption of sugar, particularly between meals and when taken in the form of sticky foods. Afonsky (1951), in a survey in China, found an extremely low incidence of dental caries among

3349 persons aged 12–27 years. Their regular diet contained no sugar in any form. In 1970 von der Fehr *et al.* reported that frequent mouth rinses between meals with 10 ml of 50% sucrose for 23 days led to significantly more incipient carious lesions than were found in controls. Seventy years previously Wallace (1900) had observed that cooks and confectioners, who frequently taste the foods they are preparing, as a rule have carious teeth.

3. Epidemiological studies

It is clear from the epidemiological evidence presented earlier that the prevalence of dental caries is high in urban communities, a common factor being a diet with a high content of sugar and refined carbohydrate foods. On the other hand the prevalence of dental caries is low among those who live in a traditional environment. These rural populations in widely separated parts of the world all appear to have a diet low in refined carbohydrate foods.

4. Heredity, race and dental caries

Although genetic factors have been suspected to be associated with the occurrence of dental caries in man (Retief *et al.*, 1973; Walker, 1973), several studies, including studies in monozygotic and dizygotic twins (Bachrach and Young, 1927; Mansbridge, 1959b) have shown clearly that environmental factors have a major influence in the pathogenesis of dental caries. That heredity, race or geography, when compared with diet and other environmental factors, plays a very small part in the aetiology of dental caries can be seen from the longitudinal studies of dental caries in people living at opposite poles of the earth. Band and Kristoffersen (1972) studied a group of Eskimos living in Anaktuvuk Pass in northern Alaska, on a diet of fish, marine mammals and birds. In 1953 "a white trader had opened a small store". During 1957–65 three more stores were opened, and sugar and other refined foods became a regular part of their diet. In 1955–57 three-quarters of the subjects had caries-free permanent teeth. By 1965 not a single person was free of dental caries. The average DMF rate per person had increased four times in these 8–10 years.

A longer dental history is available in the case of the islanders of Tristan da Cunha near the opposite pole from Alaska. When Sampson (1932) visited the island in 1932 their diet consisted chiefly of fish, potatoes, milk, eggs and green vegetables. He wrote, "They never have any bread or flour unless a ship happens to call. (Note: one year has elapsed since the last ship.)" He found that 83% had neither dental caries nor had lost any teeth. Children aged 1–5 years had no dental caries. No one under the age of 21 years had caries in permanent teeth. Between 1932 and 1937 ships called more frequently, and Barnes (1937) wrote "there has been an appreciable increase in the consumption of sugar and flour. . . . Scones and bread are made several times per week and always on Sundays." By then only 50% of the islanders had neither dental caries nor had lost any teeth. In 1942 a fishing station and a store were established. By 1952 sugar and flour had become "essential foodstuffs", average annual consumption of sugar per family was over 105 kg, and only 22% of the population had complete and caries-free dentitions. Children aged 1–5 years had dental caries in 32% of their teeth (Gamblen, 1953).

A similar trend towards increased dental caries experience on adoption of refined carbohydrate foods in regular diet has been observed among Africans in South Africa (Fricl and Shaw, 1931), East Africa (Welbourn, 1956; Emslie, 1966; Adatia, 1974) and West Africa (Akpabio, 1970; Enwonwu, 1974), among the Navajo Indians of the United States of America (Parfitt, 1959) and in the inhabitants of South Arabia (Rugg-Gunn, 1968). A positive and consistent correlation between DMF rates and frequency of candy and gum intake has been demonstrated by Hankin *et al.* (1973) among the Japanese, Hawaiian and Caucasian children in Hawaii. Hankin *et al.* (1973) concluded that the racial variation in the prevalence of dental caries was related to environmental factors rather than to genetic differences. Indeed, comparative studies in West Africa and the United States of America have shown clearly that when the environmental factors become similar, the prevalence of dental caries among Africans and their descendants is the same as that among the people of European extraction, whether they live in Africa (Enwonwu, 1974) or in the United States of America (Bagramian and Russell, 1971). Laboratory animal studies have also shown comparable caries activity in caries-susceptible and caries-resistant strains when they are caged together and subjected to the same severe cariogenic challenge (Larson, 1966; Larson *et al.*, 1968). It seems that "it is one thing to live in the same country, and quite another to live under the same conditions" (Wallace, 1900).

B. *Periodontal disease*

On the oral hygiene habits of the islanders of Tristan da Cunha, Sampson wrote in 1932 that "they never clean their teeth", yet 95% of them were free of periodontal disease. Five years later Barnes (1937) wrote, "the general habits, characteristics and dietary of the community, which were fully commented upon" by Sampson (1932) "do not appear to have undergone any radical change, except that there has been an appreciable increase in the consumption of sugar and flour". In 1937 the percentage of people free of periodontal disease had decreased to 69% (Barnes, 1937) and by 1952 only 57% of the islanders had clinically healthy periodontal tissues

(Gamblen, 1953). This suggests that a diet rich in sugar and other refined carbohydrate foods may be conducive to periodontal disease which is initiated by the accumulation of dental plaque.

Nearly three-quarters of a century ago Wallace (1900) wrote that foods "with much sugar leave the teeth with a coating". In 1970 von der Fehr *et al.* provided experimental evidence that frequent sucrose mouth rinses accelerated the rate of plaque formation in man. When sucrose was omitted from the diet of 19 members of an Antarctic expedition for 14 weeks the plaque declined significantly (Fry and Grenby, 1972). The amount of plaque formed in man on high sucrose diets is considerably greater than on high glucose or fructose diets (Carlsson and Egelberg, 1965).

More plaque and calculus are formed in experimental animals on diets containing sucrose than on sucrose-free diets (Bowen and Cornick, 1967; Frostell *et al.*, 1967; Ashley and Naylor, 1970; Shannon *et al.*, 1970). Indeed the work of Larmas and Scheinin (1967) on dogs suggests that a sugar diet may induce the activities of a number of proteolytic enzymes in the saliva.

VII. Unrefined foods and resistance of teeth against dental caries and periodontal disease

A. Dental caries

It has been supected since the beginning of the century that crude sugar cane juice is less cariogenic than refined sugar (Wallace, 1900). In 1937 Osborn *et al.* found that sugar cane juice, whole mealie meal and whole wheat, in contrast to refined flour and sugar, contained factors which reduced the solubility of enamel when incubated with saliva. These results were confirmed by Jenkins *et al.* (1959a, b), Andlaw (1960), Jenkins and Smales (1966) and Grenby (1967a, b). The solubility of enamel was apparently not lessened when it was incubated in saliva with brown sugar or honey (Jenkins *et al.*, 1959a) although they appeared to contain the solubility-reducing factors. Recently Edgar and Jenkins (1974) have shown that in the case of honey this apparent anomaly is due to the rapid degradation of the solubility-reducing agents by bacteria in saliva. In the case of raw sugar it is due to the fact that the acid produced on incubating raw sugar in saliva for more than 4 h is sufficient to overcome the effects of the solubility-reducing agents contained in the raw sugar. Factors which reduce the solubility of enamel are also present in wheat bran, wheat germ, and in hulls of oats, peanuts and pecans. These factors are water-soluble and can be extracted, from wheat at least, during normal mastication (Jenkins and Smales, 1966). The apparent cariostatic effect of unrefined flour might be due to phytates (Jenkins and Smales, 1966; Grenby, 1967b, d).

Addition of sodium phytate or phosphates to the diet results in a significant reduction in dental caries in rats (McClure, 1963; Dawes and Shaw, 1965; Luoma *et al.*, 1970, 1972; Larson *et al.*, 1972), monkeys (Bowen, 1971) and in man (Brewer *et al.*, 1970). However, Luoma *et al.* (1970) found that 4% bicarbonate–phosphate (NaH CO_3–KH_2 PO_4) combination produced calcification in the heart and kidneys in rats. It has not been determined whether all added phosphates have such long-term side-effects. Neumann *et al.* (1952) have demonstrated the cariostatic effect of chewing sugar cane once a day.

B. Periodontal disease

The beneficial effects of unrefined foods on the periodontal tissues seem to be related to the consistency of diet.

1. Animal studies

Experimental animals fed a soft diet show a marked increase in accumulation of plaque and periodontal disease (Burwasser and Hill, 1939; Mitchell, 1950; Egelberg, 1965). A diet of firm consistency, on the other hand, improves periodontal health, stimulates periodontal fibroblasts and encourages optimal growth of the jaws (Barber *et al.*, 1963; Egelberg, 1965; Weiss *et al.*, 1969). Obviously a diet which is harsh enough to damage the gingiva may be deleterious.

2. Human studies

Pelzer (1940) and Haydak *et al.* (1944) found that soft or liquid diets led to periodontal disease. Fibrous foods such as apples or oranges are effective in cleaning the mouth of fine particles such as yeast (Knighton, 1942). Eating apples after every meal and after eating anything between meals apparently benefits periodontal health (Slack and Martin, 1958). On the other hand it has been reported that chewing carrots (Lindhe and Wicen, 1969; Reece and Swallow, 1970) or apples has no significant effect on plaque formation and gingival health (Longhurst and Berman, 1973) or on reduction of plaque (Wade, 1971). Negative results in these studies may be related to the type of fibrous food chosen, the amount and frequency of consumption, chewing time, experimental period, or to all these factors.

3. Epidemiological studies

Several studies on ancient material and contemporary populations suggest that consumption of firm fibrous foods improves the periodontal tissues and jaw growth in man (Wallace, 1900; Leigh, 1929; Klatsky, 1948; Begg, 1954; Parfitt, 1959; Russell *et al.*, 1961a, b; Alexandersen, 1967; Moore *et al.*, 1968; Lavelle and Moore, 1969). An extensive review by O'Rourke (1947) had also suggested that "thorough mastication of hard, detergent foods tends to maintain the health and reserve capacity of the gingivae, periodontal membrane and alveolar bone".

VIII. Possible natural mechanism of resistance of teeth against dental caries and periodontal disease

The evidence presented above suggests the following conclusions:

1. Dental caries and periodontal disease are largely due to an imbalance between host resistance and oral environment.

2. Sucrose and other readily fermentable refined carbohydrate foods encourage accumulation of dental plaque. Excessive accumulation of microorganisms and/or their metabolites initiates dental caries and periodontal disease.

3. Unrefined carbohydrate foods contain protective factors which reduce the solubility of enamel and may afford protection against dental caries. These factors can be extracted from foods by mastication.

4. Mastication of firm fibrous foods promotes periodontal health and stimulates optimum growth of the jaws.

5. The high prevalence of dental caries in the modern western world appears to be related to the cariogenic diet and to the occurrence of dental caries at an early age. A high incidence of interstitial dental caries near the contact points is particularly noticeable.

6. Studies in populations apparently resistant to dental caries and destructive periodontal disease suggest that such resistance may be related to a lack of refined carbohydrate foods in their diet and to attrition of teeth due to vigorous mastication.

How the protective factors in unrefined foods alter the solubility of enamel is not yet clear. Madsen and Edmunds (1963) suggest that these factors may have both a systemic and a local effect. The latter appears to be due to the adsorption of these factors, probably phytates, on the surface of the calcium compounds in enamel (Jenkins *et al.*, 1959a; Grenby, 1967d; Magrill, 1973). Hallsworth *et al.* (1972) showed that the translucent zone, the first breakdown stage identifiable in a carious lesion, apparently results from demineralization associated with preferential loss of magnesium-rich material from enamel. Thus adsorption of the protective factors on the calcium compounds in enamel may increase resistance against dental caries. Darling (1963), on the other hand, argued that the apparent resistance against caries of teeth affected by conditions such as amelogenesis imperfecta and fluorosis, might be due to a relative insolubility of their organic matrix.

Magrill (1973) found a direct relationship between phytate adsorbed and reduction in solubility of calcium hydroxyapatite. It would therefore appear that the longer such factors remain in contact with teeth the more beneficial they may be. Grenby (1967d), however, found that topical application of sodium phytate to the molars of caries-susceptible rats only slightly reduced the incidence of caries. Darling (1956, 1958), Crabb (1966) and Hallsworth et al. (1972) showed that in the early stages of the dental caries process dissolution of enamel is greatest below a surface layer of relatively less affected enamel. This suggests that the effect of the protective factors, however exerted, might be increased if there were a mechanism which could actively aid their incorporation into enamel.

McCance et al. (1953) found that although bread made from low-extraction white flour took longer to pass through the alimentary tract than bread made from high-extraction wholemeal flour, the subjects took longer to eat the latter than the former. This indicates that unrefined food is chewed for a longer period, and protective factors, which are apparently extracted more thoroughly during mastication, remain in the mouth in a high concentration for a relatively longer period.

Studies on the compressibility of the enamel suggest that the protective factors might be actively incorporated into it. Following the work of Neumann (1955) and Neumann and DiSalvo (1957), Haines et al. (1963) showed that enamel at points of contact between two adjacent teeth was highly compressible at loads up to 12 lb, as would be exerted during normal mastication. It can be seen from Fig. 17.1 that forces exerted by the cusps of teeth in the opposing dental arches could be translated into compression at contact points between teeth. Haines et al. (1963) calculated the contours of the distribution of volume changes at contact points when enamel was thus compressed (Fig. 17.2). Since these resembled closely the pattern of early carious lesions demonstrated by Darling (1956), Haines et al. (1963) suggested that the pattern of penetration of the destructive agents into the enamel might be influenced by the flow of liquid within it during mastication. On the same basis it is tempting to suggest that the passage of water-soluble protective agents may also be facilitated by the movement of ions as a result of intermittent compression of enamel during mastication. It is tempting to speculate further that the mechanism whereby vigorous mastication affords resistance against dental caries (Klatsky and Klatell, 1943; Neumann, 1950; Neumann et al., 1952; Begg, 1954; Neumann and DiSalvo, 1958; Russell et al., 1961a) may be in accord with this hypothesis of active incorporation into enamel of water-soluble protective factors in unrefined foods and saliva. This may explain the increasing resistance to dental caries with advancing age. Conversely newly erupted teeth should be very vulnerable to dental caries. Cohen and Bowen (1966) found that in experimental monkeys dental caries was commoner and developed more rapidly in teeth which erupted after, or at most 6 months before, the cariogenic diet was started. An analysis of the longitudinal study of the inhabitants of Tristan da Cunha, summarized in Table 17.1, points to a similar conclusion.

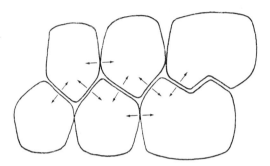

FIG. 17.1. Forces exerted by the cusps of teeth in the opposing dental arches could be translated into compression at contact points between teeth.

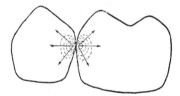

FIG. 17.2. Diagrammatic representation of the contours of distribution of volume changes in enamel when it is compressed at contact points. (Adapted from Haines *et al.*, 1963.)

Although studies by different examiners in the case of the Tristan da Cunhans cannot be considered strictly comparable, a clear pattern emerges. In 1932 the diet of these islanders was not highly cariogenic. All children between the ages of 1 and 5 years were free of dental caries. No one below the age of 21 years had caries in permanent teeth (Sampson, 1932). Children's teeth examined in 1952 had erupted in a highly cariogenic environment and Gamblen (1953) found that 32% of the teeth in children aged 1–5 years were carious. Since 1932 permanent teeth were erupting in an increasingly cariogenic environment. By 1937 caries was evident in the permanent teeth of the islanders under 21 years old. Children who were 6–13 years of age in 1937 had 1·59% permanent teeth carious (Barnes, 1937). By 1952 the incidence of dental caries in this group had risen 6-fold. On the other hand the dental caries experience of those who were 22–32 years old in 1937 had less than doubled 15 years later. The cariogenic challenge may have been greater in the younger than in the older groups, although the reports quoted do not suggest this argument.

Vigorous mastication may help to resist dental caries and periodontal disease in other ways. Foods which require to be chewed for a long period are cleared from the oral cavity more thoroughly than those not requiring much chewing. Refined carbohydrate foods such as white bread are retained for longer than wholewheat bread (Bibby et al., 1951). Secondly, mastication not only encourages salivary flow, which would have a flushing effect on teeth, but also saliva of a high buffering power (Jenkins and Kleinberg, 1956; Jenkins, 1959; Johnson and Sreebny, 1971). Thirdly, vigorous

TABLE 17.1. Dental caries experience in Tristan da Cunhans

	% Teeth carious		
Age	1932 (Sampson, 1932)	1937 (Barnes, 1937)	1952 (Gamblen, 1953)
1–5	0·0	4·3	32·02
6–13	0·19	1·59	8·30
14–21	0·0	2·15	8·52
22–32	0·50	4·76	9·7
33–45	2·61	5·66	8·39
46–55	11·8	9·0	10·22
56+	7·46	3·9	12·66

mastication would wear and flatten the cusps of teeth, reduce the depths of the fissures and eliminate potential stagnation areas on the teeth. Forward drift of teeth due to wear on their adjacent surfaces increases contact between the teeth. Increased interdental contact, friction, or both, may prevent accumulation of plaque at the contact area. Reduction in the mesio-distal dimension of teeth due to wear, and their forward drift, facilitate the accommodation of the later erupting posterior teeth (Begg, 1954; Murphy, 1964) and reduce potential stagnation areas in the mouth. Reduction in the cusp height by attrition would appear to lessen the lateral forces on the periodontal tissues (Fig. 17.3). Teeth showing signs of attrition often have little marked periodontal disease (Sampson, 1932; Klatsky, 1948; Begg, 1954; Russell et al., 1961a, b). Finally, vigorous mastication of firm fibrous foods would remove debris from the exposed areas of the teeth and help to maintain the gingival tissues in good tone. Indeed, "one of the most certain methods of inducing caries [is] to sip constantly at liquid foods and to dispense with the use of the tooth brush", wrote Wallace in 1900. That this was probably true of periodontal disease as well was shown by Haydak *et al.* in 1944.

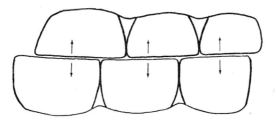

FIG. 17.3. Attrition reduces the cusp height of teeth, increases contact between adjacent teeth and decreases stagnation area. At this stage the masticatory forces are translated mainly in the axial direction.

IX. Preventive measures against dental caries and periodontal disease

It would appear that the following measures may be considered for the prevention of dental caries and periodontal disease:

1. Oral hygiene. To obtain maximum benefit this should be meticulous; teeth should be cleaned after eating anything, and have regular professional attention.

2. Use of cariostatic food additives such as fluorides which are safe in therapeutic dosage.

3. Reduction in the use of readily fermentable refined carbohydrate foods and avoidance of eating between meals.

4. Consumption of a balanced diet containing acceptable quantities of unrefined foods of firm fibrous consistency.

Civilized man's ability to refine and process his food appears to have made him independent of his dentition for the purpose of survival. It is nevertheless realized by most people that, apart from eating, a healthy dentition does have an important role in man's activities. The vast demand for dental care and replacement dentures confirms this. Although dental caries and periodontal disease rarely cause death, they do impose a considerable mental, physical and financial burden. Yet the incidence of dental disease continues to rise.

The first measure outlined above—meticulous oral hygiene and regular professional attention—requires a little but constant effort on the part of the individual. The second measure, fluoridation of individual or community water supply, has been shown to provide some protection against dental caries. Even if this measure wins general approval, periodontal disease may continue to take its terrible toll of teeth, since it would appear that a large section of our society is either unable or unwilling to make the effort required for meticulous oral hygiene and dental prophylactic care.

As far as the dentition is concerned, diminution in the use of refined carbohydrate foods would reduce the amount of fermentable substrate and discourage the accumulation of dental plaque. Inclusion in the diet of unrefined foods of firm fibrous consistency would encourage vigorous mastication which would aid digestion, induce secretion of saliva of high buffering capacity, promote periodontal health and raise resistance against dental caries. Thus measures 3 and 4 would greatly enhance the otherwise limited benefits of measures 1 and 2 (oral hygiene and food additives). It would seem not unreasonable to suggest that such a scheme of preventive dental medicine based on a natural mechanism and man's scientific dental knowledge could bring the conquest of dental caries and periodontal disease within everyone's reach. It might win general acceptance if it were realized that the dietary factors involved in the pathogenesis of dental caries and periodontal disease are also implicated in the aetiology of many fatal disorders.

It is clear that the rise in the prevalence of dental caries and periodontal disease throughout the world is almost directly related to a change in diet and eating habits. It is equally clear that these preventable dental diseases cost a great deal in terms of misery, money and man hours. While it may be difficult suddenly to reverse dietary habits they may be influenced gradually. Sufficient evidence has been presented to show that unless we apply our minds to remedy the situation the dental health of most nations will continue to deteriorate. Available evidence suggests also that promotion of dental health is only the first of several physiological benefits to be gained from retaining the fibre in our food, thereby increasing mastication. Therefore it would seem that any effort, legislation or subsidy to encourage the demand for and supply of preventive measures in dental medicine and for unrefined foods of proven value could only be to the physical and financial interest of all.

References

ADATIA, A. K. (1974). *Plant Foods for Man* **1**, 81.
AFONSKY, D. (1951). *Journal of Dental Research* **30**, 53.
AKPABIO, S. P. (1966). *Dental Practitioner and Dental Record, Bristol* **16**, 412.
AKPABIO, S. P. (1970). "Dentistry—A Public Health Service in East and West Africa." M.D.S. Thesis, University of London.
ALEXANDER, A. G. (1971). *Journal of Periodontology* **42**, 21.
ALEXANDERSEN, V. (1967). *In* "Diseases in Antiquity" (D. Brothwell and A. T. Sandison, eds), p. 551. Charles C. Thomas, Springfield, Illinois.
ANDLAW, R. J. (1960). *Journal of Dental Research* **39**, 1200.
ASHLEY, F. P. and NAYLOR, M. N. (1970). *Journal of Periodontal Research* **5**, 56.
BACHRACH, F. H. and YOUNG, M. (1927). *British Dental Journal* **48**, 1293.
BAGRAMIAN, R. A. and RUSSELL, A. L. (1971). *Journal of Dental Research* **50**, 1553

BAND, G. and KRISTOFFERSEN, T. (1972). *Scandinavian Journal of Dental Research* **80**, 440.

BARBER, C. G., GREEN, L. J. and COX, G. J. (1963). *Journal of Dental Research* **42**, 848.

BARNARD, P. D. (1956). "Dental Survey of State School Children in New South Wales" (Special Report Series No. 8). National Health and Medical Research Council, Commonwealth Government Printer, Canberra, Australia. (Quoted by Harris, R., 1963.)

BARNES, H. N. V. (1937). *British Dental Journal* **63**, 86.

BEAL, J. F. and JAMES, P. M. C. (1971). *British Dental Journal* **130**, 284.

BEGG, P. R. (1954). *American Journal of Orthodontics* **40**, 298, 373, 462, 517.

BIBBY, B. G., GOLDBERG, H. J. V. and CHEN, E. (1951). *Journal of the American Dental Association* **42**, 491.

BOWEN, W. H. (1963). *British Dental Journal* **115**, 252.

BOWEN, W. H. (1965). *International Dental Journal* **15**, 12.

BOWEN, W. H. (1971). *British Dental Journal* **131**, 266.

BOWEN, W. H. and CORNICK, D. E. (1967). *Helvetica odontologica acta* **11**, 27.

BOWEN, W. H., EASTOE, J. E. and COCK, D. J. (1966). *Archives of Oral Biology* **11**, 833.

BRABANT, H. (1967). *In* "Diseases in Antiquity" (D. Brothwell and A. T. Sandison, eds), p. 538. Charles C. Thomas, Springfield, Illinois.

BRADFORD, E. W. (1959). *Proceedings of the Nutrition Society* **18**, 75.

BRADFORD, E. W. and CRABB, H. S. M. (1961). *British Dental Journal* **111**, 273.

BREWER, H. E., STOOKEY, G. K. and MUHLER, J. C. (1970). *Journal of the American Dental Association* **80**, 121.

BROTHWELL, D. R. (1959). *Proceedings of the Nutrition Society* **18**, 59.

BRUDEVOLD, F., STEADMAN, L. T. and SMITH, F. A. (1960). *Annals of the New York Academy of Sciences* **85**, 110.

BUNYARD, M. W. (1970a). *British Dental Journal* **129**, 319.

BUNYARD, M. W. (1970b). *Caries Research* **4**, 347.

BURWASSER, P. and HILL, T. J. (1939). *Journal of Dental Research* **18**, 389.

CARLSSON, J. and EGELBERG, J. (1965). *Odontologisk Revy* **16**, 112.

CARLSSON, J., GRAHNEN, H., JONSSON, G. and WIKNER, S. (1970). *Journal of Dental Research* **49**, 415.

COHEN, B. (1959). *British Dental Journal* **107**, 31.

COHEN, B. and BOWEN, W. H. (1966). *British Dental Journal* **121**, 269.

CORNICK, D. E. R. and BOWEN, W. H. (1971). *British Dental Journal* **130**, 231.

CRABB, H. S. M. (1966). *British Dental Journal* **121**, 115, 167.

DARLING, A. I. (1956). *British Dental Journal* **101**, 289, 329.

DARLING, A. I. (1958). *British Dental Journal* **105**, 119.

DARLING, A. I. (1963). *Journal of Dental Research* **42**, 488.

DARLING, A. I. (1970). *In* "Thoma's Oral Pathology" (R. J. Gorlin and H. M. Goldman, eds), p. 239. Mosby, St Louis.

DAVIES, G. N. (1963). *Journal of Dental Research* **42**, 209.

DAWES, C. and SHAW, J. H. (1965). *Archives of Oral Biology* **10**, 567.

DAWSON, C. E. (1948). *Journal of Dental Research* **27**, 512.

DRUCKER, D. B. (1970). *In* "Dental Plaque" (W. D. McHugh, ed.), p. 241. Livingstone, Edinburgh and London.

DUANY, L. F., JABLON, J. M. and ZINNER, D. D. (1972). *Journal of Dental Research* 51, (a) 723; (b) 727.

EDGAR, W. M. and JENKINS, G. N. (1974). *British Dental Journal* 136, 7.

EGELBERG, J. (1965). *Odontologisk Revy* 16, 31.

EMSLIE, R. D. (1966). *British Dental Journal* 120, 167.

ENWONWU, C. O. (1974). *Caries Research* 8, 155.

EVERHART, D. L., GRIGSBY, W. R. and CARTER, W. H. JR. (1972). *Journal of Dental Research* 51, 1487.

FANNING, R. J., SHAW, J. H. and SOGNNAES, R. F. (1954). *Journal of the American Dental Association* 49, 668.

FITZGERALD, D. B. and FITZGERALD, R. J. (1972). *Archives of Oral Biology* 17, 215.

FITZGERALD, R. J. and LARSON, R. H. (1967). *Helvetica odontologica acta* 11, 49.

FOSDICK, L. S. (1950). *Journal of the American Dental Association* 40, 133.

FRIEL, G. and SHAW, J. C. M. (1931). *British Dental Journal* 52, 309.

FROSTELL, G. and BAER, P. N. (1971). *Acta odontologica scandinavica* 29, 401.

FROSTELL, G., KEYES, P. H. and LARSON, R. H. (1967). *Journal of Nutrition* 93, 65.

FRY, A. J. and GRENBY, T. H. (1972). *Archives of Oral Biology* 17, 873.

GAMBLEN, F. B. (1953). *Journal of the Royal Naval Medical Service* 39, 252.

GENCO, R. J. (1970). *Journal of Periodontology* 41, 196.

GIBBONS, R. J. (1964). *International Dental Journal* 14, 407.

GIBBONS, R. J., SOCRANSKY, S. S., SAWYER, S., KAPSIMALIS, B. and MACDONALD, J. B. (1963). *Archives of Oral Biology* 8, 281.

GILMORE, N. D. and RUSSELL, A. L. (1972). *Journal of Periodontal Research, Supplement* 10, 17.

GOOSE, D. H. (1967). *Caries Research* 1, 167.

GOULD, D. G. (1965). *British Dental Journal* 118, 377.

GREEN, R. M. and HARTLES, R. L. (1967). *British Journal of Nutrition* 21, (a) 225; (b) 921.

GREEN, R. M. and HARTLES, R. L. (1969). *Archives of Oral Biology* 14, 235.

GREEN, R. M., HUXLEY, H. G., DRUCKER, D. B. and BLACKMORE, D. K. (1972). *Archives of Oral Biology* 17, 903.

GREENE, J. C. (1960). *Journal of Dental Research* 39, 302.

GRENBY, T. H. (1965). *Archives of Oral Biology* 10, 433.

GRENBY, T. H. (1967). *Archives of Oral Biology* 12, (a) 513; (b) 523.

GRENBY, T. H. (1967c). *Caries Research* 1, 208.

GRENBY, T. H. (1967d). *Archives of Oral Biology* 12, 531.

GRENBY, T. H. (1969). *Archives of Oral Biology* 14, 1253.

GRENBY, T. H. and HUTCHINSON, J. B. (1969). *Archives of Oral Biology* 14, 373.

GUSTAFSON, G., STELLING, EM., ABRAMSON, E. and BRUNIUS, E. (1959). *Archives of Oral Biology* 1, 42.

GUSTAFSSON, B. E., QUENSEL, C. B., LANKE, L. S., LUNDQUIST, C., GRAHNEN, H., BONOW, B. E. and KRASSE, B. (1954). *Acta odontologica scandinavica* 11, 232.

HAINES, D. J., BERRY, D. C. and POOLE, D. F. G. (1963). *Journal of Dental Research* **42**, 885.

HALLSWORTH, A. S., ROBINSON, C. and WEATHERELL, J. A. (1972). *Caries Research* **6**, 156.

HAMP, S-E., LINDHE, J. and LÖE, H. (1972). *Journal of Periodontal Research, Supplement* **10**, 13.

HANKIN, J. H., CHUNG, C. S. and KAU, M. C. W. (1973). *Journal of Dental Research* **52**, 1079.

HARDWICK, J. L. (1960). *British Dental Journal* **108**, 9.

HARRIS, R. (1963). *Journal of Dental Research* **42**, 1387.

HAYDAK, M. H., VIVINO, A. E., BOEHRER, J. J., BJORNDAHL, O. and PALMER, L. S. (1944). *American Journal of the Medical Sciences* **207**, 209.

HEALEY, H. J. and CHEYNE, V. D. (1942). *Journal of Dental Research* **21**, 312.

HENNON, D. K., STOOKEY, G. K. and MUHLER, J. C. (1969). *Journal of the American Dental Association* **79**, 1405.

HOBDELL, M. H., SHEIHAM, A. and SLACK, G. L. (1969). *British Dental Journal* **126**, 349.

HODGE, H. C. (1943). *Journal of Dental Research* **22**, 275.

HOLLOWAY, P. J., JAMES, P. M. C. and SLACK, G. L. (1963). *British Dental Journal* **115**, 19.

HOWELL, A., RIZZO, A. and PAUL, F. (1965). *Archives of Oral Biology* **10**, 307.

IVANYI, L. and LEHNER, T. (1970). *Archives of Oral Biology* **15**, 1089.

JAMES, P. M. C. and MILLER, W. A. (1970). *British Dental Journal* **128**, 391.

JENKINS, G. N. (1959). *Proceedings of the Nutrition Scoiety* **18**, 85.

JENKINS, G. N. (1972). *International Dental Journal* **22**, 350.

JENKINS, G. N. and KLEINBERG, I. (1956). *Journal of Dental Research* **35**, 964.

JENKINS, G. N. and SMALES, F. C. (1966). *Archives of Oral Biology* **11**, 599.

JENKINS, G. N., FORSTER, M. G. and SPEIRS, R. L. (1959a). *British Dental Journal* **106**, 362.

JENKINS, G. N., FORSTER, M. G., SPEIRS, R. L. and KLEINBERG, I. (1959b). *British Dental Journal* **106**, 195.

JOHNSON, D. A. and SREEBNY, L. M. (1971). *Archives of Oral Biology* **16**, 177.

KANNER, L. (1928). "Folklore of the Teeth", p. 125. New York. Quoted by Weinberger, B. W. (1948), "An Introduction to the History of Dentistry", Vol. 1, p. 25. Mosby, St Louis.

KING, J. D., MELLANBY, M., STONES, H. H. and GREEN, H. N. (1955). "The Effect of Sugar Supplements on Dental Caries in Children." Medical Research Council Special Report Series No. 288. Her Majesty's Stationery Office, London.

KITE, O. W., SHAW, J. H. and SOGNNAES, R. F. (1950). *Journal of Nutrition* **42**, 89.

KLATSKY, M. (1948). *Journal of the American Dental Association* **36**, 385.

KLATSKY, M. and KLATELL, J. S. (1943). *Journal of Dental Research* **22**, 267.

KNIGHTON, H. T. (1942). *Journal of the American Dental Association* **29**, 2012.

KOCH, G. (1973). *International Dental Journal* **23**, 364.

KOCH, G. and LINDHE, J. (1965). *Odontologisk Revy* **16**, 327.

274 A. K. ADATIA

KRASSE, B. (1970). *In* "Dental Plaque" (W. D. McHugh, ed.), p. 199. Livingstone, Edinburgh and London.
LARJE, O. and LARSON, R. H. (1970). *Archives of Oral Biology* 15, 805.
LARMAS, M. and SCHEININ, A. (1967). *Journal of Periodontal Research* 2, 245.
LARSON, R. H. (1966). *In* "Environmental Variables in Oral Disease" (S. J. Kreshover and F. J. McClure, eds), p. 89. American Association for Advancement of Science, Washington, D.C.
LARSON, R. H. and FITZGERALD, R. J. (1964). *Archives of Oral Biology* 9, 705.
LARSON, R. H. and KEYES, P. H. (1967). *Helvetica odontologica acta* 11, 36.
LARSON, R. H., KEYES, P. H. and GOSS, B. J. (1968). *Journal of Dental Research* 47, 704.
LARSON, R. H., CLEMMER, B. and SCHERP, H. W. (1972). *Archives of Oral Biology* 17, 883.
LAVELLE, C. L. B. and MOORE, W. J. (1969). *Journal of Periodontal Research* 4, 70.
LAWRENCE, J. D. M. (1958). *Journal of the Canadian Dental Association* 24, 716.
LEACH, S. A., GREEN, R. M., HAYES, M. L. and DADA, O. A. (1969). *Journal of Dental Research* 48, 811.
LEHNER, T., WILTON, J. M. A. and WARD, R. G. (1970). *Archives of Oral Biology* 15, 481.
LEIGH, R. W. (1929). *Dental Cosmos* 71, 756, 878.
LILIENTHAL, B., AMERENA, V. and GREGORY, G. (1965). *Archives of Oral Biology* 10, 553.
LINDHE, J. and WICEN, P. (1969). *Journal of Periodontal Research* 4, 193.
LISTGARTEN, M. A. and ELLEGAARD, B. (1972). *Journal of Periodontal Research, Supplement* 10, 13.
LÖE, H. (1970). *In* "Dental Plaque" (W. D. McHugh, ed.), p. 259. Livingstone, Edinburgh and London.
LOESCHE, W. (1968). *Journal of Periodontology* 39, 45.
LOESCHE, W. J. and SYED, S. A. (1973). *Caries Research* 7, 201.
LOESCHE, W. J., HOCKETT, R. N. and SYED, S. A. (1972). *Archives of Oral Biology* 17, 1311.
LONGHURST, P. and BERMAN, D. S. (1973). *British Dental Journal* 134, 475.
LUNT, D. A. (1972). *British Dental Journal* 132, 443.
LUOMA, H., ANTONIADES, K., TURTOLA, L. O. and KUOKKA, I. M. A. (1970). *Caries Research* 4, 332.
LUOMA, H., TURTOLA, L., COLLAN, Y., MEURMAN, J. and HELMINEN, S. (1972). *Caries Research* 6, 183.
MADSEN, K. O. and EDMUNDS, E. J. (1963). *Journal of Dental Research* 42, 137.
MAGRILL, D. S. (1973). *Archives of Oral Biology* 18, 591.
MÄKINEN, K. K. (1972). *International Dental Journal* 22, 363.
MANN, A. W., DREIZEN, S., SPIES, T. D. and HUNT, F. M. (1947). *Journal of the American Dental Association* 34, 244.
MANSBRIDGE, J. N. (1959a). *Archives of Oral Biology* 1, 241.
MANSBRIDGE, J. N. (1959b). *Journal of Dental Research* 38, 337.
MANSBRIDGE, J. N. (1960). *British Dental Journal* 109, 343.
MARSHALL-DAY, C. D. (1944). *British Dental Journal* 76, 115.

MARTHALER, T. M. (1967). *Caries Research* **1**, 222.
MARTHALER, T. M. (1972). *Helvetica odontologica acta* **16**, (a) 45; (b) 69.
McCANCE, R. A., PRIOR, K. M. and WIDDOWSON, E. M. (1953). *British Journal of Nutrition* **7**, 98.
McCLURE, F. J. (1963). *Journal of Dental Research* **42**, 693.
McHUGH, W. D. (1970) (ed.). "Dental Plaque." Livingstone, Edinburgh and London.
MELLANBY, M. (1923). *British Dental Journal* **44**, 1.
MELLANBY, M. (1927). *British Dental Journal* **48**, 1481.
MILES, A. E. W. (1969). *Proceedings of the Royal Society of Medicine* **62**, 1311.
MILLER, W. D. (1890). "Micro-Organisms of the Human Mouth." The S. S. White Dental Manufacturing Co., Philadelphia.
MITCHELL, D. F. (1950). *Journal of Dental Research* **29**, 732.
MØLLER, I. J., PINDBORG, J. J. and ROED-PETERSEN, B. (1972). *Archives of Oral Biology* **17**, 9.
MOORE, W. J. and CORBETT, M. E. (1971). *Caries Research* **5**, 151.
MOORE, W. J., LAVELLE, C. L. B. and SPENCE, T. F. (1968). *Journal of Anatomy* **102**, 573.
MÜHLEMANN, H. R. and DE BOEVER, J. (1970). *In* "Dental Plaque" (W. D. McHugh, ed.), p. 179. Livingstone, Edinburgh and London.
MUMMERY, J. R. (1869). *Transactions of the Odontological Society of Great Britain* **2**, 7.
MURPHY, T. R. (1964). *British Dental Journal* **116**, 483.
NEUMANN, H. H. (1950). *British Dental Journal* **88**, 58.
NEUMANN, H. H. (1955). *Journal of Dental Research* **34**, 715.
NEUMANN, H. H. and DiSALVO, N. A. (1957). *Journal of Dental Research* **36**, 286
NEUMANN, H. H. and DiSALVO, N. A. (1958). *British Dental Journal* **104**, 13.
NEUMANN, H. H., LEFKOWITZ, W. and DiSALVO, N. A. (1952). *Journal of Dental Research* **31**, 200.
NIKIFORUK, G. (1970). *Journal of Dental Research* **49**, 1252.
NISENGARD, R. J. and BEUTNER, E. H. (1970). *Journal of Periodontology* **41**, 149.
O'ROURKE, T. T. (1947). *American Journal of Orthodontics and Oral Surgery* **33**, 687.
OSBORN, T. W. B., NORISKIN, J. N. and STAZ, J. (1937). *Journal of Dental Research* **16**, 165.
PARFITT, G. J. (1959). *Archives of Oral Biology* **1**, 193.
PARKER, R. B. and CREAMER, H. R. (1971). *Archives of Oral Biology* **16**, 855.
PEDERSEN, P. O. (1947). *Proceedings of the Royal Society of Medicine* **40**, 726.
PELZER, R. H. (1940). *Journal of the American Dental Association* **27**, 13.
POOLE, D. F. G. and NEWMAN, H. N. (1971). *Nature* **234**, 329.
POOLE, D. F. G. and SILVERSTONE, L. M. (1973). *In* "Hard Tissue Growth, Repair and Remineralization—Ciba Foundation Symposium 11 (New Series)", p. 35. ASP (Elsevier), Amsterdam.
POULSEN, S., MØLLER, I. J., NAERUM, J. and PEDERSEN, P. O. (1972). *Archives of Oral Biology* **17**, 1165.
RABKIN, S. (1942). *Journal of Dental Research* **21**, 211.
RABKIN, S. (1943). *Journal of Dental Research* **22**, 355.

REECE, J. A. and SWALLOW, J. N. (1970). *British Dental Journal* **128**, 535.
RETIEF, D. H., CLEATON-JONES, P. E. and WALKER, A. R. P. (1973). *Lancet* **2**, 1456.
RIZZO, A. A. (1970). *Journal of Periodontology* **41**, 210.
ROVIN, S., COSTICH, E. R. and GORDON, H. A. (1966). *Journal of Periodontal Research* **1**, 193.
RUGG-GUNN, A. J. (1968). *British Dental Journal* **124**, 75.
RUSSELL, A. L. (1957). *Journal of Periodontology* **28**, 286.
RUSSELL, A. L. (1963). *Journal of Dental Research* **42**, 233.
RUSSELL, A. L. (1966). *In* "Environmental Variables in Oral Disease" (S. J. Kreshover and F. J. McClure, eds), p. 21. American Association for Advancement of Science, Washington, D.C.
RUSSELL, A. L., CONSOLAZIO, C. F. and WHITE, C. L. (1961). *Journal of Dental Research* **40**, (a) 594; (b) 604.
SAMPSON, W. E. A. (1932). *British Dental Journal* **53**, 397.
SCHROEDER, H. E. (1970). *Archives of Oral Biology* **15**, 383.
SCHROEDER, H. E. and DE BOEVER, J. (1970). *In* "Dental Plaque" (W. D. McHugh, ed.), p. 49. Livingstone, Edinburgh and London.
SCHWARTZ, J. (1946). *Journal of Dental Research* **25**, 17.
SHAFER, W. G., HINE, M. K. and LEVY, B. M. (1967). "Textbook of Oral Pathology", p. 50. W. B. Saunders, Philadelphia and London.
SHANNON, I. L., CARROLL, E. C. and MADSEN, K. O. (1970). *Journal of Periodontal Research* **5**, 191.
SHAW, J. H. (1970). *Journal of Dental Research* **49**, 1238.
SHAW, J. H. and IVIMEY, J. K. (1972). *Journal of Dental Research* **51**, 1507.
SHEIHAM, A. (1969). *British Dental Journal* **126**, 115.
SHEIHAM, A. (1970). *British Dental Journal* **129**, 413.
SHIEHAM, A. and HOBDELL, M. H. (1969). *British Dental Journal* **126**, 401.
SKOUGAARD, M. R., PINDBORG, J. J. and ROED-PETERSEN, B. (1969). *Archives of Oral Biology* **14**, 707.
SLACK, G. L. and MARTIN, W. J. (1958). *British Dental Journal* **105**, 366.
SOCRANSKY, S. S., GIBBONS, R. J., DALE, A. C., BORTNICK, L., ROSENTHAL, E. and MACDONALD, J. B. (1963). *Archives of Oral Biology* **8**, 275.
SPEIRS, R. L. (1967). *Caries Research* **1**, 15.
STAHL, S. S. (1970). *Journal of Dental Research* **49**, 248.
STEPHAN, R. M. (1940). *Journal of the American Dental Association* **27**, 718.
STEPHEN, K. W. and SUTHERLAND, D. A. (1971). *British Dental Journal* **130**, 19.
SUSSMAN, H. J., BARTELS, H. A. and STAHL, S. S. (1969). *Journal of Periodontology* **40**, 210.
THEILADE, E., WRIGHT, W. H., JENSEN, S. B. and LÖE, H. (1966). *Journal of Periodontal Research* **1**, 1.
TIMMIS, J. C. (1971). *British Dental Journal* **130**, 278.
TÖTH, K. (1970). "The Epidemiology of Dental Caries in Hungary." Akademiai Kiado, Budapest.
VON DER FEHR, F. R., LÖE, H. and THEILADE, E. (1970). *Caries Research* **4**, 131.
WADE, A. B. (1971). *Dental Practitioner and Dental Record, Bristol* **21**, 194.

WAERHAUG, J. (1971). *In* "The Prevention of Periodontal Disease" (J. E. Eastoe, D. C. A. Picton and A. G. Alexander, eds), p. 1. Henry Kimpton, London.

WALKER, A. R. P. (1973). *South African Medical Journal* **47**, 1695.

WALLACE, J. S. (1900). "The Cause and Prevention of Decay in Teeth." Churchill, London.

WALTER, J. B. and ISRAEL, M. S. (1970). "General Pathology", p. 264. Churchill, London.

WEGNER, H. (1971). *Caries Research* **5**, 188.

WEISS, R., STAHL, S. S. and TONNA, E. A. (1969). *Journal of Periodontal Research* **4**, 296.

WELBOURN, H. F. (1956). *East African Medical Journal* **33**, 181.

WINTER, G. B. (1968). *British Dental Journal* **124**, 407.

WINTER, G. B., RULE, D. C., MAILER, G. P., JAMES, P. M. C. and GORDON, P. H. (1971). *British Dental Journal* **130**, 271. 434.

ZAKI, H. A. and STALLARD, R. E. (1969). *Journal of Periodontal Research, Supplement* **3**, 5.

Part VII

Chapter 18

Duodenal ulcer and diet

FRANK TOVEY

I. Introduction 279
   A. Differences between gastric and duodenal ulcers . . . 279
   B. Possible influence of refined carbohydrate foods . . . 280
   C. Varying reliability of epidemiological data 281
II. Duodenal ulcer in western countries 282
   A. Prevalence in Europe 282
   B. Prevalence in North America 284
   C. Complications 284
III. Duodenal ulcer in the Indian sub-continent 285
   A. Present distribution related to diet 286
   B. Characteristics of duodenal ulcer 289
IV. Duodenal ulcer in Africa 291
   A. Staple diets in different regions 291
   B. Earlier records 292
   C. Prevalence related to diet 293
   D. Autopsy evidence from Uganda 298
V. Possible causative factors 299
   A. Hookworms 300
   B. Stress 301
   C. Food flavourings and mastication 301
   D. Refined carbohydrate foods 302
VI. Possible protective factors. 304
VII. Conclusions 305
References 306

I. Introduction

A. Differences between gastric and duodenal ulcers

In Britain gastric ulcer commonly affected women during the nineteenth century. It began to increase in men about 1920, becoming more frequent in men than in women. The incidence increased until 1930 and thereafter it remained stationary, and has declined in recent years. It is now commonest in men over 50 years of age (Jennings, 1940; Avery Jones, 1947). Gastric ulcer is associated with chronic gastritis and usually with hyposecretion; it is possibly related to bile reflux, sometimes to gastric stasis and to dietetic or non-dietetic agents which have not yet been clearly identified. It would be difficult to correlate the rise, and even more so the fall, in gastric ulcer prevalence in Britain with the rise in the consumption of sugar and refined flour during the past century.

Increasingly gastric and duodenal ulcers are recognized as two distinct but related diseases. In the western world these two diseases differ in sex, age, social class, occupation, genetic inheritance factors, relationship to the blood groups, as well as prevalence in terms of history and geography. The causative factors, which are multiple, must therefore differ in many respects.

Duodenal ulcer is associated with hypersecretion of gastric juice, and there are probably dietetic or non-dietetic environmental agents which most workers think have not yet been identified. These agents might lower the resistance of the duodenal mucosa or alter gastric secretion or mucus formation; they might protect against ulceration.

The discussion will now be limited to duodenal ulcer, as this will simplify the presentation of complicated data, although sometimes it is interesting to show comparative figures for gastric ulcer.

This study discusses the prevalence of duodenal ulcer in the western world. It then considers in some detail the position in India, where the author (F. T.) had 16 years' surgical experience and gathered information from the whole country, especially mission hospitals in South India; it also discusses the prevalence in Africa south of the Sahara, where one editor (H. T.) had 30 years' experience and the other (D. B.) had 20 years' experience. Denis Burkitt has subsequently made frequent visits to many countries in Africa and Asia, and has received completed monthly questionnaires during 1971–74 sent to over 140 hospitals. The author and D. B. have recently made a tour of the West Coast of Africa and have collected further information from 49 hospitals and medical institutions.

B. Possible influence of refined carbohydrate foods

During the period 1870–1920 changes occurred in the consumption of the refined carbohydrates, flour and sugar. Since ischaemic heart disease and diverticular disease began to be recognized as common clinical problems in western countries in 1920, at the same time as duodenal ulcer became common, the prevalence of duodenal ulcer will be discussed in relation to changes in diet, especially those of the carbohydrate foods, both in Britain and in other countries. Wastell (1972a) stated that "low-residue refined civilized diets might possibly have contributed to the world-wide increase in duodenal ulcer in this century". It is not clear from this statement whether refined starchy foods and sugar alone were under suspicion, or whether refined fats, which have little residue and have been consumed in increased amounts in the present century, were also considered.

Cleave (1962, 1974; Cleave *et al.* 1969) propounded a hypothesis that the prime cause of peptic ulcer was the consumption of refined carbohydrate foods. He based his argument on the following points: (1) peptic ulcer occurs only in the presence of hydrochloric acid; (2) this acid is normally buffered, he considered, by protein; (3) the refining of starchy food has reduced the protein, and sugar has no protein; (4) these protein-stripped foods do not buffer the hydrochloric acid to the same extent as unrefined foods, so that the rise in gastric acidity occurs more rapidly. Cleave produced epidemiological evidence to support this hypothesis: firstly the apparent rarity of peptic ulcer among underdeveloped countries wherein unrefined carbohydrate foods were eaten; secondly the disappearance of peptic ulcers in prisoners-of-war when they ate unrefined carbohydrate foods.

C. *Varying reliability of epidemiological data*

Any hypothesis which concerns the pathogenesis of duodenal ulcer and rests on epidemiological data should recognize the possible inaccuracy and incompleteness of such data. Faced with these uncertainties, three attitudes are possible. There are those who point to all the sources of unreliability and selectivity of data so that they find it impossible to suggest any hypothesis (Pflanz, 1971). At the other extreme there are those who select data to support a particular hypothesis. The present study endeavours to follow a middle course; while admitting that all epidemiological data are subject to error, it considers there is overwhelming evidence that the prevalence of duodenal ulcer varies considerably in various parts of India and Africa and that more detailed prospective studies in chosen areas where considerable variation occurs may throw light on aetiological factors. Such studies should be primarily concerned with the incidence (number of new cases appearing during a stated period of time) and prevalence of the disease (total number of persons who have an active duodenal ulcer, or even a healed scar, at a certain time).

Mortality data offer very limited information about the prevalence of duodenal ulcer even in advanced countries, still less in developing areas of India and Africa because the disease is seldom fatal, apart from the complications of haemorrhage and perforation, both of which are considered to be less frequent in the stenosing type of duodenal ulcer encountered in tropical areas. Prevalence surveys of duodenal ulcer of any population are seldom attempted and are rarely combined with a clinical and radiological examination.

There is considerable evidence that a fair proportion of duodenal ulcers remain undetected even by the most painstaking combined examination, but can be found incidentally at operation, during endoscopy, or at autopsy. Some ulcers apparently produce no symptoms or detectable signs.

It might be assumed that necropsy records would settle the question of the prevalence of duodenal ulcer, but even in advanced countries there have been few necropsy studies offering reliable data. Ideally such data would be obtained by a carefully planned prospective study of the autopsy incidence of duodenal ulcer including both active ulcers and scars in a series of more than 1000 autopsies, age and sex being recorded in each case (Ivy *et al.*, 1950a). No necropsy series in the tropics conforms to these stipulations. Only one series of 876 autopsies in Uganda attempted to be a prospective study of the prevalence of gastric and duodenal ulcers among three African tribal groupings (Raper, 1958). It found a 3-fold increase in one group of tribes compared with another group and is discussed in detail on p. 298.

Hospital statistics—surgical, medical and radiological—are therefore almost the only indices of prevalence in most parts of India and Africa. But since men may come more easily to hospital than women, and the hospital may draw more patients from one area than another, the M : F ratio of diagnosed cases shown may not convey an accurate picture of sex incidence, nor the true local situation. Hospital statistics may be further selective in that they depend to some extent on the skill of the doctor, his ability to speak fluently with the patient and the diagnostic facilities. Thus the characteristics of duodenal ulcer rather than accurate statistics may be revealed. Many of the epidemiological data collected by the author and D. B. have come from rural hospitals of India and Africa. The picture in the larger towns is in many respects different.

II. Duodenal ulcer in western countries

A. Prevalence in Europe

Autopsy material in Europe suggests that duodenal ulcer was a rare disease until the turn of the century. In London, during the nineteenth century, two large autopsy surveys were performed specifically to determine the incidence of gastric and duodenal ulcer, whether active or healed. These showed an incidence of 0·4% duodenal ulcer (ulcers and scars) in 17,652 autopsies during 1826–92 (Perry and Shaw, 1893) and at the end of the century 0·26% in 13,055 autopsies (Fenwick and Fenwick, 1900). A comprehensive review of the incidence of active duodenal ulcer at autopsy in many European countries stated that three periods should be considered: (1) before 1900 when the incidence varied from 0·1 to 0·3%; (2) about 1900 when the incidence was 1·0%; (3) after 1913 when the incidence was 2·2–3·9%, increases which were considered to be real and not apparent (Ivy et al., 1950b). This review included autopsy data from Denmark which showed that between 1907 and 1936 the incidence of duodenal ulcer increased 5-fold in men in the age-group 20–29 years, 4-fold in the age-group 30–39 years, 3-fold in those aged 40–49 years and 2-fold in those aged 50–59 years (Ivy et al., 1950c).

In Britain, and most of northern and western Europe except France, the incidence of duodenal ulcer, whether assessed by careful population surveys or by prospective necropsy studies, has been well established in recent decades. Watkinson (1960) concluded, as a result of extensive autopsy experience at Leeds, that "the best estimate of the incidence of

TABLE 18.1. Percentage estimates of duodenal ulcer frequencies in men based on population surveys in London and York and the number of active ulcers found incidentally at necropsy in Leeds after deaths from ulcer had been excluded (Watkinson, 1961)

Age-group (years)	Population survey	Necropsy
–25	0·9	0·5
25–	1·9	2·5
35–	2·0	2·5
45–	3·2	3·8
55–	3·8	3·2
65–	2·9	3·4

ulcer in the population as a whole can be made from the frequency of ulcers found in patients dying from causes other than peptic ulcer". This approach was made to counter the criticism of earlier studies which had suggested that an undue number of patients suffering from peptic ulcer might have been attracted to the hospital for treatment and some subsequently died there. Watkinson (1961) therefore compared this data from the large necropsy series in Leeds with results obtained in the London occupation surveys of Doll et al. (1951), and in York by Pulvertaft (1959, 1968) (Table 18.1). Prevalence was found to rise during adult life until about 45 years and then to remain stationary. The rise in prevalence throughout adult life stresses the importance of recording prevalence in different age and sex groups. This has not always been done in reports from India and Africa. Doll et al. (1951) and Pulvertaft (1959) found a lower incidence of duodenal ulcer in rural than in urban populations. In the York series this difference was less in 1959 than in 1953 and had disappeared by 1968 (Pulvertaft, 1959, 1968). In the United Kingdom and North America the prevalence is higher among managers and foremen in industry than it is among lower-grade workers (Dunn and Cobb, 1962). In the 1930s duodenal ulcer was predominantly a disease of the moderately affluent, but now, like gastric ulcer, it predominantly affects the poor (Langman, 1974).

To summarize, duodenal ulcer was apparently a rare condition in Britain until about 1920; it became classifiable as a separate disease by the Registrar-General in 1921. Duodenal ulcer is commoner in the north of England and Scotland than in the southern part of England. Its prevalence increased until about 1955, since when this has steadily declined in men but has remained almost stationary in women. The sex ratio, men to women, has therefore fallen from 4·5 : 1 in 1938 to 1·9 : 1 in 1970 (Wastell, 1972b).

The ratio of duodenal ulcer to gastric ulcer has also changed. In the 1950s it was between 3 : 1 and 4 : 1 but has decreased to between 2 : 1 and 3 : 1 at the present time (Doll, 1952; Pulvertaft, 1968; Langman, 1973, 1974).

B. Prevalence in North America

The same pattern of increased incidence of duodenal ulcer probably occurred in the United States (Susser, 1967). There is, however, no direct evidence from U.S.A. autopsies concerning the prevalence of duodenal ulcer during the last century. Presumably the incidence was low, for very few duodenal ulcers were reported among 85,126 *post mortems* around the turn of the century (Ivy *et al.*, 1950b). Hospital admissions, a less satisfactory source of evidence for prevalence, indicate that duodenal ulcer was practically unknown in the American armed forces during their service in the First World War (Dunn, 1942), but was a major cause of disability in the Second World War, in both white and coloured (Boles, 1942), among whom the incidence was equal. Prior to 1936 peptic ulcer was rare in the negroes of North America (Maes and McFetbridge, 1936), but thereafter the incidence rose (Portio and Jaffe, 1938) and after 1940 the prevalence was the same as in the white population (Boland, 1942; Kirschner, 1944; U.S. Public Health Service, 1947).

C. Complications

1. Haemorrhage

In the western world haemorrhage is the commonest severe complication. About 25% of hospital admissions for peptic ulcer patients are for manifest haemorrhage. Clinical experience suggests that about 25% of peptic ulcers bleed at some time; some 7·5% of bleeding ulcers prove fatal and 1·6% of patients with peptic ulcer die from haemorrhage. It is probable that 90% of ulcer patients, provided they live for 40 years after the onset of the disease, would develop at least one haemorrhage. The frequency of haemorrhage, which increases with age, is almost similar in the sexes. Many more patients suffer from duodenal than gastric ulcer, but the frequency of manifest haemorrhage in each is comparable (Ivy *et al.*, 1950d).

2. Perforation

In the western world perforation is the second commonest complication. Its incidence has been assessed at 3–13%. Duodenal ulcers are more prone to perforate than gastric ulcers. Perforation is commonest in those aged 20–40 years and occurs more frequently in men than in women. The ratio of perforating ulcer in men and women has, however, fallen from 19 : 1 in 1928 to 5 : 1 in 1967 (Wastell, 1972c). Before 1950 in the U.S.A. perforations accounted for 13·2% of hospital admissions for peptic ulcer (Ivy *et al.*, 1950e) and in the York series up to 1959 it occurred in 11% of cases of chronic ulcer (Pulvertaft, 1959). The incidence in the United Kingdom has fallen in the last 15 years (MacKay, 1966; Sanders, 1967; I. E. Gillespie, p.c. 1970; Hospital In-Patient Enquiry for England and Wales, 1956–61.)

3. Pyloric stenosis

From hospital admission figures in the United States the incidence of some degree of stenosis has been reported as 14·6% (Emery and Monroe, Boston, 1935); 7% (Haubrick, Detroit, 1963 (period 1950–59)) and 10·5% (Kozoll and Meyer, Chicago, 1964 (period 1936–55)). Pyloric stenosis is now uncommon in the United Kindgom; the author saw only three severe and four mild cases in the last 150 cases of DU referred for a surgical opinion (4·7%) and his radiological colleague, Dr J. Parker, saw only seven cases (three marked, four moderate) in 138 barium meals positive for duodenal ulcer in a period of 12 months. Pyloric stenosis in these countries is, moreover, a late complication. Ellis (1972) reported a maximum incidence in the period 10–19 years after the onset of symptoms.

III. Duodenal ulcer in the Indian sub-continent

Duodenal ulcer as known in rural India (and Africa) presents certain unusual features. Because of the frequency of pyloric stenosis it has been called the "stenosing-type" duodenal ulcer to distinguish it from the standard "western-type" duodenal ulcer. The "stenosing-type" ulcer shows other differences such as in the sex ratio, the ratio of duodenal to gastric ulcer, the peak age incidence and the relative rarity of perforation and haemorrhage.

A. Present distribution related to diet

It is impossible to describe accurately and briefly the prevalence of duodenal ulcer, or the diet of a sub-continent as vast as India, Pakistan and Bangladesh. There are many different ethnic and social groups, and big differences between urban communities, where living conditions increasingly approximate to those of the western world, and the rural communities where life and diet still follow a traditional pattern. The staple carbohydrate foods are rice in the moister lands of the south and the east and wheat in the drier regions of the north-west. There are other carbohydrate foods such as cassava in the south and millet and leguminous seeds in the northern, western and central areas.

The traditional light stone-milling of rice has now given place to machine-milling, in villages as well as in towns. This, coupled with the additional polishing it now receives, very much reduces the fibre content of the rice.

In the rural wheat-growing areas of Rajasthan and the Punjab the wheat is used as stone-ground wholemeal flour to make chupatties. In the towns there is a tendency to use more white flour. Thus the pattern of diet emerging among the upper classes and townspeople is increasingly that of refined white polished rice in the southern and eastern areas, and of white wheat bread in the north, and much overlap in other regions. The consumption of fat, milk and protein, especially that of animal origin, is low except among certain advanced social groups; and it should be remembered that Hindus are vegetarian. Sugar intakes are, on average, still low by western standards, but rising, especially in the urban areas and among more sophisticated social groups. Spices and condiments are much in favour. The consumption of vegetables is variable and may be seasonal; that of fruit tends to be low. Vegetables tend to be cooked more in the south than in the north. Smoking is much commoner in the Punjab in North India than in the south.

Autopsy data from India are extremely scanty; no prospective study of duodenal ulcers has been traced in recent decades. For what it is worth, autopsy data at the beginning of the present century would suggest that duodenal ulcer was rare in Calcutta where Rogers (1914) reported 0·4% among 1000 autopsies, rising to 0·9% among 1600 autopsies in 1925

(Rogers, 1925). This equates with experience in the western world. No autopsy records of recent years have been traced. In any case, autopsy records in India of necessity are highly selective since some religions oppose *post mortem* examination.

It is abundantly clear from the hospital records of admissions, surgical

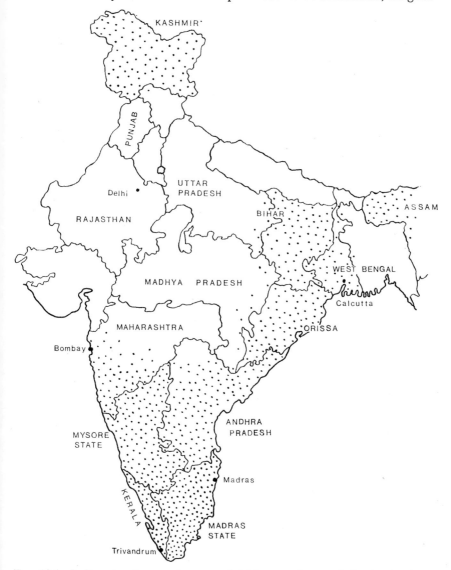

FIG. 18.1. India, showing rural areas of high prevalence of duodenal ulcer, stenosing-type. All large towns report high prevalence of duodenal ulcer, western-type.

operations and radiological examinations that duodenal ulcer is a major clinical problem in many parts of India, but not apparently in all (Fig. 18.1). This is especially true of many rural areas, where duodenal ulcer is very commonly diagnosed in some parts but infrequently in others, and a large proportion of these are of the stenosing type. (In towns duodenal ulcers of the standard western type appear to be common, although a few of the stenosing type occur.)

The areas of apparent high clinical incidence include the whole of southern India (provinces of Kerala, Mysore and Madras), also the Deccan and the provinces of Bombay, Hyderabad, Orissa, Bihar, the rice-eating areas of Kashmir, West Bengal and parts of Assam, likewise Bangladesh; taken as a whole, these are the rice-eating areas of the monsoon rainbelt. On the other hand the areas of apparent low clinical incidence, assessed in terms of hospital admissions and operations for duodenal ulcer, include most of northern India (Rajasthan and the Punjab) and some parts of Kashmir; these correspond to the areas where unrefined wheat forms the staple diet. These statements are supported by numerous references in the Indian Council of Medical Research Report No. 39 (1959). It is impossible to cite all the other references, but the following have been selected: Somervell and Orr (1936), Somervell (1942), Dogra (1940, 1941), Bradfield (1927), Hadley (1958, 1959), Chatterjee et al. (1959), Raghavan (1962, 1966), Malhotra (1964, 1967), Malhotra et al. (1964), Rao (1938), Orr and Rao (1939), McCarrison (1944), Varma (1969), Tovey (1962, 1972a), Chuttani et al. (1967), Goyal and Gupta (1966). The statements are confirmed by personal enquiries and visits to many parts of India (F. T. and D. B.).

These communications stem largely from the most experienced workers in the field, many of whom have had personal experience in several areas in India; some having worked both in areas of high incidence and of low incidence. Further, the literature on the subject is most consistent. There appears to be general agreement about the facts, bearing in mind the differences that are alleged to occur between certain rural areas, especially those of apparently low incidence, and the towns.

Dogra (1940) considered that duodenal ulcer was 15 times commoner in southern India than in the northern area already mentioned, and his was a conservative estimate compared to others (Somervell and Orr, 1936; McCarrison, 1944).

Only a few prospective population surveys have been done, but these have served to emphasize that local unexplained wide variations occur, not only between these two large areas of the north and the south of the Indian sub-continent, and not only between towns and adjoining rural areas, but also between one rural area and another. The findings of population surveys in the large cities of Delhi and Chandigarh (Chuttani et al.,

1967; Sehgal *et al.*, 1971), and in the rural areas around Chandigarh in northern India and around the town of Vellore in southern India (Benjamin and Nariewala, 1964; Plaha *et al.*, 1967) surprised the investigators, for these emphasized the problems of merely contrasting north and south India and rural and urban areas.

More prospective population studies with standardized procedures are required, especially in areas of apparently low clinical incidence. It is extremely important to establish the comparative rarity of duodenal ulcer and the concomitant diet and pattern of life before the disease becomes more frequent in these areas, as has happened elsewhere in the present century. Although it may sound paradoxical it is much more important to identify areas of proven low incidence than to study areas of high incidence.

B. *Characteristics of duodenal ulcer*

In almost all the regions of India, Pakistan and Bangladesh where peptic ulcer has been reported to have been, and still remains, a common clinical condition, surgical, radiological and medical opinion is unanimous that it is the high frequency of duodenal ulcer that dominates the scene. In 18 recently reported Indian series the average ratio of DU : GU was 19 : 1 (range 5–32 : 1). This should be compared to the ratio in America and Europe of DU : GU which is at present between 2 : 1 and 3 : 1. It is impossible to say from the Indian data whether the prevalence of duodenal ulcer has changed more than that of gastric ulcer, but it would appear likely that duodenal ulcer prevalence has increased considerably, whereas that of gastric ulcer has remained stationary or even declined. (If the Indian data concerning prevalence of all forms of peptic ulcer are correct and peptic ulcer was in fact rare in the nineteenth century, this poses an epidemiological problem of considerable magnitude. Since duodenal ulcer is common in many rural areas where the diets and the manner of life have altered least during the present century, this increases the difficulties of interpretation.)

The peak age incidence of duodenal ulcer in India occurs in men aged 30–40 years; this is a decade earlier than that encountered in the western world. Duodenal ulcer in India is much commoner in men than in women; in 11 recently reported series the sex ratio men : women was 17·6 : 1 (range 9–33 : 1). Although some reports do not mention the sex ratio for admissions of other diseases, nor the proportion of hospital beds allocated to each sex (and in many hospitals far fewer sick women attend hospital), there is sufficient information to show that in India the sex ratio of duodenal ulcer differs markedly from that of M1·9 : F1 currently prevailing in the western world, although in 1940 the sex ratio in the U.S.A. and Britain was 4·6 : 1 (Wastell, 1972b). In India duodenal ulcer is predominantly a disease of poor coolie labourers and peasants in rural areas, who often take only one meal a day. Yet these people consume much less of the refined carbohydrate foods than do other sections of the community.

There is widespread agreement in India, Bangladesh and Pakistan that in rural areas duodenal ulcer is often accompanied by severe fibrosis leading at an early stage to stenosis. The ulcer occurs most commonly on the posterior and superior aspects of the first part of the duodenum. When deep, it invades the pancreas. It is accompanied by much fibrosis around the ulcer, so that a tumour-like mass may be found at operation and stenosis often dominates the clinical picture. This stenosis may occur at an early stage of the disease, even during the first 4 years of symptoms; it does not appear to be due to a failure to obtain treatment of a long-standing ulcer (Somervell, 1942; Tovey, 1962, 1972a).

The incidence of stenosis in India has been assessed by many different surgeons at rates which vary from 24% (Tovey, 1962) to 68·5% (Varma, 1969). This should be compared with the figures from the western world.

In India surgeons are unanimous in their view that the severe complications of perforation and haemorrhage are seldom seen in the wards or operating theatre of rural hospitals in patients who display other features of the stenosing-type of duodenal ulcer (Somervell and Orr, 1936; Dogra, 1941; Gregg, 1959; Raghavachari, 1959; Rao, 1959). Somervell and Orr (1936) in Kerala province diagnosed only four cases of perforation among 2500 duodenal ulcer operations. During 16 years' surgical practice in Mysore the author diagnosed only eight perforations (1·4% of total cases) and encountered only seven haematemeses (3% of total cases).

In the larger cities of India it is considered that duodenal and gastric ulcers present all the features seen in the western world, although some cases develop stenosis from severe fibrosis. In these urban areas duodenal ulcer is not a disease predominantly of the poorer classes but of the middle and upper classes. Other features such as the sex ratio and age of peak incidence resemble the western-type ulcer. Haemorrhage is a frequent complication; it occurred in 11·2% of a hospital series in Madras (Varma, 1969) and in 25·9% of railway workers in Assam (Malhotra, 1964, 1967). Perforation too is more frequently encountered; it was noted in 25% of a hospital series in Bombay (Raghavan, 1962). Others confirm the frequency of bleeding in ulcer cases seen in city hospitals of India. In these cities recent studies indicate an increased proportion of gastric ulcer compared to duodenal ulcer, so that the DU : GU ratio is now levelling and approximating to that seen in the western world (Sen, 1945; Raghavan, 1962; Garlick and Sundar Rao, 1971).

IV. Duodenal ulcer in Africa

Discussion will be limited to duodenal ulcer among the indigenous Africans who live south of the Sahara. All reference to other ethnic groups, white South Africans and Rhodesians, Indians, coloured South Africans and Arabs will be excluded. There is considerable ethnic variation between the numerous African tribes, although certain groupings have been made, largely on a linguistic basis.

A. Staple diets in different regions

In Africa south of the Sahara rural areas predominate and, until fairly recently, urban areas were unknown except for certain cities of West Africa and the Arab towns scattered along the eastern seaboard. In sub-Saharal Africa the majority of Africans live as peasants scattered throughout the countryside; they grow their own food and consume a large amount of various starchy foods (Chapter 3), which vary from one locality to another, and reflect varying conditions of climate, especially rainfall, and of soil fertility. The millets were the ancient traditional cereal of Africa, especially in the drier areas; they store well and are usually eaten as a type of porridge; if milled they are only lightly processed and still contain much fibre. Starchy roots, tubers and fruits, such as sweet potato, yams and plantains are grown, especially where rainfall is plentiful. Maize has become the dominant cereal in the drier areas of southern and east Africa; it is taken lightly milled and contains 2% of fibre. Rice, usually eaten as white polished rice, low in fibre, is grown in only a few areas of Africa, but may be eaten as the staple carbohydrate food by special groups, such as the Arabs, Indians and coastal groups of Africans in East and West Africa. It is also consumed by the higher social African groups throughout the continent. Wheat is grown in moderate amounts in the cooler and drier parts of southern and eastern Africa; more white bread is being eaten as a subsidiary food in all urban areas, especially by upper social groups. Cassava is grown often as a famine crop in the drier areas and on poor soils of most African countries.

A small amount of sugar cane was grown throughout tropical Africa; it was used in the preparation of alcoholic drink, and a small amount was chewed, the fibrous pith being spat out. Manufactured sugar is a new item of diet; only a modest amount of it is eaten in many rural areas of tropical Africa, where it may be used only to sweeten tea. Sugar consumption rises rapidly as soon as technological development occurs and towns grow up. Consumption is moderately high among South African Bantu; in 1970 it was assessed to average 65–75 g/day per person in their rural areas and 55–85 g/day per person in urban areas. White South Africans in the higher socio-economic groups then averaged 80–100 g/day per person and in the lower income groups 120–140 g/day per person. Indians in South Africa consumed 70–90 g/day per person (Walker *et al.*, 1971).

Except in a few pastoral tribes fat consumption is low throughout Africa, but it rises with sophistication and wealth, especially in urban areas. In West Africa and the Congo basin oil seeds and nuts contribute a fair amount of fat and palm oil to the diet. The consumption of protein, especially animal protein, tends to be low among poorer socio-economic groups. The intake of green leafy vegetables, which is seldom large, varies considerably from one area to another and from season to season, as does the method of cooking and preparation. Fruit is taken in variable amounts, but is usually very limited.

B. Earlier records

1. South and East Africa

Records from South and East Africa all indicated an apparent rarity of duodenal and gastric ulcers. Only eight peptic ulcers and two perforations were found in 8328 Bantu medico-legal *post mortems* in Johannesburg during 1928–37 (Eagle and Gillman, 1938). In this series the specific number of duodenal and gastric ulcers was not given. At about the same time only four patients among 18,000 Bantu hospital admissions in Johannesburg were diagnosed as peptic ulcer (Beyers, 1927). In East Africa Vint (1936–37), who performed 1000 hospital and medico-legal *post mortems*, found no active peptic ulcer; he searched his material well, for he recorded one healed gastric ulcer scar and three gastric carcinomata.

In some countries of eastern Africa surgeons recognized that duodenal ulcer, frequently associated with pyloric stenosis, might be common in certain areas, but apparently rare in others long before there were any radiological facilities. Brainbridge, the first surgical specialist in Kenya, worked there for 10 years before he operated on his first case of duodenal ulcer in an African, a male from Uganda, although he remembered having seen one perforation "some years ago" (Brainbridge and Trowell, 1933–34). F. J. Wright (p.c., 1972), who worked in Kenya from 1936 to 1954, recalls only one acute and one chronic ulcer amongst the unsophisticated rural population. Duodenal ulcer has become commoner in recent years in sophisticated Africans in Nairobi. Mowat (1934–35), the first surgical specialist in Uganda, considered duodenal ulcer to be at that time a relatively common complaint. In Zanzibar, Vassallo (1934–35) reported that peptic ulcer, especially duodenal ulcer, was common not only in Arabs but also in the Swahili and other indigenous African tribes. Enzer (1937–38) reported the infrequent occurrence of DU in Mombasa.

Bergsma (1931), a surgeon in Addis Ababa, Abyssinia, reported 200 cases of peptic ulcer in 2 years in a 70-bed hospital; many of these were stenosing duodenal ulcers. Surgeons in Burundi and Rwanda have reported a high frequency of duodenal ulcer in that region since 1933 (Goodchild, 1949; Ceuterick, 1955). Further studies in East Africa have entirely vindicated the view that the prevalence of duodenal ulcer was high in some rural areas and low in others.

2. West Africa

The picture in West Africa was very similar. Surgeons reported that duodenal ulcer, often of the stenosing type, was commonly encountered in the hospitals of the larger coastal towns of the West Coast, such as Lagos, Nigeria (Aitken, 1933). Before there were radiological facilities, in 6 years Ellis (1948) diagnosed and operated on 123 duodenal ulcers in that city, many of which were complicated by much fibrosis and stenosis. Three of these had perforated. There was only one gastric ulcer. The frequency of duodenal ulcer not only in the towns but also in the rural areas of the southern part of many West African countries was confirmed by later surgical experience (Konstam, 1954; Joly, 1956). The high frequency in the coastal belt of western Nigeria was emphasized by the fact that more abdominal operations were performed for stenosing duodenal ulcer than all other surgical abdominal conditions, excluding emergencies and gynaecological conditions (Konstam, 1966). This has been set out in some detail, to demonstrate that clinical workers, unaided by radiology, are able to recognize areas of high and low frequency.

C. Prevalence related to diet

An attempt will now be made to define *rural* areas with high and low prevalence of duodenal ulcer at the present time in Africans (Fig. 18.2). As will be discussed shortly, duodenal ulcer, often acute, and of the "western type", is commonly diagnosed in all the larger towns of tropical Africa. In the rural areas where the incidence is high, duodenal ulceration is of the "stenosing type" resembling that found in the high incidence rural areas of India. In studying the information available it has been borne in mind that patients from rural areas, lacking medical and surgical facilities, often travel to the nearest large town hospital and consequently appear in the hospital statistics of an urban area (Raper, 1958).

1. West Africa

One of the clearest zones of demarcation between areas of high and low clinical frequency of duodenal ulcer, often of the stenosing-type, is found in West Africa. The frequency is high in the hot humid coastal and rain forest zones of West Africa, wherein starchy roots, tubers and fruits are the main crops. Some 20 communications from West Africa testify to this frequency of ulcer in the southern region with its high rainfall, and to the apparent low frequency in the northern inland arid regions (savannah), where the diet is predominantly millet, sorghum, maize and groundnuts; Nigeria (Bohrer *et al.*, 1964; Lewis and Bohrer, 1970), Dahomey (Tournier-Lasserve *et al.*, 1961), Togoland (H. Gögler, p.c. 1973), Ghana (Badoe, 1972; E. Q. Achampong and A. van Enk, p.c. 1972), Ivory Coast (P. Wragg,

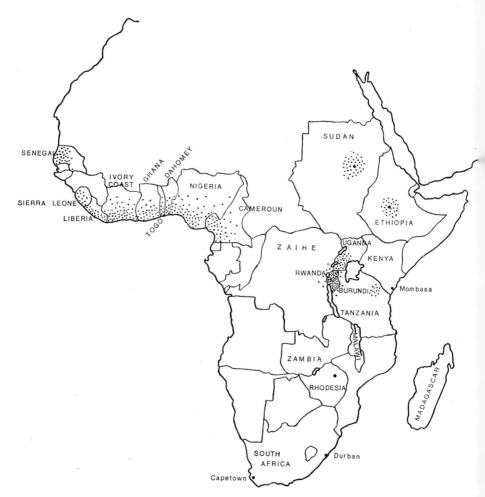

Fig. 18.2. Africa, showing rural areas of high prevalence of duodenal ulcer, stenosing-type. Many towns record rising prevalence of duodenal ulcer, western-type.

p.c. 1972), Senegal (Payet *et al.*, 1959; Cave *et al.*, 1963; Izarn, 1969; Chabal and Izarn, 1970); Sierra Leone (L. Wilkinson, p.c. 1973) and in South Cameroon (Touze, 1960). This pattern was confirmed during a recent visit by the author and D. B. to hospitals and medical institutions in Ghana, Ivory Coast, Liberia, Sierra Leone and Togoland. In addition to a low incidence in the northern savannah areas, a low incidence was also found in some of the coastal savannah areas, such as Adidome in Ghana and in the part of Senegal lying south of Gambia. A. van Enk (p.c., 1947) has recently visited all hospitals in Ghana and is of the opinion that duodenal ulcer is more common in the rain forest than in the coastal plains. He has also confirmed its rarity in the northern savannah regions. Although rare 20 years ago, duodenal ulcer is now being increasingly reported in large towns such as Zaria in the north of Nigeria; this is considered to be a true increase, not merely one of increased recognition (E. T. Mess and T. West, p.c. 1972). In the coastal belt chronic duodenal ulcer is predominantly a disease of the poorer male peasants. Stenosis is a prominent early feature; haemorrhage and perforation are less frequently encountered. The peak age is around 30. Gastric ulcer is uncommon.

2. *Nile–Congo watershed*

The most pronounced area of high clinical frequency of duodenal ulcer, often of the "stenosing type", appears to be centred on the fertile upland countries that constitute the watershed between the Nile and Congo rivers. Hamber and Bergen (1971, 1973) have reviewed the extensive African literature and traced the growth of knowledge since the first reports in 1933. Raper (1958), as will be discussed shortly, has confirmed the large number of duodenal ulcers found at autopsy in tribes from this region. Hospital records suggest that the highest admission rates for duodenal ulcer are towards the south in Burundi and that its prevalence may decrease northward to Rwanda and Uganda, and eastwards to Tanzania. The high prevalence area extends westward into the Congo basin. Frequency appears to decrease rapidly on entering the drier regions of northern Uganda which merge with the southern Sudan. It is also low in the highlands of Kenya and the drier central regions of Tanzania.

It would be unwise to regard the region of high prevalence as sharply defined, since this now appears to be more extensive than was previously estimated. In many rural hospitals in this area stenosing duodenal ulcer is the major surgical illness; thus at Matana, Burundi, in a 58-bedded hospital, 79% of the major operations were for peptic ulcer, mostly the stenosing duodenal variety, 780 such operations being performed in 10 years (G. Hamber, p.c. 1972). At Buye, a 72-bedded hospital, 404 peptic ulcer operations were done in a period of 2 years 8 months. Gastric ulcer is also seen, but the DU : GU ratio is 12 : 1. Males predominate. Compli-cations other than stenosis occur, perhaps more commonly than was previously considered. Hamber (p.c., 1972) reported six perforations (1%) but more haematemeses (15%) in 625 cases of peptic ulcer at Buye hospital. The prevalence of duodenal ulcer appears similar in the Nilohamitic Tutsi and the Bantu Hutu tribes who live in Burundi and Rwanda.

Duodenal ulcer is also very common among the Wachagga around Mount Kilimanjaro and other hilly, well watered areas of northern Tanzania (J. Taylor and F. Wright, p.c. 1972).

3. *Ethiopia*

The picture is incomplete, but there are reports from widely scattered areas of an apparently high prevalence of stenosing duodenal ulcer.

4. *Low incidence areas*

To complete the picture all available reports are consistent in confirming the low incidence of duodenal ulcer in rural areas of Kenya, Zambia, most of Tanzania, Rhodesia, most of Zaire, Malawi, Lesotho, Natal and Transvaal. This is discussed in greater detail later.

5. *Prevalence in more westernized Africans*

In recent years experienced clinicians in many East African towns and urban areas have been diagnosing more cases of acute "western-type" duodenal ulcer. They consider that this represents a true increase and is not merely due to improved diagnostic facilities. In Nairobi Whittaker (1966) reported that 22·2% of 1000 consecutive upper gastrointestinal tract radiological examinations showed evidence of acute duodenal ulcera-tion. In 1966, some 60 operations for peptic ulcer were performed at his hospital, half of which were for stenosing duodenal ulcer. Both acute and chronic ulcers were seen; 15% of all peptic ulcer patients had a history of bleeding, and about six perforations were seen annually (Miller, 1966). A similar but more confused picture of both varieties of ulcer was seen at that time at Dar-es-Salaam, Tanzania (Greech, 1965) and at Kampala, Uganda (Moore, 1967). In all three East African capitals gastric ulcer was still uncommon and especially at Kampala, where the ratio DU : GU was 50 : 1. A notable feature of the more acute duodenal ulcer is its occurrence in young educated African men who have adopted a western way of life. During 2 years' observation of 400 East African college students who were eating western-type diets, 19 duodenal ulcers were found (2·1% of new cases per year). There was one case of haematemesis, but no perforation (Allbrook, 1958). Many were in fact relapses, having had ulcer histories of up to 6 years, which illustrates that it is sometimes difficult to differentiate between the chronic stenosing and the western more acute type of duodenal ulcer which is characterized by a shorter history and a greater tendency for the patients to be admitted to hospital for haemorrhage or perforation. It is also difficult to assess the proportion developing stenosis; surgeons tend to give a high figure. Miller (1966) in Nairobi considered that 50% developed stenosis, but Moore (1967), who conducted a radiological examination in Kampala, found only 12% stenosis, 24 out of 197 cases of DU.

Both clinical and autopsy evidence indicates a low but increasing incidence of peptic ulcer in South African Bantu in urban areas. In 1927 Beyers reported that only four cases of peptic ulcer were diagnosed in 18,000 Bantu hospital admissions in Johannesburg. McKenzie (1957) reported that only 25 male and two female cases were diagnosed among over 14,000 hospital admissions in a 2 year period at Durban, less than 0·1%. Kark (1961) also reported from Durban an incidence of 0·028% in hospital admissions among urban Bantu from 1950–59 compared with 1·0% in a far smaller Indian community—the latter, originating mainly from South India and Bengal, having preserved their traditional dietary pattern. Features of the acute western-type duodenal ulcer were appearing among Bantu, since perforations were diagnosed in 14% and haemorrhage in 15% of their admissions.

The most convincing evidence of the rarity of duodenal ulcer among South African Bantu in former times is derived from 2367 Bantu autopsies at Johannesburg. Duodenal ulcers were found in only eight men and two women during a deliberate search of all material (Higginson and Simson, 1958).

In the non-white section of Johannesburg General Hospital, Bremner (1972) reported an admission rate of 0·00016% for duodenal ulcer in the period 1921–26 and of 0·0027% in the period, 1964–71. The incidence of complications was perforation 47%, stenosis 22% and haemorrhage 9%.

After 30 years' medical experience in Rhodesia, Gelfand (1963) considered that the incidence of the acute western-type duodenal ulcer was rising in urban Bantu and that more haemorrhages were being seen. Wapnick and Gelfand (1973) reported 75 cases of duodenal ulcer and 18 of gastric ulcer in urban Bantu in 4 years, and maintained that peptic ulcer was still very uncommon in Rhodesian Africans in their traditional environment. In the 75 cases of duodenal ulcer there were the following complications: 31 haemorrhages, 30 perforations and five cases of pyloric stenosis. This agrees with the experience of Barker at Nqutu, a rural area of Natal;

he diagnosed only two cases of peptic ulcer among 25,000 in-patients during 1950–60 (Cleave et al., 1969; Cleave, 1962, 1974).

D. Autopsy evidence from Uganda

Clinical and radiological evidence in Kampala, Uganda, has suggested that this is an area of relatively high prevalence of duodenal ulcer (Shaper and Williams, 1959; Moore, 1967). At the medical school, Kampala, Raper and his two colleagues, during the 6 year period 1951–56, made a prospective study of duodenal ulcer and gastric ulcer among 554 consecutive hospital autopsies on Africans (454 men and 100 women) and 222 (193 men and 29 women) consecutive medico-legal autopsies (Raper, 1958). The hospital had 500 beds and served several hundred thousand Africans. It drew patients from the Nile–Congo watershed countries of Burundi and Rwanda. Of the 55–60% deaths occurring in the hospital who came to autopsy, it was recognized that they were not from a representative cross-section of the community, and comprised mostly poor patients whose relatives had not refused permission for autopsy.

Only chronic ulcers with a definite crater and macroscopic fibrosis were analysed, scars being recorded separately. No particulars of the size of the ulcer or scar were given but many were apparently small and relatively shallow, which the author suggests "may have some bearing both on the apparent absence of symptoms and on the clinical rarity of perforation". During this 6 year period only four autopsies were performed on patients with perforated ulcers, two duodenal and two gastric.

Since, as has already been said, in all tropical African countries more men than women attend hospital and come to autopsy, emphasis will be placed on the men. African tribes were considered in four groups: (1) poor immigrant labourers from Burundi and Rwanda and neighbouring tribes (253 male autopsies); (2) local Bantu-speaking tribes of Uganda (263 male autopsies), small peasant farmers living under conditions of moderate wealth in their own small farms in the countryside; (3) Nilotic tribes (74 male autopsies) from the northern drier areas in Uganda who lived in Kampala and had regular employment; (4) Kenya immigrants (57 male autopsies). In men there were 43 duodenal ulcers; some 42 bodies showed duodenal scars. Many who had an active overt duodenal ulcer had single or multiple scars of healed lesions, but these were not listed separately. Among men the ratio DU : GU average 6·6 : 1 (hospital), 6·7 : 1 (medio-legal).

The incidence of duodenal ulcer, including scars, varied considerably among the tribal groups: (1) poor immigrants 17·9%; (2) local Bantu 12%;

(3) Nilotic town workmen 4·7%. These differences were reflected in the clinical experience of doctors in these three regions. The highest incidence, as will be discussed later, was amongst the poorest social group who mostly ate unprocessed starchy carbohydrate foods and took very little sugar.

The Kampala mean figure for duodenal ulcer and scars (men) was 13·4%. This should be compared to figures from prospective studies in Europe, such as those for duodenal ulcer and scars (men) at Leeds 9·6% (Watkinson, 1960), in Germany 9·0%, the Netherlands 7·1% (Pflanz, 1971). At Leeds the frequency of active duodenal ulcer in male autopsies was 2·4% and of scars 7·2%; at Kampala the prevalence of duodenal ulcers (43) was almost equal to that of scars (42). The prevalence of active duodenal ulcer in Kampala was therefore 6·8%, almost three times as high as that obtained in Leeds, and the highest prevalence of duodenal ulcers recorded anywhere in the world.

Raper commented on the mildness of these duodenal ulcers; few had penetrated the pancreas, perforated the peritoneum or caused haemorrhage. Only five out of the 76 hospital patients had complained of symptoms sufficiently marked to seek treatment. This gross disparity between clinical detection during life and autopsy incidence is disconcerting. No comments were made on the prevalence of pyloric stenosis, fibrosis or the formation of adhesions.

It was noted that "no adequate record of the presence of hookworms or strongyloides was kept; but these infections are commoner as well as more intense in the poorer subjects". Personal experience (H. T.) suggests that many of these poor subjects would have had any number of hookworms, from a few score to a few hundred in the duodenum and upper jejunum. These loosen soon after death and can be counted only if the entire bowel contents are flushed out.

V. Possible causative factors

There are inherent difficulties in determining the prevalence of duodenal ulcer, whether by hospital admissions or *post mortems*, for both are selective. Prevalence at autopsy exceeds that determined by clinical assessment, and even community surveys cannot offer conclusive results, for a fair proportion of ulcers remain undetected, even by radiology. It is also difficult to determine what diet has been eaten. In spite of all these uncertainties, however, the striking differences in duodenal ulcer prevalence in various parts of India and Africa, even at the same prospective *post mortem* study (Raper, 1958), have led local clinical workers to search for environmental factors which may be responsible for these differences.

It seems unlikely that a firm distinction can be made between two varieties of duodenal ulcer, the standard western-type and the stenosing variety, characteristic of many seen in rural areas of India and Africa. It is not possible at present to state the proportion of patients in the tropics who develop stenosis. The patients probably seek more surgical aid than uncomplicated cases and therefore constitute an undue proportion of ulcer operations. But perforation and haemorrhage would equally call for urgent attention. After studying all aspects of the problem it is considered that there is only one disease—chronic duodenal ulcer—but that in certain regions of India and Africa a fair proportion of patients frequently, but not invariably, develop early fibrosis and stenosis and apparently have less tendency to perforation and haemorrhage. In these areas duodenal ulcer shows marked male predominance, gastric ulcer is relatively uncommon, and the peak age incidence is about 10 years younger than in the west. This suggests some local superimposed factor affecting the clinical course.

A. Hookworms

Chandler (1928, 1929) suggested that hookworms were more prevalent in those areas of India which had a high prevalence of duodenal ulcer, but any association of hookworm infestation and duodenal ulcer prevalence was not substantiated in a survey of patients and controls by Raju and Narielwala (1965) or by Leslie and Tovey (1955). Both occur commonly in many warm rural areas in tropical India and Africa, where the soil is moist because of a good rainfall. Latrines are primitive among peasant communities. In Africa, hookworm infestation is low in Rwanda/Burundi and high in southern Uganda, both areas in which duodenal ulcer is common. It is high in the coastal region of West Africa where duodenal ulcer is common and in the northern areas where duodenal ulcer is rare. Hookworm infestation is prevalent in much of Zaire where duodenal ulcer is uncommon. It is therefore possible that, while hookworms may not affect the prevalence of duodenal ulcer, they may be a factor in the development of early fibrosis and stenosis in patients suffering from an ulcer. Konstam (1970) reported Nigerian children who, though diagnosed both clinically and radiologically as having duodenal ulcer, had no ulcer at operation but had hookworms in the duodenum and enlarged lymph glands behind the doudenal cap. This factor should possibly receive more attention because of the close association of duodenal ulcer, often of the stenosing type, and ancylostomiasis.

B. Stress

The rise in prevalence in England during 1920–55, the decrease in prevalence after 1955, particularly in the south, together with the rises and falls that have occurred in other European countries and America, must count heavily against any theory that the strains of modern urban life in advanced technological countries are primary aetiological factors.

Peasants in India and Africa have many anxieties, even if these differ from those encountered in the western world, and such anxieties are present in both the high and low incidence areas. It is possible, however, that the stress caused by the increased pace of living in urban areas, and in western countries, may be a factor in the more acute type of ulcer found there.

C. Food flavourings and mastication

It must be emphasized that chronic duodenal ulcer is extremely common among the least advanced social groups in large areas of southern India and central Africa. Workers in these tropical regions have suggested certain aetiological factors, but none of these has gained widespread support. Among these have been spices and peppers, the consumption of which is high in South India and along the coast of West Africa, where duodenal ulcer is common. But these flavourings are also widely used in the areas where duodenal ulcer is uncommon—North India, the northern savannah regions of the west coast of Africa, and Zaire. Spices and peppers are not a feature of the diet in the very high incidence areas of Rwanda and Burundi. Caffeine, alcohol and tobacco have also been suggested, but their consumption bears no relationship to the geographical distribution of duodenal ulcer. Long intervals between meals occur in both high and low incidence areas. Malhotra (1964) suggested that the amount of mastication required to consume staple carbohydrate food may be important. Chupatties, the staple diet of the low incidence areas of the Punjab and Rajasthan, require a lot of mastication with increased production of saliva. This contrasts with the sloppier rice diet of South India which requires little mastication. He suggests that the alkaline and mucus content of the saliva will protect the gastric mucosa. The physiological reasoning behind this is a little doubtful because, after temporarily lowering the acidity, alkali acts as an antral stimulant, and also intraluminal mucus has no protective action on the mucosa. Nor does Malhotra's theory fit in with the situation in Africa, where a sloppy diet is consumed in both high and low incidence areas.

D. Refined carbohydrate foods

The picture with regard to any association between the incidence of duodenal ulceration and the consumption of refined carbohydrate foods is confused. On the west coast of Africa the diet is a mixture of rice, yams, plantains and sweet potatoes with an increasing amount of white bread and flour. A certain quantity of cassava may be eaten all the year round. The diet in Rwanda and Burundi is seasonal and largely made up of plantains, maize, sweet potatoes, millet, beans and peas. Cassava is taken only seasonally in times of shortage. The staple diet around Kilimanjaro is maize and in Ethiopia a millet (teff).

Probably the most important step would be to establish areas of very low prevalence of duodenal ulcer and watch the events that accompany a rising incidence. The Bantu in South Africa and Rhodesia (p. 296) continue to have a low prevalence, even in urban areas where sugar consumption (80–100 g/day) (p. 291) approximates to that taken by the lower socio-economic South African whites (p. 292), but Bantu still consume much lightly milled maize meal (p. 291). The consumption of bread has been rising in recent years in all Bantu urban townships, although the actual amount eaten is not known. Diverticular disease, which reflects many years of low-fibre diets, is still very rare in South African Bantu (p. 103).

As mentioned earlier, the evidence of hospital admissions and radiological examination over a wide area of South Africa, Rhodesia, Lesotho, Malawi, Zambia, north-west Uganda, Kenya, most of Tanzania, and Zaire, together with the drier northern inland belt in the West African countries, suggests that duodenal ulcer has a low prevalence in most of their rural areas. The more acute type of duodenal ulcer is, however, being diagnosed with increased frequency in all the large towns in these areas. This is considered to be a real difference. In these rural areas, most of which are comparatively dry, unrefined carbohydrates in the form of maize, various millets and guinea corn are the staple food. They are often stone-ground or only lightly milled as a meal still containing much fibre (p. 291). In India the lowest prevalence of duodenal ulcer is in the Punjab and Rajasthan, areas where chupatties are still made of wholemeal wheat, and fibre-rich leguminous seeds are eaten. In the southern area of India, where duodenal ulcer is most prevalent, the diet is largely rice, usually of the white fibre-depleted variety, with cassava in the extreme south-west. The picture suggests that unrefined wheat and other grains may be protective, but the evidence is confusing. Millet (*Eleusine coracana*), crude fibre 3·0 g/100 g, but not an allied grain (*Sorghum vulgare*), crude fibre 2·0 g/100 g (both unrefined), appear to be protective in one area of India (Tovey, 1962, 1972a).

As mentioned, in African towns a reported rise in the prevalence of a more acute type of duodenal ulcer has been considered by clinicians to be a possible result of the westernization of diet (Allbrook, 1958; Gelfand, 1963). A similar rise has been noted in Indian cities (Sen, 1945; Garlick and Sundar Rao, 1971) and this is comparable to the earlier incidence in Europe and North America. The aetiological factors of this world-wide increase remain uncertain, but could be due to the increased consumption of refined carbohydrates.

Cassava, which when refined loses what little protein it contains, although its fibre content remains high, is a feature of the diet in the areas of high duodenal ulcer incidence of Kerala in South India and along the coastal zone of West Africa. In the low incidence areas to the north of West Africa its consumption is only seasonal. It is consumed only in small amounts and at certain seasons in Burundi and Rwanda, countries with a high prevalence of duodenal ulcer; more is consumed in the West Nile region of Uganda where duodenal ulcer was less prevalent (Raper, 1958). The situation is the same in Zaire and western Zambia. In much of tropical and semi-tropical Africa cassava is in fact a famine crop. Cleave (1974) makes a point that the amount of protein remaining in cassava after its preparation depends on whether or not it requires peeling and whether it is leached before or after the peeling. The cassava in western Zambia, where duodenal ulcer incidence is low, has a higher protein content (approx. 1·4%) than the cassava in southern Nigeria (approx. 0·8%), where the DU incidence is high.

Cleave (1962, 1974), also suggested that the increasing incidence of duodenal ulcer (of the western type) in the coloured population of North America after 1930 (p. 284) might have been related to the change from hominy (unrefined maize) to more sophisticated refined carbohydrate foods.

The evidence presented by Cleave (1962, 1974) and Cleave et al. (1969) concerning the effect of unrefined carbohydrate foods on duodenal ulcer sufferers in prisoner-of-war camps during the Second World War is convincing. For instance, they recorded that prisoners with duodenal ulcers were symptom-free in Singapore from 1942 to the end of 1943, when an issue of rice bran was added to their normal diet of polished rice. The issue ceased at the end of 1943 and was followed by "a plague of duodenal ulcers".

The author, in an uncontrolled trial, gave a supplement of 40 g of rice bran for 3 months to 45 patients with chronic unremitting duodenal ulcer symptoms on two tea estates in South India and obtained a remission in approximately 50% (Tovey, 1972b, c).

On the other hand evidence against the role of refined carbohydrates (sugar and flour) as aetiological factors in duodenal ulcer comes from Britain during the years in which the higher fibre National flour was compulsory 1942–53 and the availability of sugar was reduced 20–25% for part of the time. Before the war deaths from duodenal ulcer were rising on a wave of increased prevalence in men and women. Mortality per million men was 66 in 1937 and rose to a plateau of 85–104 during 1945–1955. Since 1954 mortality has been dropping fairly steadily to 50 in 1970.

It is possible that improved treatment has contributed to this decreased mortality in the last two decades, and that war strain and bombing contributed to the marked rise in 1940–45, but no fall in mortality occurred during 1942–53 comparable to that which occurred in the case of diabetes mellitus (Chapter 16) or diverticular disease (Chapter 9), both of which were considered to be related to the increased consumption of fibre in the "National Loaf".

Unrefined carbohydrates and bran have quite marked though variable buffer content (Tovey, 1974) compared with refined carbohydrates. The buffering is due to both the higher mineral and protein content. Experimental studies demonstrate that the gastric response to various foods is complex. Higher pH levels were found after white bread was eaten than after brown bread (Lennard-Jones et al., 1968). On the other hand Tovey (1974), employing a wide variety of foods (polished and unpolished rice, rice bran, millet, etc.), showed that foods containing more protein or mineral buffer resulted after a short fall in acidity in a greater acid concentration because they were more powerful antral stimulants. He suggested that the buffer content of food in normal quantities probably has little effect on ultimate pH levels, for the antrum responds with a greater production of acid when stimulated by alkali or protein; this however is self-limiting, and secretion is cut off as soon as pH reaches a low level. In in vitro experiments, Tovey (1974) did not detect any powerful pepsin inhibitor in a variety of carbohydrate foods, and found no difference between refined and unrefined carbohydrates.

VI. Possible protective factors

Experimental studies have suggested that protective factors present in some foods may increase mucosal resistance. This has led to the use of liquorice products and gefarnate, a vitamin K analogue discovered during research work on cabbage. Several workers (Cheney, 1950a, b, c; Singh et al., 1962) have demonstrated that certain foodstuffs give protection against ulcer produced experimentally, and Tovey et al. (1975) have confirmed the marked protection offered by certain uncooked vegetables, especially cabbage, dhal and brinjal. These factors are thermolabile and destroyed by cooking. It is possible that the consumption of these, or similar vegetables, and their method of preparation, may influence duodenal ulcer prevalence in the tropics. P. Jayaraj (p.c. 1974) showed that Punjabi diet protected rats against ulcers following pyloric ligation and that South Indian diet gave no protection.

The picture with regard to the consumption of green vegetables, cooked and uncooked, and the distribution of duodenal ulcer is confusing. More fresh vegetables were eaten in the low incidence areas of the Punjab than in the high incidence areas of South India where all vegetables tend to receive prolonged cooking in the curry. In the high incidence areas of Burundi and Rwanda very few fresh green vegetables are eaten. Along the west coast of Africa, in Zaire and in Rhodesia green leaves of various sorts including cassava leaves are eaten in the sauce, usually after prolonged cooking, but no differences have been shown between high and low incidence areas except in the low incidence areas of northern Ghana where the quantity consumed is greater and the amount of cooking is less.

In their rat experiments Tovey *et al.* (1975) found no protective action against ulceration by pre-feeding with wheat or rice bran, or maize or millet (ragi).

VII. Conclusions

The present geographical distribution of duodenal ulcer in the rural areas of India and Africa and the habits of the people in these areas do not suggest that there is any association between the occurrence of duodenal ulcer and such factors as alcohol, caffeine, smoking, spices, infrequent meals, malnutrition or hookworm. While the situation in India supports Cleave's hypothesis, the distribution in Africa does not entirely support his concept that the incidence is related to the consumption of refined carbohydrate foods, nor does it support Malhotra's theory that the prevalence is related to mastication. The localization of high and low incidence areas does, however, support the existence of local environmental factors which may well be dietary. In the past attention has been focused on possible ulcerogenic factors and it may now be more rewarding to investigate the presence or absence in the diet of protective factors. These may take the form of buffers as in unrefined foods, or they may exert a protective action on the mucosal cells akin to that of carbenoxolone.

The evidence suggests that the type of ulcer occurring in high prevalence rural areas of India and Africa differs from that found in urban areas and in the "West". It is associated with early fibrosis often progressing to stenosis; haemorrhage and perforation are rare; there is a marked male predominance and gastric ulcer is relatively uncommon. This suggests that different factors operate in the two areas—it may be that dietary factors combined with hookworm in the rural areas produces more fibrosis and that stress related to the pace of city life results in a more acute ulcer in urban areas.

Finally, although there is little established knowledge concerning ulcerogenic and protective factors in the environment, the changing prevalence of duodenal ulcer in terms of place and also in terms of time, renders it certain that environmental factors must operate.

References

AITKEN, A. B. (1933). *West African Medical Journal* **6**, 63.
ALLBROOK, D. B. (1958). *East African Medical Journal* **35**, 97.
AVERY JONES, F. (1947). *British Medical Journal* **2**, 441, 477.
BADOE, E. A. (1972). *Ghana Medical Journal* **2**, 248.
BENJAMIN, V. and NARIEWALA, F. M. (1964). *Proceedings Second Asian Congress Gastroenterology*, p. 44.
BERGSMA, S. (1931). *Archives of Internal Medicine* **47**, 144.
BEYERS, C. F. (1927). *Journal of the Medical Association of South Africa* **6**, 33.
BOHRER, S. P., SOLANTA, T. F. and WILLIAMS, D. A. (1964). *British Medical Journal* **4**, 515.
BOLAND, F. (1942). *Annals of Surgery* **115**, 939.
BOLES, R. S. (1942). *American Journal of Digestive Diseases* **9**, 241.
BRADFIELD, E. W. C. (1927). *Transactions VII Congress Far Eastern Association for Tropical Medicine* **1**, 221.
BRAINBRIDGE, C. V. and TROWELL, H. C. (1933–34). *East African Medical Journal* **10**, 365.
BREMNER, C. G. (1972). *South African Journal of Surgery* **10**, 139.
CAVE, L., SANKALE, M. and FERAL, J. (1963). *Médecine Africaine Noire* **10**, 385.
CEUTERICK, J. (1955). *Annales Société belge médecine tropicale* **35**, 119.
CHABAL, J. and IZARN, R. L. M. (1970). *West African Medical Journal* **19**, 30.
CHANDLER, A. C. (1928). *Indian Journal of Medical Research* **14**, 185.
CHANDLER, A. C. (1929). *Ibid.* **15**, 143.
CHATTERJEE, S. C., DAS, D. and SEN GUPTA, S. N. (1959). *Journal of the Indian Medical Association* **30**, 35.
CHENEY, G. (1950a). *American Dietetic Association Journal* **26**, 668.
CHENEY, G. (1950b). *California Medicine* **77**, 248.
CHENEY, G. (1950c). *Stanford Medical Bulletin* **8**, 144.
CHUTTANI, S., WIG, K. L., CHABBRA, T. D., VASUDEVA, Y. L., GADEGAR, N. G. and CHUTTANI, H. K. (1967). *Indian Journal of Medical Research* **55**, 1121.
CLEAVE, T. L. (1962). "Peptic Ulcer." John Wright, Bristol.
CLEAVE, T. L. (1974). "The Saccharine Disease." John Wright, Bristol.
CLEAVE, T. L., CAMPBELL, G. D. and PAINTER, N. S. (1969). "Diabetes, Coronary Thrombosis and the Saccharine Disease", pp. 87–112. John Wright, Bristol.
DOGRA, J. R. (1940). *Indian Journal of Medical Research* **28**, 146.
DOGRA, J. R. (1941). *Ibid.* **29**, 311, 665.
DOLL, R. (1952). *In* "Modern Trends in Gastroenterology" (F. Avery Jones, ed.), p. 361. Butterworth, London.
DOLL, R., JONES, F. A. and BUCKATZSCH, M. M. (1951). "Occupational Factors in the Aetiology of Gastric and Duodenal Ulcers." Medical Research Council Special Report Series No. 276. Her Majesty's Stationery Office, London.
DUNN, J. P. and COBB, J. S. (1962). *Journal of Occupational Medicine* **4**, 343.
DUNN, W. H. (1942). *War Medicine* **2**, 967.
EAGLE, P. C. and GILLMAN, J. (1938). *South African Journal of Medical Science* **3**, 1.
ELLIS, H. (1972). *In* "Chronic Duodenal Ulcer" (C. Wastell, ed.), p. 255. Butterworth, London.

ELLIS, M. (1948). *British Journal of Surgery* **36**, 60.

EMERY, E. S., JR. and MONROE, R. T. (1935). *Archives of Internal Medicine* **55**, 271.

ENZER, J. (1937–38). *East African Medical Journal* **14**, 91.

FENWICK, S. and FENWICK W. S. (1900). "Ulcer of the Stomach and Duodenum." Churchill, London. (Cited by Ivy *et al.*, 1950, p. 472.)

GARLICK, F. H. and SUNDAR RAO, P. S. S. (1971). *British Journal of Surgery* **58**, 905.

GELFAND, M. (1963). *Central African Journal of Medicine* **12**, 366.

GOODCHILD, R. T. S. (1949). *East African Medical Journal* **26**, 137.

GOYAL, R. K. and GUPTA, P. S. (1966). *Journal of the Association of Physicians of India* **14**, 181.

GREECH, P. (1965). *East African Medical Journal* **42**, 106.

GREGG, I. A. (1959). *Indian Council for Medical Research* Report No. 39.

HADLEY, G. C. (1958). *Schweizerische Zeitschrift für Pathologie* **21**, 472.

HADLEY, G. C. (1959). *Indian Council for Medical Research* Report No. 39.

HAMBER, G. and VON BERGEN, M. (1971). *Tropical and Geographical Medicine* **23**, 213.

HAMBER, G. and VON BERGEN, M. (1973). *Ibid.* **25**, 1.

HAUBRICK, W. S. (1963). *In* "Gastroenterology", 2nd edition (H. C. Bockus, ed.), Vol. 1, p. 592. W. B. Saunders, Philadelphia.

HIGGINSON, J. and SIMSON, I. (1958). *Schweizerische Zeitschrift Pathologie Bakteriologie* **21**, 577.

HOSPITAL IN-PATIENT ENQUIRY FOR ENGLAND AND WALES 1956–67. Unpublished Data, quoted by Langman, 1973 (q.v.).

INDIAN COUNCIL FOR MEDICAL RESEARCH (1959). Report No. 39.

IVY, A. C., GROSSMANN, M. I. and BACHRACH, W. H. (1950). "Peptic Ulcer." Churchill, London. (a) p. 456; (b) 473; (c) p. 475; (d) p. 557; (e) p. 542.

IZARN, R. L. M. (1969). "La Therapeutique Chirurgicale de l'Ulcère Gastro-duodenale à Dakar de 1963 à 1968." Thesis, Faculté de Médecine, Paris 1969. (Cited by Hamber and von Bergen, 1973.)

JENNINGS, D. (1940). *Lancet* **1**, 395 and 444.

JOLY, B. M. (1956). *West African Medical Journal* **5**, 55.

KARK, A. E. (1961). *Gut* **2**, 363.

KIRSCHNER, A. A. (1944). *Review of Gastroenterology* **11**, 397.

KONSTAM, P. G. (1954). *Lancet* **2**, 1039.

KONSTAM, P. G. (1966). *American Journal of Surgery* **112**, 864.

KONSTAM, P. (1970). *In* "Alimentary and Haematological Aspects of Tropical Disease" (A. W. Woodruff, ed.), p. 55. Edward Arnold, London.

KOZOLL, D. D. and MEYER, K. A. (1964). *Archives of Surgery* **89**, 491.

LANGMAN, M. J. S. (1973). *In* "Clinics in Gastroenterology," Vol. 2. (W. Sircus, ed.), p. 219. W. B. Saunders, London.

LANGMANN, M. J. S., (1974). *In* "Chronic Duodenal Ulcer" (C. Wastell, ed.), p. 9. Butterworth, London.

LENNARD-JONES, J., FLETCHER, J. and SHAW, D. G. (1968). *Gut* **9**, 177.

LESLIE, H. and TOVEY, F. I. (1955). *Journal of the Indian Medical Association* **25**, 548.

LEWIS, E. A. and BOHRER, S. P. (1970). *West African Medical Journal* **19**, 59.

McCARRISON, R. (1944). "Nutrition and National Health." Faber, London.

MACKAY, C. (1966). *British Medical Journal* **1**, 701.

McKENZIE, M. B. (1957). *South African Medical Journal* **31**, 1041.

MAES, U. and McFETBRIDGE, E. M. (1936). *American Journal of Surgery* **33**, 13.

MALHOTRA, S. L. (1964). *Gut* **5**, 412.

MALHOTRA, S. L. (1967). *Gut* **8**, 180.

MALHOTRA, S. L., MAJAMDAR, C. T. and BARDOLI, P. C. (1964). *Gut* **5**, 355.

MILLER, J. R. M. (1966). *East African Medical Journal* **43**, 258.

MOORE, E. W. (1967). *East African Medical Journal* **44**, 513.

MOWAT, A. J. (1934–35). *East African Medical Journal* **11**, 62.

ORR, I. M. and RAO, M. V. R. (1939). *Indian Journal of Medical Research* **27**, 159.

PAYET, M., PELLEGRINO, A. and D'ASSOMPTION, V. (1959). *Bulletin Société Médecine Africa Noire Langue Française* **4**, 369.

PERRY, E. C. and SHAW, L. E. (1893). *Guy's Hospital Reports* **50**, 171.

PFLANZ, M. (1971). *In* "Duodenal Ulcer" (H. Weiner, ed.), p. 121. Karger, Basel.

PLAHA, S. K., SEHGAL, A. K., GUPTA, B. R., MALIK, K. and CHUTTANI, P. N. (1967). *Proceedings Annual Conference Indian Society Gastroenterology*. Simla.

PORTIO, S. A. and JAFFE, R. H. (1938). *Journal of the American Medical Association* **110**, 6.

PULVERTAFT, C. N. (1959). *British Journal of Preventive Social Medicine* **13**, 131.

PULVERTAFT, C. N. (1968). *Postgraduate Medical Journal* **44**, 597.

RAGHAVACHARI, A. C. (1959). *Indian Council for Medical Research* Report No. 39.

RAGHAVAN, P. (1962). *Gastroenterology* **42**, 130.

RAGHAVAN, P. (1966). *Proceedings 3rd World Congress Gastroenterology* Tokyo **2**, 18.

RAJU, S. and NARIELWALA, F. M. (1965). *Gut* **6**, 546.

RAO, M. N. (1938). *Indian Medical Gazette* **73**, 454.

RAO, V. G. (1959). *Indian Council for Medical Research* Report No. 39.

RAPER, A. B. (1958). *Transactions of the Royal Society of Tropical Medicine and Hygiene* **52**, 535.

ROGERS, I. (1914). *Indian Medical Gazette* **49**, 41.

ROGERS, I. (1925). *Glasgow Medical Journal* **103**, 1.

SANDERS, R. (1967). *Gut* **8**, 58.

SEHGAL, A. K., CHUTTANI, P. N., GUPTA, B. B., MALIK, K. and GUPTA, H. D. (1971). *Indian Journal of Medical Research* **59**, 1612.

SEN, P. K. (1945). *Indian Physician* **4**, 7.

SHAPER, A. G. and WILLIAMS, A. W. (1959). *British Medical Journal* **2**, 757.

SINGH, G. B., ZAIDI, S. H. and BAJPAL, R. P. (1962). *Indian Journal of Medical Research* **50**, 741.

SOMERVELL, T. H. (1942). *British Journal of Surgery* **30**, 113.

SOMERVELL, T. H. and ORR, I. M. (1936). *British Journal of Surgery* **24**, 227.

SUSSER, M. (1967). *Journal of Chronic Diseases* **20**, 435.

TOURNIER-LASSERVE, C., GESOME M. and BADAROU, (1961). *Médecine tropicale* **21**, 554.

TOUZE, M. E. (1960). *Médecine Africaine Noire* **7**, 381.

TOVEY, F. I. (1962). "Nutritional Aspects of Peptic Ulcer and its Surgery in India." Ch.M. Thesis, University of Liverpool.

TOVEY, F. I. (1972a). *Tropical and Geographical Medicine* **24**, 107.

TOVEY, F. I. (1972b). *British Medical Journal* **2**, 532.

TOVEY, F. I. (1972c). *Journal of the Christian Medical Association of India* **47**, 312.

TOVEY, F. I. (1974). *Postgraduate Medical Journal* **50**, 683.

TOVEY, F. I., JAYARAJ, P. and CLARK, C. G. (1975) *Postgraduate Medical Journal* (in press).

U.S. PUBLIC HEALTH SERVICE (1947). "Vital Statistic Rates in the United States 1900–1940." United States Government Printing Office, Washington.

VARMA, R. A. (1969). *In* "After Vagotomy" (A. Williams and A. G. Cox, eds). Butterworth, London.

VASSALLO, S. M. (1934–35). *East African Medical Journal* **11**, 62.

VINT, F. W. (1936–37). *East African Medical Journal* **13**, 332.

WALKER, A. R. P., HOLDSWORTH, O. M. and WALKER, E. J. (1971). *South African Medical Journal* **45**, 515.

WAPNICK, S. and GELFAND, M. (1973). *South African Medical Journal* **47**, 625.

WASTELL, C. (1972). "Chronic Duodenal Ulcer." (a) p. 5; (b) p. 35; (c) p. 6. Butterworth, London.

WATKINSON, G. (1960). *Gut* **1**, 14.

WATKINSON, G. (1961). *In* "Modern Trends in Gastroenterology" (W. I. Card, ed.), p. 23. Butterworth, London.

WHITTAKER, L. R. (1966). *East African Medical Journal* **43**, 336.

Part VIII

Chapter 19

Some diseases characteristic of western civilisation prevalent in wild and domestic animals

ROBERT W. LEADER and DAVID W. HAYDEN

I. Introduction 311
II. Atherosclerosis 311
III. Venous thrombosis and pulmonary embolism 313
IV. Peptic ulceration 313
V. Cholelithiasis. 314
VI. Diabetes 315
VII. Dental caries 315
VIII. Obesity. 315
IX. Intestinal neoplasia. 315
X. Conclusion 316
References 316

I. Introduction

Statistics concerning the relative incidence of diseases of animals other than man, as they relate to environment, would be most valuable. Unfortunately, there has never been a satisfactory recording system, and all reports discussed in this chapter are fragmentary. Hopefully, in the future, as man comes to appreciate more fully the potential benefits of using the animal population as sentinels of biological, physical and environmental dangers, a system will be perfected and applied.

II. Atherosclerosis

There have been fairly extensive efforts to capitalize on the incidence of various types of arteriosclerosis in animals to increase our knowledge about

311

this important disease of man. Many experimental studies have involved the administration of abnormal rations to animals such as chickens, rabbits, or dogs, and because of these artificial circumstances the relevance of comparing the disease produced to human atherosclerosis is questionable. During the past few years, however, new approaches to the study of animal atherosclerosis have yielded more significant results.

Aged pigs spontaneously develop lesions very similar to those of human atherosclerosis and the recent development of miniature swine, which reach about the same body weight in adulthood as man, has provided a convenient model. Lee et al. (1970) have reported that when atherogenic diets are fed to swine they will develop occlusive coronary artery disease and myocardial infarction.

Luginbuhl and Detweiler (1968) described cerebral infarction associated with atherosclerosis in swine that closely resembles cerebral vascular disease of man. Hypertensive encephalopathies and related conditions are not known to occur in animals other than man.

Studies of certain breeds of pigeons by Clarkson et al. (1959) have shown that naturally occurring atherosclerosis and indeed even coronary infarctions occur in these animals. Breed differences could not be correlated with age, sex, diet or physical activity, and the authors suggested that atherogenesis may be controlled by genetic factors. The lesions closely resemble those seen in man.

Non-human primates have recently been useful in the study of atherosclerosis. They are more closely related to man than other animals, and studies of the metabolism, absorption, and excretion of blood lipids indicate close similarities to man.

Wissler and Vesselinovitch (1968) in their review emphasized two important points about the pathogenesis of atherosclerosis: (1) species vary remarkably in development of atherosclerosis when apparently similar "stimuli" are applied; and (2) any species will eventually develop atheromatous lesions if subjected to a sustained elevation of blood lipids.

Atherosclerosis is reported in wild animals and birds. However, complications such as thrombosis or myocardial infarction are rare. Evaluation of this information presents considerable difficulty because, apart from the work of a few investigators, examination of arteries does not appear to have been made on a systematic basis, and incidence rates are therefore lacking.

Ratcliffe and Cronin (1958) and Ratcliffe et al. (1960) believe there is ample evidence that psychological stress is a factor in inducing atherosclerosis in captive wild animals. The chief evidence was that growing populations and crowding in cages, plus ever greater numbers of human visitors, seemed to contribute to an increase in arterial disease. Dietary methods were reformed to eliminate the possibility of deficiencies, but the incidence of cardiovascular disease continued to rise.

One inevitably gains the impression that the incidence of true atherosclerosis in any mammal apart from man is low. It is higher in birds than in mammals. When it occurs, there appears to be some correlation of incidence of lesions with age, but not necessarily with blood cholesterol levels.

All these studies suggest that a variety of animals can be manipulated either genetically or by being subjected to dietary regimes differing significantly from those to which the species has been naturally adapted, so as to become prone to develop atherosclerosis.

Lee *et al.* (1970), for instance, specifically prescribed high-cholesterol diets and in addition X-irradiated their animals, and Clarkson *et al.* (1959) limited their pigeons to a choice of certain grains. The studies of Ratcliffe and Cronin (1958) and Ratcliffe *et al.* (1960) again indicate that atherosclerosis is the result of an unnatural environment, though in this case specifically imposed stress is suggested as a causative factor. These studies suggest, as do human epidemiological investigations, that atherosclerosis is related to a somehow abnormal environment, without indicating the specific factors responsible.

III. Venous thrombosis and pulmonary embolism

In animals spontaneous venous thrombosis and pulmonary embolism are very rare, but have occasionally been observed in cattle following prolonged recumbency and in horses suffering from an anaemia caused by a virus infection. There is nothing comparable to the deep vein thrombosis which so frequently occurs in hospitalized patients in the western world.

IV. Peptic ulceration

Gastric ulcers have been recognized in all domestic and many captive wild animals and birds. However, only the pig has received considerable attention. Gastric ulcers in swine have a world-wide distribution and are of increasing economic importance. Stomach ulcers in swine are frequently multiple and appear to favour the non-glandular area around the cardia. Fatal gastric haemorrhage commonly occurs.

Oesophagogastric ulcers of swine have morphological similarities to peptic ulcers in man (Kernkamp, 1945), and investigation of ulcerogenesis in this species may contribute information applicable to man.

The incidence of gastric ulceration in swine is unknown, although studies of packing house material show rates as high as 16–25% (Kowalczyk *et al.*, 1960; Hoekstra, 1962). This is much higher than the prevalence of 2·5%

in pigs examined at necropsy because of obvious illness (Muggenburg *et al.*, 1964).

In swine, the appearance of gastric ulcers in epizootic proportions frequently coincides with the introduction of new management practices which include the use of high-protein diets, transportation stress, and trends toward intensive rearing conditions with more confinement. Not only is the content of the food important but also the form in which it is presented. Pelleting of food increased the incidence of ulcers from 4·4% to 13·8% when compared to meal feed (Griffing, 1963). Also, pigs fed 2·5% coarsely ground straw meal grew faster than those fed the same amount of finely ground straw, and the latter group had a greater incidence of ulcers (Baustad and Nafstad, 1969). These results indicate that modern milling practices which produce concentrated and refined feed ingredients may be important factors in the diet of swine which contribute to ulcerogenesis.

As in the case of atherosclerosis, peptic ulceration in animals appears to be related to environmental factors differing from those to which the species is adapted, and again both dietary and psychological factors have been incriminated. There is nothing comparable to the chronic duodenal ulceration which is so common in certain human communities.

V. Cholelithiasis

Gallstones are infrequent in animals compared to their occurrence in man. Calculi recovered from horses, cattle and birds are largely composed of calcium salts and bile pigments with varying but limited amounts of cholesterol (Bol' and Bol', 1954). They must therefore be considered to be caused by factors different from those responsible for the high incidence of cholesterol stones in modern western man.

Gallstones are seen most often in the horse (which has no gallbladder) and cow, more rarely in the dog, and are seldom observed in cats, pigs or sheep (Hutyra *et al.*, 1949). An incidence of 0·4% was noted in slaughterhouse cattle (Feldman, 1928). Among 21 adult female baboons, gallstones were found in two animals (Glenn and McSherry, 1970). These animals were in captivity and on a dietary regime different from that to which they would normally be accustomed. There is no evidence that primates develop gallstones other than in captivity. It may be significant that diverticular disease, which in man is related to cholelithiasis, has been observed at autopsy in a zoo primate (N. S. Painter, p.c. 1972).

The cholesterol content of these stones ranged from 86% to 97%, thereby closely approximating that which is seen in human gallstones, since the cholesterol content of human bile is greater than that found in most other species.

VI. Diabetes

Diabetes mellitus is observed, but only occasionally, in a wide range of species. Certain inbred strains of mice, however, do develop diabetes. Spontaneous diabetes of the Chinese hamster bears the closest resemblance to juvenile insulin deficiency diabetes in man. Less marked similarities to human diabetes are seen in other species of rodents in which diabetes is frequently coupled with obesity. The sand rat (*Psammomys obesus*) has been described by Hackel *et al.* (1965) as a valuable model for the study of diabetes. These animals show severe diabetes with pancreatic islet cell degranulation and glycogen nephrosis.

VII. Dental caries

Dental decay of the type seen in man is virtually unknown in other animals. Among domestic animals dental caries are common only in the horse, where it has been estimated that about 12% have evidence of decay (Gorlin, *et al.*, 1959). Examination of 200 dogs revealed only two animals with caries of the type seen in man (Gardner *et al.*, 1962). The cat appears to be unusually free of dental disease, while sheep show a predisposition for developing cervical caries.

The relative absence of fermentable carbohydrates in the diet, shape of the teeth, high saliva pH, and urea content all have been cited as factors in animals which may explain these differences.

VIII. Obesity

The incidence of obesity among wild animals is probably very low. Among domesticated dogs and cats obesity is relatively common. These animals enjoy the niceties of an affluent society, are often overfed with totally unsuitable foods, and are in addition under-exercised.

Aged dogs are the animals most prone to obesity.

IX. Intestinal neoplasia

Neoplasms of the digestive tract occur infrequently in animals when compared to man.

In the United States Department of Agriculture's (USDA) 2 year survey (Monlux and Monlux, 1972), 1952–53, of neoplasms found in Denver abattoirs, 0·1% of tumours found in cattle were intestinal adenocarcinomas. None was found in swine or sheep. Most of these intestinal malignancies involved the small intestine. The colon, caecum and rectum were seldom involved.

Tumours have been demonstrated in many species, but only in the domestic dog and cat do they occur with any notable frequency. Canine tumours have been studied and characterized to an extent which allows some valid comparisons with similar neoplasms in man. The incidence of all tumours in dogs was reported as 4·2% among over 7000 canine neoplasms (Ontario Veterinary College, 1968). Ten adenomatous polyps were found in the alimentary canal of dogs in records covering a 15 year period by Hayden and Nielsen (1973). The dog has the greatest incidence of large bowel malignancy.

Since the domestic dog intimately shares man's environment, including his food, one might expect intestinal tumours to occur more frequently in this species in the western world than in other animals if, as seems likely, diet is an important causative factor.

Among other animals, Dodd (1960) has reported a high frequency of small bowel adenocarcinomas of sheep in some New Zealand flocks. These neoplasms, like those in dogs and cats, occur in older sheep.

Polyps and adenomas of the large bowel are infrequently reported in animals other than the dog.

X. Conclusion

For reasons previously mentioned, one can readily appreciate the difficulty in obtaining incidence rates for diseases in wild and domestic animals, for comparison with those in man. Yet this approach appears justified if we are to understand better the pathogenesis of disease in both man and animals.

All the diseases mentioned, which have a characteristically high prevalence in modern western civilization, are rare in undomesticated animals, and only a few are now relatively common in those that have been selectively bred and domesticated.

References

BAUSTAD, B. and NAFSTAD, I. (1969). *Pathologica veterinaria* 6, 546.

BOL', K. G. and BOL', B. K. (1954). Cited by Glenn and McSherry (1970).

CLARKSON, T. B., PRICHARD, R. W., NETSKY, M. G. and LOFLAND, H. B. (1959). *American Medical Association Archives of Pathology* 68, 143.

DODD, D. C. (1960). *New Zealand Veterinary Journal* 8, 109.

FELDMAN, W. H. (1928). *Journal of Cancer Research* 12, 188.

GARDNER, A. F., DARKE, B. H. and KEARY, G. T. (1962). *Journal of the American Veterinary Medical Association* 140, 433.

GLENN, F. and McSHERRY, C. K. (1970). *Archives of Surgery* 100, 105.

GORLIN, R. J., BARRON, C. N. and CHAUDHRY, A. P. (1959). *American Journal of Veterinary Research* 20, 1032.

GRIFFING, W. J. (1963). *Veterinary Medicine Letter, Iowa State University* **34,** 286.

HACKEL, D. B., SCHMIDT-NIELSEN, K., HAINES, H. B. and MIKAT, E. (1965). *Laboratory Investigation* **14**, 200.

HAYDEN, D. W. and NIELSEN, S. W. (1973). *Zentralblatt für Veterinärm Medizin, A* **20**, 1.

HOEKSTRA, W. G. (1962). *Feed Stuffs* **34**, 1.

HUTYRA, F., MAREK, J. and MANNINGER, R. (1949). "Special Pathology and Therapeutics of Domestic Animals", 5th edition, Vol II, p. 367. Alexander Eger, Chicago.

KERNKAMP, H. C. H. (1945). *American Journal of Pathology* **21**, 111.

KOWALCZYK, T., HOEKSTRA, W. G., PUESTON, K. L., SMITH, I. D. and GRUMMER, R. H. (1960). *Journal of the American Veterinary Medical Association* **137**, 339.

LEE, K. T., KIM, D. N. and THOMAS, W. A. (1970). *Circulation* **41**, Supplement 3, 111.

LUGINBUHL, H. and DETWEILER, D. K. (1968). *In* "Animal Models for Medical Research". Proceedings of a Symposium, National Academy of Sciences, Washington, D.C.

MONLUX, W. S. and MONLUX, A. W. (1972). Atlas of Meat Inspection Pathology. Agricultural Handbook No. 367, United States Department of Agriculture.

MUGGENBURG, B. A., REESE, N., KOWALCYZK, T., GRUMMER, R. H. and HOEKSTRA, W. G. (1964). *American Journal of Veterinary Research* **25**, 1673.

Ontario Veterinary College Graduate Symposium, 21 June, 1968.

RATCLIFFE, H. L. and CRONIN, M. T. I. (1958). *Circulation* **18**, 41.

RATCLIFFE, H. L., YERASIMIDES, T. G. and ELLIOTT, G. A. (1960). *Circulation* **21**, 730.

WISSLER, R. W. and VESSELINOVITCH, D. (1968). *Advances in Lipid Research* **6**, 181.

Part IX

Chapter 20

Disorders of unknown aetiology showing certain epidemiological associations

HUGH TROWELL

I. Introduction	319
II. Auto-immune diseases	320
A. General consideration	320
B. South Africa and East Africa	321
C. Nigeria	321
D. Auto-immune diseases of joints and connective tissues	322
E. Multiple sclerosis	323
III. Variations in endocrines and leucocytes	325
A. Thyroid gland	325
B. Adrenal gland	326
C. Neutropenia	327
References	329

I. Introduction

All diseases mentioned in the preceding Chapters 8–18 have been discussed in terms of their epidemiology and the data derived from experiments. Articles in which it has been suggested that refined starchy carbohydrates should be considered as one of the aetiological factors in each of these diseases have already been published in medical journals. There are also some other diseases which show, at least in Africa, striking epidemiological association with those already mentioned.

Fourteen years ago a review of all the diseases to be discussed in this chapter suggested that their incidence was affected by environmental factors, possibly dietetic ones (Trowell, 1960a). A prolonged search of the medical literature 1960–1973 of Africa has added fresh supporting data concerning environmental factors. Considerable progress has been made in unravelling mechanisms involved in pathogenesis, especially those involved in auto-immune diseases, but standard teaching remains adamant that the aetiology of all these diseases is unknown.

II. Auto-immune diseases

A. General consideration

Research in Nigeria (Greenwood and Francis, 1967; Greenwood, 1968) and South Africa (Gear, 1946; Zoutendyk, 1970) has demonstrated that Africans, at least in those areas, developed less auto-immune bodies in the blood than did Europeans and seldom suffered from auto-immune diseases. Comparison was made with the incidence of these diseases in Europe and North America and with the auto-immune bodies present in normal persons in those continents or in South African whites.

The plasma proteins of South African whites and South African Bantu are similar at birth with respect to the concentration of albumin and globulin. After 6 months of age the concentration of the plasma proteins of Bantu infants starts to differ from that of white infants. This change occurs in all parts of Africa south of the Sahara and it has been called the African pattern of plasma proteins. Many South African Bantu infants are breast-fed for many months, and food such as maize meal porridge is not introduced until 6–12 months of age. Many South African white infants are breast-fed for only a short period of time and then are fed cow's milk mixtures. They are introduced at an early age to refined carbohydrates in the form of sugar in various feeds and low-fibre starchy carbohydrates. Nevertheless it has not been proved that the African pattern of serum proteins is a response to diet.

The most significant change in the development of the African pattern of plasma proteins is the rise of the γ-globulins (immunoglobulins). This pattern of plasma proteins emerges early in life and from the standpoint of auto-immune disease the most important change is the high level of γ-globulin. Cape Town white adults had plasma γ-globulin 0·8 g/100 ml, whereas Cape Town Bantu adults had 1·4 g/100 ml (Ahrens and Brock. 1954). In Pretoria, electrophoresis estimations of Bantu adult γ-globulin recorded 1·3 g/100 ml (Kinnear, 1956). Higher levels of γ-globulin have been recorded in the tropics, together with a reduced plasma albumin. These changes have been ascribed largely to malaria. Malaria will not, however, explain the high γ-globulin levels encountered in African Bantu in non-malarious regions such as Pretoria, Cape Town and Johannesburg. In Johannesburg Zoutendyk (1970) has made a detailed study of the characteristically high levels of immunoglobulins with unique properties which persist for many years, especially in rural Africans. Walker (1972) has suggested that the levels tend to fall again after urbanization. It is not known what features of urban life are responsible for this change and the role of diet has not been examined critically.

B. South Africa and East Africa

Auto-immune acquired haemolytic anaemia of the conventional type is uncommon in South African Bantu. Zoutendyk (1970) reported that in 808 consecutive specimens of Bantu blood submitted for direct Coombs' test 1·5% were positive compared with 4·7% positive in 1460 specimens from whites. Thyroid auto-antibodies were detected in 0·55% of 180 Bantu patients manifesting thyroid pathology, compared with 9% positive in 1112 whites.

Clinical evidence also suggested that auto-immune disease was uncommon in Johannesburg Bantu; lupus erythematosus was uncommon, and a positive direct Coombs' test, frequently present in white patients, had not been detected among Bantu. Among South African Bantu Zoutendyk (1970) knew of only one reported case of ulcerative colitis, and one of Hashimoto's thyroiditis. Pernicious anaemia, myasthenia gravis and Addison's disease were all extremely rare, and multiple sclerosis had not been detected. Other studies in South Africa, Rhodesia and East Africa confirm the rarity of pernicious anaemia (Trowell, 1960b; Mngola, 1968; Forbes and Gordon, 1969), and only two cases of subacute combined degeneration have been described (Woods and Rymer, 1955).

C. Nigeria

Greenwood (1968) has studied auto-immune diseases at Ibadan, Nigeria. He confirmed that the γ-globulin levels of apparently healthy Africans were higher than those of healthy Europeans. This was due to an increase of IgG and IgM (Rowe et al., 1968). The occurrence of rheumatoid factor and heterophile agglutinins in a high proportion of Africans was further evidence of altered immunological status. U.S.A. negroes, the descendants of West Africans, had lower γ-globulin levels than West Africans (Lichtman et al., 1965). In West Africa it is considered that malarial and helminthic infections alter γ-globulin levels, but the role of diet, suggested by experience at Cape Town, has not been investigated.

At the University College Hospital, Ibadan, Nigeria, Greenwood reported on the prevalence of auto-immune diseases during 1956–66. During this period there were only 66 cases of connective tissue diseases (rheumatoid arthritis 42, Still's disease 21, systemic lupus erythematosus 2, systemic sclerosis 1); 20 cases of thyroid disease (primary thyrotoxicosis 19,

Hashimoto's thyroiditis 1); and 18 cases of other diseases (pernicious anaemia 4 (of whom 3 were Europeans), ulcerative colitis 8, myasthenia gravis 6), a total of only 104 patients with auto-immune disease out of a total of 98,454 admissions. Greenwood (1968) also reviewed the literature of all auto-immune diseases in Africa, but it is proposed to limit discussion in the following sections specifically to those disorders which are more common.

D. Auto-immune diseases of joints and connective tissues

1. Rheumatoid arthritis

Rheumatoid arthritis has been studied in Kenya (Hall, 1966), Uganda (Kanyerezi, 1969), Nigeria (Greenwood, 1968; Greenwood and Herrick, 1970), Nigeria and Liberia (Muller et al., 1972), Rhodesia (Gelfand, 1969) and South Africa (Anderson, 1970). The majority of these investigators had special experience of rheumatoid arthritis in other countries and so were able to compare the disease as seen in Africans with that encountered in Europe and North America. Without exception all reports emphasize that the disease as seen in Africans presents certain unusual features. Thus in Africans rheumatoid arthritis is less common, it is a less severe disease, shows less radiological signs, responds more readily to treatment and has a better prognosis (Greenwood, 1968; Anderson, 1970; Muller et al., 1972). Nodules and vascular lesions are rare.

Considerable dissatisfaction has been expressed by all investigators with the criteria of diagnosis as laid down by the Committee of the American Rheumatism Association 1959 (Greenwood and Herrick, 1970; Muller et al., 1972). Surveys which have employed modern methods of examination and adopted the standard criteria of diagnosis have suggested that the prevalence of rheumatoid arthritis in West Africa in comparison with the prevalence in England was about 1 : 3 in women and 1 : 2 in men (Muller et al., 1972). It is impossible to make a valid comparison because the standard tests have not proved reliable in Africa. This cannot be due to race, since in the U.S.A. the tests have proved that American negroes have the same prevalence of rheumatoid arthritis as whites (Engel and Birch, 1967). Investigators of rheumatoid arthritis in Europe and North America do not consider that climate influences the prevalence of the disease.

2. Still's disease

This disease, although uncommon, has been reported in Nigeria (Greenwood, 1968).

3. Ankylosing spondylitis

This is very rare among Africans. Gelfand (1969) saw only one case during an 8 year study of arthritis in Rhodesia; Hall (1966) reported a single case only in a 2 year study of polyarthritis in Kenya; he also described three patients suffering from Reiter's disease.

Few investigators have offered any opinion concerning possible reasons for the unusual features of these arthritic diseases in Africans. Environmental factors were suggested in Nigeria (Greenwood and Herrick, 1970). Malaria and other tropical infections modify the immunoglobulins and might alter the response to rheumatoid arthritis, but these tropical infections are far less frequent at Pretoria, South Africa, where Anderson (1970) described similar anomalous features but offered no explanation. As in other auto-immune diseases in Africa, it is important to examine all aspects of the diet, including fibre, and to bear in mind the variation in the structure and function of certain endocrine glands in Africans (p. 325).

E. Multiple sclerosis

Multiple sclerosis (MS) is a disease of unknown aetiology, but there is considerable support for the proposition that auto-immune factors operate in its pathogenesis. MS has a unique epidemiology (Acheson, 1972). In the northern hemisphere of Europe and America, and possibly in the southern hemisphere, there is a correlation with latitude. High-risk areas occur above 40°N; the risk is lower in warmer, semi-tropical latitudes. This broad generalization does not, however, explain the relatively low prevalence of MS in Japan, which is bisected by the 40°N line of latitude. In that country epidemiological data is plentiful, but the disease, even including all possible variations, is rare, as it is in China, North Korea and the eastern U.S.S.R. (Spillane, 1972).

It has been suggested that MS may be due to a slow-acting virus or be a sequel of some universal virus such as that causing measles. The virus might, along with myelin auto-antigens, initiate a myelin sensitization process, which is a manifestation of auto-immunity (Lumsden, 1972). Although symptoms are delayed for many years and usually do not appear until adolescence or later, the disease originates in early life. Careful studies of MS among immigrant populations have shown that the place where childhood and adolescence is spent influences subsequent development of the disease; unknown factors operate at that time either to increase the risk in certain groups or to act as protective factors in others (Dean and Kurtzke, 1971; Brody, 1972).

Studies of immigrants to Israel, Dutch Antilles, Hawaii and South Africa have demonstrated that these groups retain the prevalence rates of the country in which they were born, but if immigration occurs before 15 years of age the risk is altered and approximates to that of the country into which immigration has occurred. In Israel MS was, for instance, found to be five times commoner among 664,581 immigrants from Europe than among 527,000 immigrants from Africa and Asia, indicating that environmental factors altered prevalence (Leibowitz *et al.*, 1969). Since some of the most detailed studies have been performed in Israel, it may be appropriate to note that similar decreased prevalence of other diseases has been detected in immigrants. Ischaemic heart disease (Chapter 15) and diabetes mellitus (Chapter 16) have been less prevalent among Israeli immigrants from Africa and Asia than among those coming from Europe and America. Among many other differences it should be noted that the former ate large amounts of high-fibre carbohydrates, the latter ate moderate amounts of low-fibre carbohydrates.

In South Africa the extensive studies of Dean (1967) indicated a low MS prevalence in South African whites, and showed the disease to be commoner in the South Africa-born English-speaking community (12·7/100,000) than in the South Africa-born Afrikaans-speaking community (3·6/100,000). Not a single case of MS has been diagnosed among the 15 million Bantu, almost all of whom would have received much fibre-rich maize meal during childhood and adolescence. No data has been traced on fibre intakes in the South Africa-born Afrikaans-speaking community, the majority of whom live in rural areas. Personal experience suggests that many still take fibre-rich maize meal porridge, but that the South Africa-born English-speaking community prefer low-fibre breakfast cereals.

In the United States the U.S. whites have only slightly higher prevalence rates of MS than U.S. negroes at all latitudes (Brody, 1972). In Africa, however, MS is extremely rare in all indigenous Africans. No case had been described among Africans south of the Sahara when the matter was reviewed previously (Trowell, 1960c). Recently at Nairobi, Kenya, two cases have been described. On the basis of the histories and neurological examination, including that of the cerebrospinal fluid, the diagnosis was considered to be established "beyond reasonable doubt" (Harries and Foster, 1970).

The evidence suggests that two or three factors may operate in the pathogenesis of MS. The auto-immune process may be initiated by an infective agent such as a virus and the role of latitude and climate may operate either in promoting the development of the disease or the prevalence of the infective agent. Among Africans socio-economic factors may favour infection at an early age in childhood. The possibility that a high-fibre diet may act as a protective factor, or that changes in endocrine structure and function (p. 325) may influence pathogenesis should also be considered. In any study of the role of fibre, attention should be paid not to crude fibre, but to dietary fibre, especially that associated with the starchy foods, since sugar intakes in South African Bantu are almost as high as those in upper-class South African whites (Walker, 1972).

III. Variations in endocrines and leucocytes

A. Thyroid gland

1. Normal African thyroid gland

Compared with Europeans, certain differences have been detected in the normal thyroid gland, examined at autopsy from Africans whose diet and manner of life were still largely traditional. In Cameroun (Olivier, 1945) and Nigeria (Taylor, 1968a), the weight of the normal adult African thyroid gland was about half that considered normal in other continents. This reduction of size and weight did not appear to be explained by the slightly lower body weight. Extravascular aggregates of lymphocytes were seen far less frequently in Nigerian thyroids than would be expected from experience elsewhere; they were seen only twice in more than 1000 sections (Taylor, 1968a).

2. Colloid goitre

In certain areas of Africa colloid goitre is common; it is due to a deficiency of iodine in the water supply. In these areas colloid goitre may be almost the only thyroid disease demanding surgery (Nevill and Kungu, 1969).

3. Thyrotoxicosis

It has been stated that the incidence of thyrotoxicosis is similar in U.S.A. whites and negroes at the present time, but all reports from Africa south of the Sahara emphasize that it is a rare disease among indigenous Africans (Taylor, 1968b), but not among those of Caucasian descent (Trowell, 1960d). According to the surgical records of the Groote Schuur Hospital, Cape Town, 1952–55, a partial thyroidectomy for thyrotoxicosis was performed on 52 South African white women and five white men, and on only a single South African Bantu woman and on no Bantu man. Although white admissions were six times those of the Bantu, this did not explain the great disparity (Kihn, 1957). No recent studies concerning the prevalence of thyrotoxicosis have been traced from South Africa. In Bulawayo, Rhodesia, during 1950–60, thyrotoxicosis was diagnosed in 124 Rhodesian whites, never in the far more numerous Rhodesian Africans (Shee and Houston, 1963). In that country Gelfand (1962) had diagnosed the condition only once in some 30 years of medical experience in that country.

Although the disease was very rare in Nairobi, Kenya, from 1940 to 1959, some nine cases were diagnosed during 1967 and confirmed by the detection of hyperplasia in the portion of gland removed at operation. It was considered that the disease was increasing among Africans at Nairobi, and other towns in Kenya (Wright, 1967; Nevill and Kungu, 1969).

In Nigeria thyroglobulin antibodies at a titre of 1 : 25 or more were detected in 2·5% of Nigerian women over 35 years of age, compared to the value of 19% obtained in a series of English women of the same age living in England (Greenwood and Herrick, 1970). Thyroid auto-antibodies are less common among South African Bantu than among South African whites (p. 321) (Zoutendyk, 1970).

4. Other thyroid diseases

Primary adult myxoedema has not been described in an African (Greenwood, 1968; Taylor, 1968b). Hashimoto's thyroiditis has been diagnosed once in 10 years at the University Hospital, Ibadan, Nigeria (Greenwood, 1968), and one doubtful case in a Bantu has been reported at Johannesburg (Zoutendyk, 1970).

B. Adrenal gland

1. Normal adrenal gland

Detailed studies of the adrenal gland have been made in Uganda males at Kampala (Allbrook, 1956). Twenty-four fresh adrenal glands were removed from men who had suffered sudden traumatic death. The mean adrenal gland-weight was low, 3·8 g (range 2·2–5·3 g), and the adrenal cortex was much smaller than in Europeans; there was no correlation between the weight of this gland and that of the body. In a comparable study in Jamaica a similar decrease in adrenal gland-weight was found (Stirling and Keating, 1958). In both series significantly lower weights were reported than those encountered in U.S.A. negroes, whose adrenal gland weights are comparable to those accepted as normal in the U.S.A. and Europe, the mean weight being 6·9 g in adult men (Swinyard, 1940). The adrenal cortex was considerably smaller in both Uganda Africans and Jamaica negroes than in U.S.A. whites and non-whites.

2. 17-oxosteroid and 17-oxogenic steroid excretions

The 17-oxosteroids in the urine include metabolites of 17-hydroxycorticosteroids formed by the adrenal cortex. In the normal adult male two-thirds of 17-oxosteroid excretion comes from adrenal (cortisol) metabolism, one-third from the testis. In women 17-oxosteroid excretion comes from the adrenal gland alone. In Nigeria the urinary excretions of 17-oxosteroid and oxogenic steroids were studied in two groups of African women (30 nurses and 25 wives of labourers), and in two groups of African men (20 laboratory staff and 25 labourers (Edozien, 1960). The mean excretion of 17-oxosteroids in the urine was 8·5 mg/24 h in nurses and 5·8 mg/24 h in labourers' wives. 17-oxogenic steroid excretion showed comparable changes. The male laboratory assistants also excreted more 17-oxosteroids and more 17-oxogenic steroids in the urine than the labourers. The differences were statistically significant, $P < 0·01$ (17-oxosteroid excretion), $P < 0·001$ (17-oxogenic steroid excretion). European male laboratory assistants in Nigeria had higher excretion of both urinary steroids than had the African male laboratory assistants. Edozien (1960) speculated that the differences in urinary steroid excretion between the Europeans, African technicians and African labourers might relate to the diets characteristic of each group. Among the many differences in their respective diets, the dietary fibre content would increase from the first group to the last.

Similarly, low urinary excretion of 17-oxosteroids has been demonstrated in Chinese and Malay subjects in Malaysia, where Europeans had urinary excretion comparable to that found in Europe and North America, $16·0 ± 4·82$ (range 10·5–27·9) mg/24 h (Lugg and Bowness, 1954). Similar low urinary excretions have been detected in Indians in India (Balasundaram and Naganna, 1972). These corticosteroids influence many aspects of metabolism in the body and may well influence the prevalence and the character of certain chronic non-infective diseases.

3. Addison's disease (and Cushing's syndrome)

No case of Addison's disease had been reported in an African when the matter was reviewed previously (Trowell, 1960e). In the subsequent 6 years only two cases were reported in East Africa, but recently six typical cases have been described in Kenya Africans (Bagshawe and Forrester, 1966).

C. Neutropenia

There have been several reviews of the difficult question of the marked neutropenia present in many Africans (Trowell, 1960f; Shaper and Lewis, 1971). Evidence is accumulating that low neutrophil counts are environmental in origin and are probably caused by diet (Ezeilo, 1972a). Although the polymorph count is low in healthy African subjects, neutrophilic leucocytosis occurs normally in response to infections or during pregnancy (Ezeilo, 1972b).

Ezeilo (1972a) investigated the effect of diet on the neutrophil count of four different groups of healthy persons aged 18–35 years (Fig. 20.1). Two groups (A and B) were Zambians living at Lusaka. Group A comprised 77 Zambian civil servants (68 men, 9 women); they ate a traditional high-fibre maize meal diet. Group B were 87 Zambian students (72 male university students, 15 female nurses); they took semi-westernized food during the term but traditional Zambian meals in the vacation. Group C comprised 47 African male students who had lived in Glasgow for periods varying from 1 day to 12 years. They ate typical British food, as did members of Group D, 30 male European and Asian Glasgow residents.

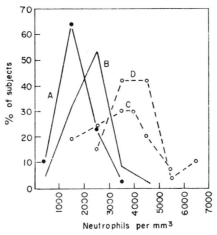

Fig. 20.1. Influence of diet on distribution of neutrophil counts (Ezeilo, 1972a). (A) 77 Zambian civil servants eating traditional high-fibre diets. (B) 87 Zambian students eating semi-westernized diets. (C) 47 Zambian students eating low-fibre British diets. (D) 30 European and Asian students eating low-fibre British diets.

Much neutropenia was found in both African groups in Zambia; 88% of Group A (traditional diet) and 55% of Group B (semi-western diet) had neutrophil counts below 2500/mm³. Only 25% of Groups C and D (both eating British diets) had similarly low neutrophil counts. It is desirable that these observations be submitted to controlled experiments on fully specified diets.

Before these observations of Ezeilo (1972a) had been published, Shaper and Lewis (1971) suggested that the characteristic African neutropenia might be genetic in origin. They had reported some neutropenia in 26 West Indian out-patients and in six West African in-patients in a British hospital, and they referred to the neutropenia detected in American negro men compared to American whites over 30 years ago (Forbes et al., 1941). Clearly more observations are needed on larger numbers of Africans who come to reside in Britain, noting the diet taken before leaving Africa and the duration of stay in Britain. In the U.S.A. in recent years little significant difference has been reported in neutrophil counts in white and negro groups (Broun *et al.*, 1966), indicating that as with other diseases discussed in this book, past differences between these racial groups has almost disappeared. It has been stressed several times in this book that the diet and pattern of disease in American negroes 30 years ago differed from that encountered at the present time. In Africa all investigators agree that neutropenia is not a manifestation of ill-health, that a physiological leucocytosis occurs in response to infections and that there is no correlation between leucopenia, malaria parasite rates, malaria antibodies, or serum protein levels.

Ezeilo (1972a) considered that the African neutropenia was not genetic, but environmental in origin, because (1) neonatal cord blood neutrophil counts were similar in African and European infants born at Lusaka (Ezeilo, 1972b), and (2) western diets decreased the African neutropenia. Yemenite Jews, who also have a lower prevalence of many western diseases than those brought up in Israel, displayed a similar neutropenia (Alkan and Feinaro, 1967). In South Africa, rural Venda men had a lower mean neutrophil count ($3189/mm^3$) than urban Venda men ($3564/mm^3$). One of the many factors distinguishing the rural Yemenite from Israeli Jews and the rural from the urban Venda was the higher dietary fibre content of the diet of the rural groups (Groen *et al.*, 1966; Lubbe, 1971). There is, however, no evidence at present to incriminate this as influencing leucopenia.

References

ACHESON, E. D. (1972). *In* "Multiple Sclerosis" (D. McAlpine, C. E. Lumsden and E. D. Acheson, eds), pp. 3–80. Churchill Livingstone, Edinburgh.

AHRENS, L. and BROCK, J. P. (1954). *South African Journal of Clinical Sciences* 5, 20.

ALKAN, W. J. and FEINARO, M. (1967). *Israel Economist* 23, 81.

ALLBROOK, D. (1956). *Lancet* 2, 606.

ANDERSON, I. F. (1970). *South African Medical Journal* 44, 1227.

BAGSHAWE, A. F. and FORRESTER, A. T. T. (1966). *East African Medical Journal* 43, 525.

BALASUNDARAM, D. and NAGANNA, A. (1972). *Journal of the Indian Medical Association* 59, 6.

BRODY, J. (1972). *British Medical Journal* 2, 173.

BROUN, G. O. Jr., HERBIG, F. K. and HAMILTON, J. R. (1966). *New England Journal of Medicine* 275, 1410.

DEAN, G. (1967). *British Medical Journal* 1, 724.

DEAN, G. and KURTZKE, J. F. (1971). *British Medical Journal* 2, 725.

EDOZIEN, J. C. (1960). *Lancet* **1**, 258.

ENGEL, A. and BIRCH, T. A. (1967). *Arthritis and Rheumatism* **10**, 61.

EZEILO, G. C. (1972a). *Lancet* **2**, 1003.

EZEILO, G. C. (1972b). *Tropical and Geographical Medicine* **24**, 152.

FORBES, J. I. and GORDON, J. A. (1969). *Central African Journal of Medicine* **15**, 92.

FORBES, W. H., JOHNSON, R. E. and CONSOLAZIO, F. (1941). *American Journal of Medical Science* **201**, 407.

GEAR, J. H. (1946). *Transactions Royal Society of Tropical Medicine and Hygiene* **39**, 301.

GELFAND, M. (1962). *Central African Journal of Medicine* **8**, 123.

GELFAND, M. (1969). *Central African Journal of Medicine* **15**, 131.

GREENWOOD, B. M. (1968). *Lancet* **2**, 380.

GREENWOOD, B. M. and FRANCIS, T. I. (1967). *West African Medical Journal* **16**, 97.

GREENWOOD, B. M. and HERRICK, E. M. (1970). *British Medical Journal* **1**, 70.

GROEN, J. J., BALOGH, M. and YARRON, E. (1966). *Israel Journal of Medical Science* **2**, 196.

HALL, L. (1966). *East African Medical Journal* **44**, 161.

HARRIES, J. R. and FOSTER, R. M. (1970). *East African Medical Journal* **47**, 693.

KANYEREZI, B. R. (1969). *East African Medical Journal* **46**, 71.

KIHN, R. B. (1957). *South African Journal of Laboratory and Clinical Medicine* **3**, 71.

KINNEAR, A. A. (1956). *South African Journal of Laboratory and Clinical Medicine* **2**, 263.

LEIBOWITZ, U., KAHANA, E. and ALTER, M. (1969). *Lancet* **2**, 1323.

LICHTMAN, M. A., HAMES, C. G. and McDONOUGH, J. R. (1965). *American Journal of Clinical Nutrition* **16**, 492.

LUBBE, A. M. (1971). *South African Medical Journal* **45**, 1289.

LUGG, J. W. H. and BOWNESS, J. M. (1954). *Nature* **174**, 1147.

LUMSDEN, C. E. (1972). *In* "Multiple Sclerosis" (D. McAlpine, C. E. Lumsden and E. D. Acheson, eds), pp. 311–621. Churchill Livingstone, Edinburgh.

MNGOLA, E. N. (1968). *East African Medical Journal* **45**, 669.

MULLER, A. S., VALKENBURG, H. A. and GREENWOOD, B. A. (1972). *East African Medical Journal* **49**, 75.

NEVILL, G. and KUNGU, A. (1969). *East African Medical Journal* **46**, 598.

OLIVIER, G. (1945). *Bulletins et mémoires de la Société anatomique de Paris* **6**, 146.

ROWE, D. S., MACGREGOR, I. A., SMITH, S. J., HALL, P. and WILLIAMS, K. (1968). *Clinical and Experimental Immunology* **3**, 63.

SHAPER, A. G. and LEWIS, P. (1971). *Lancet* **2**, 1021.

SHEE, C. J. and HOUSTON, W. (1963). *Central African Journal of Medicine* **9**, 267.

SPILLANE, J. D. (1972). *British Medical Journal* **1**, 506.

STIRLING, G. A. and KEATING, V. J. (1958). *British Medical Journal* **2**, 1016.

SWINYARD, C. A. (1940). *Anatomical Record* **76**, 69.

TAYLOR, J. R. (1968). *East African Medical Journal* **45**, (a) p. 383; (b) p. 390.

TROWELL, H. (1960). "Non-infective Disease in Africa." Edward Arnold, London. (a) pp. 461–472; (b) p. 387; (c) pp. 258–261; (d) pp. 286–289; (e) p. 2; (f) pp. 428–429.
WALKER, A. R. P. (1972). *South African Medical Journal* **46**, 1127.
WOODS, J. D. and RYMER, J. J. H. (1955). *Lancet* **2**, 1274.
WRIGHT, C. J. (1967). *East African Medical Journal* **44**, 455.
ZOUTENDYK, A. (1970). *South African Medical Journal* **44**, 469.

Part X

Chapter 21

Concluding considerations

HUGH TROWELL and DENIS BURKITT

I. The overall picture. 333
II. Processing carbohydrate foods 334
   A. Starch 334
   B. Sugar 335
III. Processing fats 335
IV. Modern western diets 336
   A. Characteristics 336
   B. Rising sugar intakes 336
   C. Rising fat intakes 337
V. Inter-relationships between some non-infective diseases of the large bowel (appendicitis, constipation, diverticular disease, irritable colon, polyps, carcinoma) 337
VI. Fibre 338
   A. The connecting link in the inter-relationships of certain diseases 338
   B. Definitions of crude fibre and dietary fibre 340
   C. Fibre requirements 340
VII. Epidemiological observations and postulated mechanisms . . 342
   A. Epidemiology 342
   B. Relative times of emergence 342
   C. Mechanisms 343
VIII. Any other hypothesis? 343
IX. Some practical considerations of diet 344
References 345

I. The overall picture

Various results, which are considered to be attributable to refined carbohydrate foods, have been described in the chapters of this book. Separately they can be viewed as trees which collectively comprise a wood. This wood must be surveyed as a whole in order to examine adequately the fundamental concept, which was set forth first by Cleave (1956) and elaborated in later studies (Cleave and Campbell, 1966; Cleave et al., 1969) that the refining of carbohydrate foods has three different aspects, each of which could be responsible for a raised prevalence of different diseases: (1) concentration of the carbohydrate component leading to over-consumption of food, (2) removal of fibre, (3) removal of protein. Cleave considered that each of the diseases discussed were examples of what he called "The Saccharine Disease", meaning "related to sugar". Stimulated by this hypothesis and also by his far-reaching epidemiological studies in Africa and Asia, we undertook our present enquiry.

II. Processing carbohydrate foods

A. Starch

When wheat is milled to form white refined flour three changes occur:

(1) fibre content is considerably reduced;
(2) some of the starch granules are separated physically from their close proximity to fibre, celluloses, hemicelluloses and lignin;
(3) absorbable nutrients—protein, fat, mineral salts, vitamins and trace elements—are somewhat reduced.

Research has concentrated on the identification of these absorbable nutrients which, if deemed advisable, can be returned to the flour for its enrichment. Almost no attention has been paid by nutritionalists to the other changes which result in (1) a reduced intake of all the constituents of fibre, (2) the presence of fibre-depleted starch, (3) the possibility of consuming large amounts of calorie-rich sugar and vegetable fat, both devoid of fibre.

The milling of wheat divides the grain into two main portions, (1) white flour 70% extraction, (2) the remainder, some 30%, which contains the bran. White flour contains 5% more calories and 9% less protein than an equal weight of wholemeal flour. It is therefore a misuse of the word "concentrated", as often used, to refer to white flour as a concentrated food, which suggests that it could easily be over-consumed because it is concentrated. Statements to this effect have carried little weight with nutritionalists. White flour, 70% extraction, can be truthfully described as fibre-depleted starch, its crude fibre having been reduced 95% compared with wholemeal flour. In Britain by about 1870 ordinary white flour probably contained crude fibre 0·2–0·5%; at the present time it contains about 0·1%.

Since not only the fibre content but also the consumption of bread and cereal products has fallen considerably during the past hundred years, the intake of cereal crude fibre has probably fallen to about one-sixth of the 1870 level. Fruit and vegetables contain fibre, but this differs in chemical composition and in some of its actions on the gastrointestinal tract of man, and it surrounds little starch. Since *refining* is usually taken to mean removing impurities, it is incorrect to speak of white flour as refined flour, that is, free of impurities. It should be called *highly milled* flour.

B. Sugar

It is correct to speak of sugar as a refined food, for many impurities have been removed from the unrefined sugar juice, produced by crushing the cane. Whether sugar cane is crushed by machinery, as in Europe, or by human teeth, as in Africa, the unrefined juice contains negligible amounts of fibre. Although manufactured sugar has been concentrated six times from the unrefined juice, its chemical composition remains almost unchanged. As sugar is palatable, cheap and soluble, large amounts can be added as an invisible constituent of food and drink. This change is usually the first to occur in the westernization of diets in Africa and Asia. Sugar consumption then rises rapidly until it approaches that of western diets, providing nearly 20% of daily calories. Consumption levels then tend to remain stationary, as in Britain since 1957, or decline slightly, as has occurred in the U.S.A. since the 1930s. Sugar is a high-energy concentrated food containing 400 kcal/100 g.

III. Processing fats

Fats and oils are actually the highest energy foods, containing 900 kcal/100 g. In the northern countries of Europe and America during the nineteenth century, butter and animal fats, but little vegetable oil and no margarine, were available. The processing of vegetable oils and subsequent hydrogenation is a modern phenomenon; it has only been done in the present century. All vegetable oils are concentrated some three to five times from sources such as olives, soya beans and peanuts in which they are contained within cell-walls of fibre. Vegetable fats and oils contain no fibre. The consumption of fat, sugar and protein (especially animal protein) is usually low in underdeveloped countries in which the diet contains much fibre-rich lightly processed starchy food. This provides the total energy intake which, by western standards, is low, but the stature of people in these countries is often smaller than that of westerners, and the body weight remains relatively stationary throughout life, even though there might be greater physical activity.

IV. Modern western diets

A. Characteristics

When the diet of people in an underdeveloped country becomes urbanized or "westernized", the result is usually an increased consumption of sugar, then of fat (both of which are fibre-free), accompanied by a reduction in starchy carbohydrate food, and if this becomes more highly milled there is a consequent reduction in fibre intake, as shown in the diet of urbanized Bantu (Fig. 21.1).

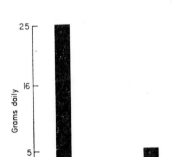

FIG. 21.1. The reduction in the fibre content of the diet that occurs when Africans move from a rural to an urban situation. (From Lubbe, 1971.)

B. Rising sugar intakes

All contributors view with much misgiving the present high level of sugar consumption in western nations. As regards dental caries, one might advise that very little sugar should be taken in the diet, especially between meals, but otherwise no firm basis has been established concerning recommended levels of sugar in the diet of adults. The problem appears to have two aspects: the possible injurious effects of sugar, and effects attributed to the reduced consumption of starchy carbohydrate and its fibre.

It is suggested that sugar and white flour are both implicated as factors in the production of gallstones. It is also considered that high intake of sugar is one of many factors that promotes obesity in some but by no means all persons. Any dietary factors that promote obesity, such as sugar, and to a lesser extent fats and alcohol, will increase the severity of many diseases, and may influence directly the development of some, such as maturity-onset diabetes. Obesity is also commonly associated with gall-stones, hypertension, possibly ischaemic heart disease, arthritis of the weight-bearing joints and other conditions. Many animal experiments can be cited in which diets containing sucrose, 50–80% of the energy, have led to pathological processes. Such diets are highly artificial, especially in animals unaccustomed to eating any manufactured sucrose in their natural diet; it does not follow that sucrose, 20% of the energy, promotes these diseases in man.

It is felt that the whole weight of evidence is in favour of a reduced intake of sugar and an increased consumption of whole cereal products in the diet at all ages. The editors started their enquiry considerably stimulated by Cleave's hypothesis of the major role of sugar. As their investigations proceeded, quite independently, they began to lay more emphasis on the beneficial effects of adequate fibre intake and the ill-effects of fibre deficiency.

C. Rising fat intakes

This study was planned to consider only refined carbohydrate foods, but at times it has been considered that the increased consumption of fat, or certain varieties of fat, has probably been conducive to the development of obesity, maturity-onset diabetes and other diseases associated with obesity. Saturated fat raises serum cholesterol levels and probably increases the risk of ischaemic heart disease.

V. Inter-relationships between some non-infective diseases of the large bowel (appendicitis, constipation, diverticular disease, irritable colon, polyps, carcinoma)

The geographical and, where it can be determined, socio-economic distribution of these non-infective diseases of the bowel, is closely similar when allowance is made for the fact that some may require a longer exposure to a new environment than do others before becoming clinically apparent. Appendicitis even in economically advanced countries is primarily a disease of younger age-groups. It became prominent in the western world several decades before an appreciable rise in the prevalence of diverticular disease. Although the time of emergence of benign or malignant tumours of the bowel as important clinical problems in the western world is uncertain, the prevalence of these diseases has not been observed to rise in developing countries until some decades after a rise in appendicitis. Apart from appendicitis, all these illnesses are characteristic of later life. It is significant that appendicitis (Boland, 1942), diverticular disease (Kocour, 1937), bowel cancer (Quinland and Cuff, 1940; Steiner, 1954) and adenomatous polyps (Helwig, 1947) were all significantly less frequent in American negroes than in whites some 30–40 years ago, but that approximate parity in incidence between these groups has since been reached. The geographical association between these non-infective diseases of the bowel is illustrated by the fact that in more industrialized Sweden both bowel cancer (Doll et al., 1966) and diverticular disease (Kohler, 1963) are three times as prevalent as they are in southern Finland.

All these considerations suggest that there is some causative factor common to each of these non-infective diseases of the large bowel. This does not imply that the common factor postulated is the sole factor, or even the major factor. Probably all diseases, especially chronic non-infective disorders, are multifactorial, and result from interaction of genetic inheritance and sex with various environmental factors. It is suggested, however, that fibre-depleted starchy carbohydrates play an important role in the pathogenesis of each of these diseases of the large bowel and that this may be the factor that links them so closely epidemiologically.

Sucrose is normally digested and absorbed in the small intestine and is unlikely to influence these diseases of the large bowel unless there is a failure of either of these functions. Variations in the fat and protein content of the diet may play a part, but both of these are normally largely digested and absorbed in the small intestine. Fibre is not digested in the small intestine but is partially hydrolysed by bacteria in the large bowel. Dietary fibre, a complex of celluloses, hemicelluloses and lignin, varies in its composition; a deficiency or absence of some elements may have a greater influence than others on the production of certain diseases. The possible protective role of fibre in the pathogenesis of diseases of the large bowel is not a new suggestion; it has been advanced by workers in England (Dimock, 1937), South Africa (Walker, 1947, 1961; Bersohn et al., 1956) and East Africa (Trowell, 1960).

VI. Fibre

A. The connecting link in the inter-relationships of certain diseases

An attempt has been made to depict diagrammatically the inter-relationships of many diseases so as to illustrate the suggested links between the postulated fundamental cause—fibre deficiency—and the diseases thereby produced (Fig. 21.2). The diseases have been classified according to whether the major causative factor is postulated to be (1) deficiency of dietary fibre, (2) the presence of fibre-depleted starch, or (3) a high consumption of refined sugar. Considerable simplification has been necessary in order to emphasize the main points in the general hypothesis, and the possible role of refined fats has been omitted. This hypothesis must be considered tentative, and further investigation will doubtless lead to its modification. It must be emphasized that at all stages of each pathological process other factors, largely unidentified, certainly contribute, and modify the disease.

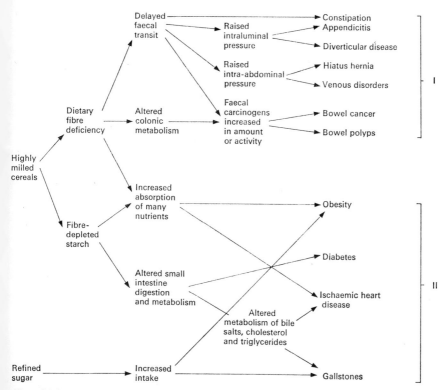

FIG. 21.2. Diagrammatic representation of the mechanisms whereby the diseases listed are postulated to result from the consumption of fibre-depleted carbohydrate foods.

It will be noted that in all diseases discussed in Chapters 8–17 of this book, dietary fibre is considered to play an important role. This appears most manifest in diseases of the colon and those associated with constipation (Group I). These stand on the right at the head of the list, and certain mechanisms have been clearly defined. The role of fibre and/or fibre-depleted carbohydrates in altering digestion and metabolism within the small intestine is suggested (Group II), but requires further evaluation by experiments in animals and man.

The diagram does not include duodenal ulcer (Chapter 18), as its relationship to diet remains uncertain. The auto-immune and endocrine diseases discussed in Chapter 20 have not been included in Fig. 21.2 because the epidemiological data is scanty, and no metabolic mechanisms can be suggested, nor animal experiments cited, which link these diseases to diet. Nevertheless there is strong evidence that they are extremely rare or mild in Africans consuming traditional diets, that they are beginning to appear in urban groups, and their incidence in U.S. negroes is almost similar to that in the U.S. white population. The aetiology of these diseases remains unknown.

B. Definitions of crude fibre and dietary fibre

The term "crude fibre" has come from the farmers and agricultural chemists who by international agreement have defined it as the portion of flour that resists digestion by dilute acid and dilute alkali. The confusion concerning the meaning of "fibre" is increased because most food tables refer to fibre as "carbohydrate by difference". This includes the celluloses, hemicelluloses and lignin that are derived from the cell-walls. It has been suggested that this group of substances be called dietary fibre. Dietary fibre is very similar to the unavailable carbohydrate and lignin. The crude fibre of wheat wholemeal is 2·0%, but its dietary fibre (celluloses, hemicelluloses and lignin) is 11·0%. In the context of human nutrition fibre has not been adequately defined. Food tables do not report the amounts of celluloses, hemicelluloses and lignin present in food. Analysis is time-consuming and involves numerous technical difficulties. The dietary fibre content of most foods has not been estimated.

C. Fibre requirements

The threshold of fibre requirements to protect against different diseases is still unknown and is likely to remain so for a long time. It is not a single substance, cellulose, but a group of substances. All analyses of the various constituents of dietary fibre stress that it differs considerably in chemical composition and physical structure according to its sources. It is a common observation that bran is laxative, and an equal amount of crude fibre derived from many fruits and vegetables does not often have a similar effect.

During the period 1925–50 the relatively sudden emergence as important clinical conditions of such diseases as diverticular disease and ischaemic heart disease in persons usually aged 50–70 years suggests that the required threshold in the case of these diseases may have been reached some 40–50 years previously, say about 1880–90, since it requires several decades of exposure in susceptible individuals before these diseases become clinically apparent. Although the daily intake of fibre associated with starchy foods, cereals and potatoes, had been falling for most of the eighteenth and nineteenth centuries, but the evident rarity of ischaemic heart disease and diverticular disease at that time suggests that there was sufficient dietary fibre to satisfy requirements and prevent these diseases in most persons. The great change appeared to occur towards the end of the nineteenth century.

Many may be tempted to feel that the addition of a small amount of bran to the daily food will correct any deficiency. While it is true that the arrival of more hemicellulose and cellulose once or twice a day into the large bowel might benefit certain colonic disorders, such as constipation and diverticular disease, it is unlikely to alter much the digestion of fibre-depleted starch granules and many other chemical and physical conditions in the small intestine. Experimental evidence, albeit on the cholesterol-fed rat, suggests that bran added to the diet is far less effective than an equal amount of crude fibre in whole cereals in reducing serum cholesterol levels (Vijayagopalan and Kurup, 1970). Possibly the chief action will be found to lie in the influence of fibre-rich foods on triglyceride metabolism. All this adds another element of uncertainty in any attempt to state requirements of dietary fibre. It will probably be more important to envisage requirements of fibre-rich carbohydrate foods. The concept of threshold requirements is depicted in Fig. 21.3.

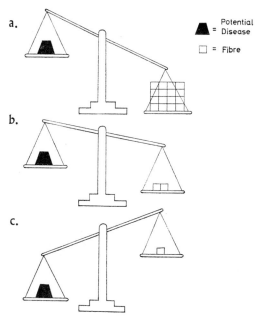

FIG. 21.3. Postulated thresholds of fibre requirements sufficient to protect from disease: (a) much more fibre than required; (b) great reduction but sufficient for requirements; (c) insufficient to avoid disease.

VII. Epidemiological observations and postulated mechanisms

A. Epidemiology

The epidemiology of the characteristically western diseases outlined in this book appears factual, although additional information may well necessitate substantial modifications and demonstrate local variations. More data from different countries and communities are required, especially with reference to changes that occur on migration. Careful prospective studies of the prevalence of disease in relation to age and sex are specially desirable. The geographical distribution and inter-relationships and chronological emergence of these diseases can be observed, as can inter-relationships both in clinical and autopsy studies. These should be related to the diet that has been eaten throughout life.

B. Relative times of emergence

Some of these diseases apparently depend on a lesser intensity of, or a shorter exposure to, complex dietary factors than do others, and as a result of this the prevalence of certain diseases appears always to rise before that of others (Fig. 21.4). Not only does the incidence of appendicitis always

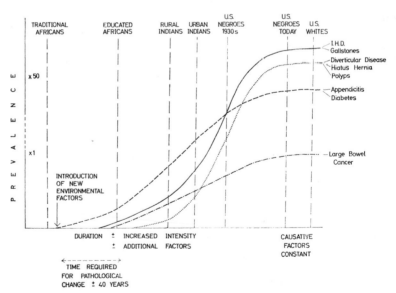

FIG. 21.4. Diagrammatic representation of the fact that different diseases, postulated to result in part from common causative factors, emerge as important clinical entities at varying times after the introduction of the new environmental factor, and subsequently increase in prevalence at different rates.

rise some decades before that of the other non-infective diseases of the large bowel but no situation has been found wherein varicose veins have become common while haemorrhoids are still rare, although the reverse frequently occurs.

C. Mechanisms

The epidemiological association of many of these diseases with dietary fibre intakes appears factual; this, however, does not prove that the relationship is causative; it may be a purely fortuitous association. The suggested mechanisms of pathogenesis must in most instances be deemed to be only speculative. They are, however, consistent with epidemiology, dietary intakes and suggestions derived from the results of animal experiments. In constipation, diverticular disease, perhaps obesity, and even gallstones, the supporting evidence seems to have passed beyond the stage of mere "hypothesis" and justifies the title of "theory". In other diseases mentioned in Chapters 8–17, the basic concept rests on a modicum of epidemiological data and a few clues suggested by animal experiments. The role of a deficiency of fibre in the alimentary tract and/or that of the consumption of fibre-depleted carbohydrate foods has been considered as a possible cause, or causes, common to each disease, but not as exclusively responsible for any. The possible common factor of fibre has been diagrammatically represented as a connecting link which might explain the associations between these diseases (Fig. 21.5).

VIII. Any other hypothesis?

This approach, which may be considered as a major modification of Cleave's original hypothesis, is bound to meet with criticism. Its very simplicity has been offensive to some, as if complicated explanations were more likely to be valid than simple ones. In its defence the question may be asked, "What alternative hypothesis is there to explain the epidemiology and inter-relationships of the diseases in question?"

To others it will appear as if we have modified this hypothesis beyond recognition. With due apologies to Surgeon Captain T. L. Cleave, R.N., we can only say that this is nothing compared to the modification that will be produced by our successors. Doubtless many conclusions drawn will require amendment even before the book is published. Certain fundamental aspects of the hypothesis outlined in this book are diagrammatically represented in Fig. 21.2. This diagram represents a gross simplification; it illustrates only one facet of a complex picture of causation.

Multiple causes of diseases

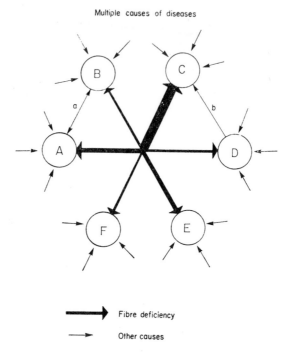

→ Fibre deficiency

→ Other causes

Fig. 21.5. Diagrammatic representation of the fact that a number of different diseases, each resulting from multiple causes, many have one causative factor in common. This may be a more or less predominant factor in different diseases, and would result in an association between these diseases. Two or more diseases may have a causative influence on one another (a), or one disease may play a causative role on another without the reverse being true (b).

IX. Some practical considerations of diet

It seems fitting to conclude with a few essentially practical comments. It is important to recognize that fibre varies according to its source; that derived from cereals is different in many respects from that of fruit and vegetables. The question is often asked, "What, in practice, is a high-fibre diet, and what are the most important changes recommended in eating habits?" A counsel of perfection is usually unacceptable and unnecessary. It is desirable to increase the consumption of all unprocessed or lightly processed cereal products. These are rich in cereal fibre, and include wholemeal bread, oatmeal porridge, whole cereal wafers, high-fibre breakfast cereals such as All-Bran and Weetabix, also potatoes. Leguminous seeds and cabbage are also rich in fibre and are laxative. These foods have a high satiety value, i.e. a high satiety/energy (calorie) ratio (Heaton, 1973), or a high fibre/energy (calorie) ratio, and do not normally predispose to obesity. At the same time it is desirable to decrease the consumption of such refined carbohydrate foods as white flour, white rice and sugar, which include sweets, confectionery, white bread, cake and biscuits; also sweetened drinks and alcohol. The addition of sugar to tea and coffee should be curtailed. If extra sweetness is required, artificial sweetners can be used, as they are, in the small amounts taken, believed to be safer than sugar. All these foods have a low satiety/energy (calorie) ratio, or a low fibre/energy (calorie) ratio.

Since it is unlikely that refined carbohydrate foods will be totally avoided, and only unrefined carbohydrate foods consumed, it is advised that cereal fibre, preferably in the form of bran, be added to food in sufficient quantities to ensure the passage of at least one soft stool daily. Needs vary considerably, but most people require one to three dessertspoonsful a day which can be readily taken with breakfast cereals or soup or mixed with fruit juice or milk.

References

BERSOHN, I., WALKER, A. R. P. and HIGGINSON, J. (1956). *South African Medical Journal* 30, 411.

BOLAND, F. K. (1942). *Annals of Surgery* 115, 939.

CLEAVE, T. L. (1956). *Journal of the Royal Naval Medical Service* 40, 116.

CLEAVE, T. L. and CAMPBELL, G. D. (1966). "Diabetes, Coronary Thrombosis and the Saccharine Disease." John Wright, Bristol.

CLEAVE, T. L., CAMPBELL, G. D. and PAINTER, N. S. (1969). "Diabetes, Coronary Thrombosis and the Saccharine Disease", 2nd edition. John Wright, Bristol.

DIMOCK, E. M. (1937). *British Medical Journal* 1, 906.

DOLL, R., PAYNE, P. and WATERHOUSE, J. (1966). "Cancer Incidence in Five Continents", pp. 162, 192. International Union Against Cancer. Springer-Verlag, Berlin.

HEATON, K. W. (1973). *Lancet* 2, 1418.

HELWIG, E. B. (1947). *Surgery, Gynecology and Obstetrics* 84, 36.

KOCOUR, E. J. (1937). *American Journal of Surgery* 37, 430.

KOHLER, R. (1963). *Acta chirurgica scandinavica* 126, 148.

LUBBE, A. M. (1971). *South African Medical Journal* 45, 1289.

QUINLAND, W. S. and CUFF, J. R. (1940). *Archives of Surgery* 30, 393.

STEINER, P. E. (1954). "Cancer. Race and Geography", pp. 75–81. Williams and Wilkins, Baltimore.

TROWELL, H. (1960). "Non-infective Disease in Africa", pp. 216–219. Edward Arnold, London.

VIJAYAGOPALAN, P. and KURUP, P. A. (1970). *Atherosclerosis* 11, 257.

WALKER, A. R. P. (1947). *South African Medical Journal* 21, 590.

WALKER, A. R. P. (1961). *South African Medical Journal* 35, 114.

Index

A

Aborigines, 54, 229, 241
Absorption, 59, 61
Addison's disease, 321, 327
Agar-agar, 206
Agricultural Revolution, 241
Alcohol, 198, 244, 291, 305, 345
Aleurone, 25, 48
Amelogenesis imperfecta, 266
Amylase, 23
Amylopectin, 28
Angina pectoris, 201, 202
Ankylosing spondylitis, 323
Apocholic acid, 128
Appendicitis, 37, 38, 337, 339, 342,
   Chapter 8
Apricots, 27
Arabinans, 28, 34
Arabinoxylans, 28, 34
Aristotle, 255
Artichokes, 30
Astronauts, 78
Auto-immune bodies, 320
Auto-immune diseases, 320–322, 339
Avicenna, 228

B

Balloons, 79, 80
Bananas, 27, 31
Barley, 24, 25, 31, 34, 43, 44, 207, 238
Beans, 32, 63, 91, 127, 208, 214, 236,
   302
Beetroot, 27, 240
Bengal gram, 210

Beri-beri, 36
Bran, 24, 25, 31, 37, 44, 48–50, 65, 66,
   69, 77, 78, 108, 110, 111, 113,
   189, 205, 206, 213, 215, 263,
   303–305, 334, 341, 345
Bowel cancer, 38, 316, 337-339, 342,
   Chapter 10
Bread
   brown, 24, 69, 78, 242, 304
   National, 54, 304
   white, 24, 37, 54–56, 60–64, 77,
   78, 93, 111, 112, 137, 199, 207,
   213, 215, 237, 242–244, 268, 302,
   304, 345
   wholemeal, 27, 36, 37, 60–63, 64,
   77, 78, 111, 195, 199–201, 209,
   242, 268
Brinjal, 304
Bushmen, 54, 229
Butter, 25, 53, 77, 112, 211, 214, 242,
   243

C

Cabbage, 63, 304
Calculi, renal, 50
Carbohydrate intolerance, 138
Carmine capsules, 70–72, 78
Cassava, 26, 31, 45, 179, 286, 291,
   302, 303
Chaff, 24, 48
Chalk, 24, 50
Cheese, 32, 53
Chenodeoxycholate, 65, 186, 188
Cholate (cholic acid), 65, 183, 210
Cholecystitis, 37

Cholestyramine, 127
Chupatties, 69, 199–201, 236, 286, 301, 302
Cineradiography, 80, 81, 107
Constipation, 38, 337, 339
Corn, *see* Maize
Corn flakes, 24
Coronary heart disease, 180, 181, Chapter 15
Crohn's disease, 64, Chapter 11

D

Darwin, Charles, 241
Dates, 27, 32, 240
Deep vein thrombosis (DVT), 38, 167, 313, Chapter 12
Dental caries, 38, 54, 315, Chapter 17
Deoxycholate (deoxycholic acid) 65, 127, 128, 188–190, 210
Dextrin, 28
Dhal, 304
Diabetes, 35, 37, 38, 47, 54, 61, 180, 181, 189, 195, 196, 212, 216, 220, 221, 315, 324, 337, 339, Chapter 16
Diabetes insipidus, 228
Digestion, 59, 61, 63
Diverticular disease, 38, 47, 155, 167, 168, 202, 243, 280, 302, 304, 337–343, Chapter 9

E

Eggs, 32, 243
Embryo, *see* Germ
Endosperm, 24, 25, 44, 48, 49
Energy/fibre ratio, 243–245, 344, 345
Energy/satiety ratio, 180, 344, 345
Eskimos, 1, 54, 177, 179, 221, 229, 261

F

Fenugreek, 32
Fibre, dietary, 27-30, 33, 48, 63-65, 70, 92, 93, 110, 130, 182, 200, 206, 207, 211, 214, 216, 218, 305, 338, 340, 341
Fibrinolysis, 217–220
Fish, 32
Flour,
　National, 50, 202, 231–233, 304
　white, 25, 37, 44, 49–51, 53, 54, 56, 93, 94, 138, 205, 213, 214, 231–233, 236, 239, 241, 286, 302, 334, 335, 345
　wholemeal, 24, 44, 49, 50, 213, 334, 340
Fluorides (fluoridation), 252, 258, 259, 269
Fluorosis, 266

G

Galactans, 30, 34
Galactose, 34
Gallstones, 38, 66, 167, 168, 216, 314, 336, 337, 339, 342, 343, Chapter 14
Gcfarnate, 304
Germ (embryo), 48, 49, 263
Glucans, 34
Glycuronans, 35
Goitre, colloid, 325
Grapes, 27
Groundnuts, 32, 127, 295
Guinea corn, 302
Gum (arabic) 30, 206

H

Haemorrhoids, 38, 343, Chapter 12
Hashimoto's thyroiditis, 321, 322, 326
Heartburn, 61
Hemicellusoses (pentosans), 24, 27–30, 33, 34, 48, 63, 110, 127, 130, 206. 210, 214, 338, 340, 341
Hiatus hernia, 38, 339, 342, Chapter 13
Hinton's method, 71, 73

Hippocrates, 69
Hominy, 45
Hookworms, 299, 300, 305
Horse gram, 32
Hottentots, 229
Hypertension, 195, 196, 221, 337
Hyperuricaemia, 196
Hypothalamus, 242

I

Immunoglobulins, 320
Ingestion, 59, 60
Iron, 24, 50
Irritable colon, 38, 113, 337, Chapter 9
Ischaemic heart disease (IHD), 35–38, 47, 54, 61, 130, 131, 167, 233, 280, 324, 337, 339, 340, 342, Chapter 15

K

Kurd Jews, 238
Kwashiorkor, 55

L

Laplanders, 229
Lecithin, 183, 184
Lentil, 32
Lichen, 54
Lignin, 27–29, 30, 32, 33, 35, 214, 216, 338, 340
Liquorice, 304
Lithocholate, Chapter 14
Lupus erythematosus, 321

M

Maize (corn) 24, 31, 45, 50, 54, 55, 61, 91, 179, 199, 201, 208, 209, 217, 236, 237, 241, 244, 263, 291, 295, 302, 305, 320, 324, 328
Maltose, 23

Manioc, see Cassava
Mannans, 34
Maoris, 55
Masai, 7, 79, 179
Melon seeds, 70, 78
Methyl-cellulose, 112, 183, 206
Milk, 25, 32, 37, 53, 112, 179, 242–245, 261, 286
Millet, 24, 25, 31, 45, 70, 179, 201, 205, 236, 238, 286, 291, 295, 302, 304, 305
Moss, 54
Multiple sclerosis, 323, 324
Myasthenia gravis, 321, 322
Myocardial infarction, see Ischaemic heart disease
Myxoedema, 326

N

Navajo Indians, 254, 262
Neutropenia, 327, 329
Niacin, 24, 45, 49
Nomads, 78, 79

O

Oatmeal, 24, 51, 179
Oats, 24, 25, 31, 34, 45, 207, 208, 214, 216, 263
Obesity, 25, 35–38, 53, 54, 64, 165–168, 179, 180, 188, 189, 196, 212, 216, 221, 315, 336, 337, 339, 343, Chapter 16
Oesophagitis, 161
Osteoporosis, 50

P

Peanuts, 34, 263
Peas, 27, 32, 302
Pecans, 263
Pectin, 206, 207, 210, 211
Pellagra, 45

Pentosans, *see* Hemicelluloses
Peptides, 63
Pericarp, 25, 48
Perityphlitis, 91
Pernicious anaemia, 321, 322
Phleboliths, 156
Phosphates, 264
Phytate (phytic acid), 50, 263–266
Pima Indians, 54, 175, 181, 241
Plantain, 31, 127, 201, 291, 302
Polyps, 316, 337–339, 342, Chapter 10
Polyuronides, 35
Porridge, 51
Potatoes, 26, 31, 45, 51–53, 179, 196, 198, 201, 207, 208, 242, 261, 340
Potatoes, sweet, 27, 31, 45, 91, 291, 302
Pressures, intracolonic, 79–82, 111–113, 155
Pro-Banthine, 82, 113
Prostigmin, 82, 112
Pulmonary embolism, 144, 148, 152, 217, 218, 313

R

Red Indians, 54
Reflux, 61, 165
Regurgitation, 61, 161
Reilly's operation, 111
Reiter's disease, 323
Rheumatic heart disease, 202
Rheumatoid arthritis, 321–323
Riboflavin, 24, 49
Rice, 25, 31, 36, 45, 55, 91, 93, 199, 200, 205, 206, 208, 214, 235, 236, 239, 286, 288, 291, 302, 304, 345
  parboiled, 25, 235
Rickets, 50
Roots, 26, 27
Ruminants, 29
Rye, 24, 31, 44

S

Saccharine disease, 37, 38, 334
Sago, 31
Saliva, 60, 62, 63, 263, 301
Scurvy, 258
Seaweeds, 206
Segmentation, 81, 82, 108, 110, 113
Sieves, 43, 44, 238
Smoking, 196, 198, 202, 221, 286, 305
Sorghum, 31, 205, 295, 302
Spinach, 206
Starch, 23, 24, 28, 43, 44, 47, 48, 50, 63, 168, 215, 221, 257, 334
Still's disease, 321, 322
Stool consistency, 72, 78, 79
Subacute combined degeneration, 321
Sugar beet, 25, 34, 46
Sugar cane, 25, 31, 46, 291, 335
Systemic sclerosis, 321

T

Tapioca, 205
Taurocholate, 189
Thiamin, 24, 36, 49, 50
Thyrotoxicosis, 321, 325
Transit times, 37, 38, 64, 94, 110, 129, Chapter 7
Tristan da Cunha, 261, 262, 267
Trypsin, 63
Tubers, 26, 27

U

Ulcerative colitis, 38, 321, 322, Chapter 11

V

Varicose veins, 38, 167, 200, 343, Chapter 12
Vegans, 77

Vegetarians, 76, 77, 126, 286
Venus of Willendorf, 241

W

Wheat, wholemeal (*see also* Flour, wholemeal), 24, 31, 55, 302, 340

X

Xylans, 28, 34

Y

Yams, 26, 31, 291, 302
Yemenite Jews, 200, 229, 238, 329

Postscript

DENIS BURKITT and HUGH TROWELL

The literature of this book was with few exceptions closed in 1973, and this postscript summarizes some more recent additional information and altered concepts. The most recent statement on Cleave's concept "The Saccharine Disease" was published in 1974.

I Definition of dietary fibre

Many consider that the definition of dietary fibre has been over simplified, and that it cannot be confined, as in this book, to the structural polymers of the plant cell-wall that resist hydrolysis by human alimentary enzymes. There are in addition other substances that are naturally concentrated in the plant cell-wall and which are considerably reduced in quantity by the modern refining of cereals (Trowell, 1974a, b).

1. Structural polymers

(a) polysaccharides—celluloses and hemicelluloses; (b) lignins.

2. Associated cell-wall substances

(a) Lipids; (b) unavailable nitrogen associated with lignin (Van Soest and McQueen, 1973); (c) trace elements such as chromium, zinc and manganese; (d) phytates; (e) other identified and unidentified associated substances.

In order to preserve existing definitions there is much to be said in favour of restricting the term *dietary fibre* to the structural polymers (1) and to refer to the wider group (1) and (2) as the *dietary fibre complex*. This decision must be left to others. If they choose to use the term dietary fibre to include the *whole* complex group of substances (1) and (2), it is not for us to object. It corresponds to the realities of the situation, whether assessed in terms of the gastrointestinal contents or in terms of the refined cereal flours. It must be clearly recognized that if either of the terms dietary fibre or dietary fibre complex is extended to include *all* substances that are reduced by modern refining of cereals and other plant foods, then that term will have lost all clarity of definition. For instance, many B vitamins, also tocopherols, minerals and proteins are partially removed when cereals are milled or processed.

It must also be clearly recognized that present knowledge indicates that the nutrient substances in the cell contents of plant foods traditionally eaten by man are capable of being digested by his alimentary enzymes. The reserve poly-saccharide inulin may be a partial exception. Almost the only natural food that is rich in inulin is the Jerusalem artichoke in which, it has been suggested, 50% of the inulin is available, that is, digested by man (McCance and Widdowson, 1960). For all practical purposes the dietary fibre complex is derived entirely from plant cell walls.

II Varicose veins

The pathogenesis of varicose veins suggested in Chapter 12 fails to explain cases in which incompetence of communications between the deep and super-ficial vein appears to be the initial defect. Raised intra-abdominal pressures may affect the veins in ways not yet understood, or other unrecognised factors may play more or less major roles in some patients.

III Haemorrhoids

The most convincing argument incriminating raised intra-abdominal pressures in the pathogenesis of haemorrhoids is that of Graham-Stewart (1963). He showed that such pressures caused retrograde flow of blood down the superior haemorrhoidal veins, thus increasing the pressures within the superior haemor-rhoidal plexus. During attempts at stool evacuation these raised intravenous pressures are associated with reflex relaxation of the anal sphincters so that the pressures are unopposed and tend to cause dilatation of the veins (Fig. 1). With all other forms of abdominal straining the raised pressures in the superior haemorrhoidal plexus are associated with reflex contraction of the anal sphincters

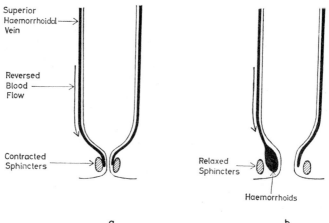

Fig. 1. (a) The increased pressure in haemorrhoidal plexus of veins caused by reversed blood-flow resulting from abdominal straining compensated for by contraction of anal sphincters; (b) Increased pressure caused by straining not compensated for by anal contraction. (Reproduced by kind permission from *Journal of the Royal College of Physicians of London* **9**, 138, 1975.)

which support the plexus from without, thus compensating for the raised intravenous pressures. These mechanisms operate whether or not the rectum contains faeces; and it could be that even the straining associated with the diarrhoea of chronic bowel infections might predispose to haemorrhoids in a similar manner. This could help to explain a relatively high prevalence of haemorrhoids in some communities in developing countries.

IV Ischaemic heart disease

A. Epidemiological studies

In 27 countries there is a significant correlation between national mortality rates for ischaemic heart disease and cancer of the colon. Six prospective studies of ischaemic heart disease yielded 90 cases of colonic cancer, but in them blood cholesterol levels were lower than expected. This was surprising in view of the influence of dietary saturated fat intakes in raising blood cholesterol levels. It was suggested, therefore, that further study was needed to evaluate the dietary intake of polyunsaturated fat and fibre (Rose et al., 1974). Another study of the epidemiology of diverticular disease and ischaemic heart disease provided new data concerning the prevalence of the former disease from 9 radiologists and 173 hospitals scattered throughout many countries in Africa and Asia. It appeared that where one disease was rare the other disease was rare, and where one disease was common the other disease was common. It was suggested that fibre deficiency was a factor in both diseases (Trowell et al., 1974). In all this there is no suggestion that fibre deficiency is the only risk factor in either disease.

B. Experimental studies

Planned experiments have demonstrated that fibre influences cholesterol metabolism in animals. In vitro experiments have shown that natural sources of fibre, such as alfalfa, wheat straw, bran, oat hulls and sugar cane pulp, bind the bile salts, sodium taurocholate and glycholate. Synthetic cellulose proved inactive (Kritchevsky and Story, 1974).

In vivo experiments have been performed in baboons. Those fed fibre-free semi-synthetic cholesterol-free diets had higher levels of serum cholesterol and triglycerides than those eating fibre in fruit, vegetables and bread (Kritchevsky et al., 1974). Rats fed ground cereal diets, supplemented with cholesterol and cholic acid, had lower plasma cholesterol levels and increased faecal excretion of steroids compared with rats fed fibre-free semi-synthetic diets (Balmer and Zilversmit, 1974). A similar diet of ground cereals exerted a comparable effect in hamsters; even brand and Fusarium mould, the latter rich in cutins, proved hypocholesterolaemic in rats (Owen et al., 1974). Bran, however, did not lower serum cholesterol levels in rats fed diets supplemented with cholesterol but not with cholic acid (Kay and Truswell, 1974). Observers stress that fibre from different sources varies in its effects on cholesterol metabolism in animals. Bagasse, a waste produce from the manufacture of sugar, is rich in fibre, especially lignin. Rats fed *ad libitum* diets supplemented with bagasse excreted more bile acids than those fed a fibre-free synthetic diet. These diets were not supplemented with cholesterol or cholic acid. The serum cholesterol levels of these groups of rats were unchanged (Morgan *et al.*, 1974).

Two groups of human volunteers ate ordinary western-type diets supplemented either with bagasse or with wheat bran for many months. There was no change in their serum cholesterol or triglyceride levels attributable to either fibre supplement. Faecal acid steroid excretion was increased by bagasse but not by bran (I. McLean Baird, personal communication, 1974). Other young adults ate wholemeal bread instead of white bread for many months, but there was no change in serum cholesterol or triglyceride levels (K. W. Heaton, personal communication, 1974). He commented on the desirability of extending the trial to older age-groups having hyperlipidaemia. Little is known of the long-term effect of consuming wheat wholemeal bread. The possible effects of oatmeal, brown rice, other whole cereals, leguminous seeds, starchy staples such as potatoes, also vegetables and fruit on lipid metabolism of man have seldom been investigated. It is suggested that the question of fibrinolysis, triglyceride metabolism and blood insulin levels, and carbohydrate tolerance, may prove profitable lines of investigation in ischaemic heart disease and in diabetes mellitus.

References

BALMER, J. and ZILVERSMIT, D. B. (1974). *Journal of Nutrition* **104**, 1319.

CLEAVE, T. L. (1974). "The Saccharine Disease." John Wright, Bristol; and The Keats Publishing Company, Connecticut (in press).

GRAHAM-STEWART, C. W. (1963). *Diseases of the Colon and Rectum* **6**, 333.

KAY, R. M. and TRUSWELL, A. S. (1974). *Proceedings of the Nutrition Society*, Abstracts, 17A.

KRITCHEVSKY, D. and STORY, J. A. (1974). *Journal of Nutrition* **104**, 458.

KRITCHEVSKY, D., DAVIDSON, L. M., SHAPIRO, I. L., KIM, H. K., KITAGARVA, M., MALHOTRA, S., NAIR, P. P., CLARKSON, T. B., BERSOHN, I. and WINTER, P. A. D. (1974). *American Journal of Clinical Nutritition* **27**, 29.

McCANCE, R. A. and WIDDOWSON, E. M. (1960). "The Composition of Foods", Medical Research Council Special Report Series No. 297, p. 91. Her Majesty's Stationery Office, London.

MORGAN, B., HEALD, M., ATKIN, S. D., GREEN, J. and CHAIN, E. B. (1974). *British Journal of Nutrition* **32**, 447.

OWEN, D. E., MUNDAY, K. A., TAYLOR, T. G. and TURNER, M. (1974). *Proceedings of the Nutrition Society*, Abstracts, 16A.

ROSE, G., BLACKBURN, H., KEYS, A., TAYLOR, H. L., KANNEL, W. B., OGLESBY, P., REID, D. D. and STAMLER, J. (1974). *Lancet* **1**, 181.

TROWELL, H. C. (1974a). *Lancet* **1**, 503.

TROWELL, H. C. (1974b). *Lancet* **2**, 1510.

TROWELL, H., PAINTER, N. and BURKITT, D. (1974). *American Journal of Digestive Diseases* **19**, 864.

VAN SOEST, P. J. and McQUEEN, R. W. (1973). *Proceedings of the Nutrition Society* **32**, 123.